THE
COMPLETE
BOOK
OF
SWIMMING

THE COMPLETE BOOK OF SWIMMING

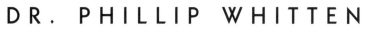

DR. PHILLIP WHITTEN

ILLUSTRATIONS BY ETHAN BERRY

RANDOM HOUSE / NEW YORK

Library of Congress Cataloging-in-Publication Data

Whitten, Phillip.
The complete book of swimming / Phillip Whitten.
p. cm.
Includes bibliographical references and index.
ISBN 0-679-74667-6
1. Swimming. I. Title.
GV834.W55 1994
797.2′1—dc20 92-56805

Manufactured in the United States of America
98765

Book design by Jo Anne Metsch
Book layout by Barbara Marks

To my son, Russell,

an inspiration since the day he was born,
a source of immense happiness
and pride

with love and appreciation

ACKNOWLEDGMENTS

I'VE BEEN SWIMMING ever since I was a little boy, and swimming for fitness, health, and competition since I was fifteen. So this could be like an Academy Awards ceremony, with me thanking everyone in the last half century who encouraged both my swimming and my writing. But there is neither time nor space for such a project.

There are, however, a number of people without whose support this book literally would not have been possible. And there are others whose advice greatly enhanced the quality of this work.

First of all I am deeply indebted to my mother, Sylvia, who first taught me to swim; and to my father, Clifton, who was my most enthusiastic fan when I was in high school and who spent countless weekends at age-group meets serving tirelessly as a swimming official.

I also want to express my appreciation to the many coaches—Don Couch, George Haines, Mr. A., Tom O'Neill, Peter Farragher, and others—who taught and coached me over the years, especially those who put up with me when I was a teenager.

Those of us who love the sport owe a great debt of gratitude to Ransom Arthur, M.D., former dean of the School of Medicine at the University of Oregon. It was his vision and persistence that led to the creation of Masters swimming and to the concept of swimming as a lifelong means of maintaining optimal fitness and health.

Specifically, I would like to express my gratitude to the following individuals, who not only provided in-depth critiques of each of the stroke chapters but also provided specific suggestions for improving the book: Judy Bonning, 1990 U.S. Masters Swimming Coach of the Year and head coach at Billabong Aquatics in Coral Gables, Florida; Skip Kenney, U.S. Olympic coach and head men's coach at Stanford University; Gerry Rodrigues, 1992 U.S. Masters Swimming Coach of the Year (along with Clay Evans) and former coach at Southern California Aquatics Masters Swim Club (SCAQ); and Dr. Manuel Sanguily, former Olympian, one of the world's greatest Masters swimmers and a friend for over thirty years.

Others who provided insight and assistance include Dick Deal, publisher of *SWIM* and *Swimming World* magazines; Dr. David Hunter, my friend and colleague; Bob Ingram, senior editor of *Swimming World;* Bill Mulliken, 1960 Olympic champion, friend, and rival; and Dr. Barry Sears, a leading figure in the field of dietary endocrinology, who patiently helped me understand the hormonal component of how foods affect athletic performance, the building of lean body mass, and resistance to illness and disease.

Above all, I'd like to thank all my swimming companions and competitors over the years for their indispensable assistance. Usually without knowing it, they offered ideas, inspiration, and themselves as role models, helping to make this book a reality.

I also want to acknowledge with great appreciation: Jill Kneerim, my agent and managing director of the Palmer & Dodge Agency in Boston, who first saw the potential of this book and helped keep it moving at several critical junctures; my editor at Random House, who had a vision of the importance of this book and offered encouragement and editorial guidance; Lawrence LaRose, who was always helpful and efficient; Ethan Berry, my illustrator, about whose work I have more to say in the introduction; and the sports medicine researchers, cardiologists, gerontologists, psychologists, sociologists, sex researchers, nutritionists, swim coaches, and pioneers in the scientific study of swimming, whose research and writings provide the scientific basis for our understanding of the profound benefits conferred by swimming.

Several individuals and publications generously allowed me to reprint their work in this book: *SWIM* magazine; Gerry Rodrigues, Clay Evans, and the rest of the coaching staff at Southern California Aquatics Masters (SCAQ); Coach Mike Collins of the Davis (California)

Acknowledgments

Aquatic Masters (DAM); and Coach Scott Rabalais of the Crawfish Masters Swim Team, Baton Rouge, Louisiana, whose workouts were adapted and included in Appendix A; and Diana S. Woodruff, whose life-expectancy test was adapted in Chapter 5.

I would also like to thank the editorial staff at Random House, and in particular my copy editor, Susan Brown, who helped me say what I wanted to say better; Bernie Klein, the design director, and Jo Metsch and Barbara Marks for their work on the design of the book; Susan Shapiro, who designed the cover and listened patiently to my seemingly endless suggestions; Benjamin Dreyer, the production editor; Joel Lipton, who shot and reshot the cover of the book, and who was inspired by the book to start swimming himself; and Alex Middaugh and Chris Hall, both Masters swimmers with Southern California Aquatics Masters, who generously agreed to serve as the cover models for the book.

Finally, I'd like to express my profound gratitude to my son, Russell, and my wife, Donna, who were with me all the way on this project. Their countless suggestions, always offered with love, proved incalculable in improving the book. In addition, they provided emotional support and a much-needed sense of humor in the dark days when it seemed the book might never be finished.

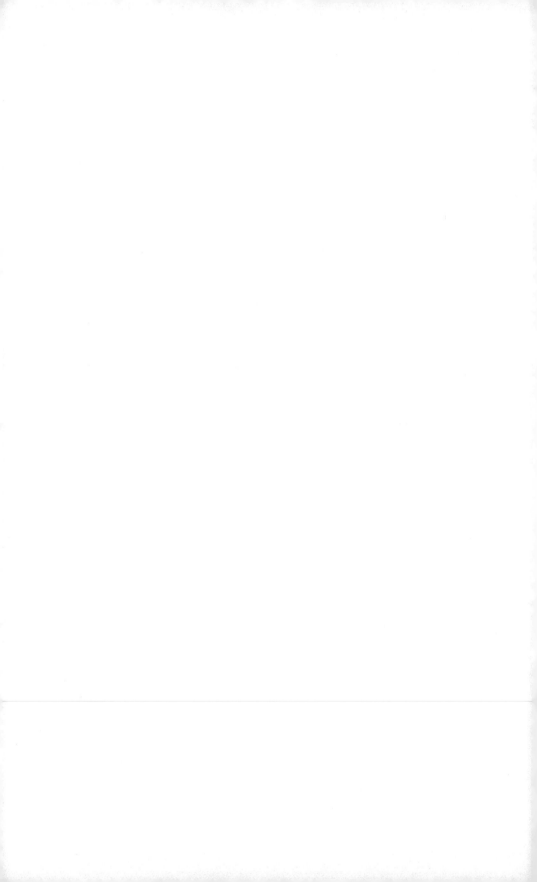

CONTENTS

Acknowledgments   vii
Introduction   xiii

I. SWIM FOR YOUR LIFE   1
 1. Swimming and Health   3
 2. Swimming: The Best Form of Exercise   13
 3. Getting to the Heart of the Matter   20
 4. Swim and Be Trim   39
 5. The Fountain of Youth Discovered:
     Swimming and Longevity   59

II. GETTING IN THE SWIM   87
 6. How to Begin Swimming:
     Different Strokes for Different Folks   89
 7. The Freestyle   101
 8. The Backstroke   119
 9. The Breaststroke   134
10. The Butterfly   156

III. BECOMING FIT   173

11.   Swimming and Sexuality:
      How to Enhance Your Love Life   175
12.   Women and Swimming   187
13.   The Sport of a Lifetime: Swimming from 8 to 108   199
14.   Getting in Shape: The Ins and Outs of Training   216

APPENDIX A   Sample Training Programs   239
APPENDIX B   The Swimmer's Marketplace   290
APPENDIX C   How to Calculate Your Life Expectancy   298
APPENDIX D   How to Calculate Your Percent Body Fat   305
APPENDIX E   For the Record   318
APPENDIX F   The Swimmer's Address Book   345
APPENDIX G   Sources for Learning More About Swimming   347
APPENDIX H   Meals with Protein-to-Carbohydrate Balance   356

      Index   361

INTRODUCTION

SINCE THE EARLY 1970s, as a by-product of the booming concern with self-improvement and personal growth and development, America has rediscovered physical fitness. One consequence has been that Americans—long dismissed as pampered and spoiled by more vigorous peoples—have become the leaders of a worldwide fitness revolution. In the process, there has been a marked improvement in our national health: for the first time in this century, death rates from heart disease and stroke have declined, while the incidence of lung cancer among men has leveled off and begun to decline.

Another result is that new industries related to health and physical fitness have been born, while existing industries have expanded and prospered:

- Health and "natural" foods have become Big Business.
- Sports apparel and equipment companies produce thousands of successful products to help us become more effective in our athletic endeavors—and look stylish while doing so.
- Multifaceted health and fitness clubs—with swimming pools, aerobics classes, Nautilus and Universal weight equipment, Nordic-Track, and racquetball courts—have mushroomed in communities

around the country, as well as in thousands of corporations and resorts.

- Medical specialists in athletic injuries have set up shop in every city and town in the United States.
- Experts dispense training and fitness advice on radio spots and television shows, while celebrities produce best-selling exercise videocassettes.
- Dozens of sports and recreation expositions are held in major cities each year.
- Scores of new sports and fitness magazines have appeared and prospered while existing health and fitness magazines have undergone rapid increases in circulation.

Americans have become concerned with the *quality* of their lives. They are convinced that one way, perhaps the best way, to improve the quality of their lives is to get in shape. And, as almost all experts agree, there is no better way to get in shape—and stay in shape—than swimming. That is why I have written *The Complete Book of Swimming.*

WHY SWIMMING?

It's not just the experts who recognize the value of swimming. It's everyone! I don't know how many times I've been at parties and, in the course of a conversation, revealed that I am a lifelong swimmer. The next thing I know, my interlocutor will be telling *me,* "You know, swimming is really the best all-around exercise there is . . . especially as you grow older." And so it is.

This observation is borne out by the fact that virtually every poll on physical activities conducted in the last thirty years has shown that swimming is America's most popular recreational/athletic activity.

Swimmers are less visible than joggers because they are not on public roads or in parks. They do their activity away from the public eye, in pools (and lakes and oceans). But make no mistake about it: they are out there, churning up the laps, in numbers estimated by the polls at between *30 and 120 million people*! And their numbers are growing.

In large measure, the fitness boom has been faddish. First tennis was the "in" activity; then it was jogging; then racquetball and aerobics. All of these are worthy and healthful activities, but all have their downsides as well. Swimming has all their virtues and more. And it has no downside.

Virtually all experts now recognize that *swimming is the best and most complete form of exercise there is.* It provides the same aerobic benefits that running and other activities do. But, unlike running and other forms of exercise, it works *all* the muscles of the body; since it does not put the strain on connective tissues that running and jogging do, it rarely leads to injury; and it provides numerous psychological benefits as well—from increased self-esteem to an enriched love life. According to recent stories in such bellwethers as *The New York Times* and the *Los Angeles Times,* swimming is destined to be the sport of the late 1990s and the twenty-first century.

WHOM THIS BOOK IS FOR

Part of the reason for swimming's continuing appeal is demographic. While the sport is ideal for people of all ages, it is especially suited for an aging population. There is no doubt that Americans are steadily growing older. But we find it hard to picture ourselves as retiring to the rocking chair on the front porch. We plan on remaining vigorous and healthy well into old age.

The Complete Book of Swimming is written for those folks who want to become physically fit and stay physically fit for the rest of their lives; for folks who are seeking a way to enhance their lives. There are chapters on the different strokes that provide the "how-to" information people need to get started. Equally important are the chapters that answer such questions as Why should I swim? Why swimming and not some other sport? How can swimming improve my health? How can it enhance my life? How will I become a better person—more vital, competent, vigorous, sexy . . . *alive* by swimming?

Above all, this book is meant to be accessible and interesting to a large audience. There are other swimming books on the market, but these are concerned, almost entirely, with stroke technique and training programs. They preach to the converted, failing to ask the question *Why* should I swim? They don't explore the benefits of swimming beyond immediate aerobic fitness. They don't relate stories of people with whom the reader can identify, people whose lives were transformed by swimming. *The Complete Book of Swimming* was written to do all of that—and more. My goal in writing this book is nothing less than to introduce you to the world of swimming and to change your life.

If you are not a swimmer, it will show you how to become healthier and happier than you ever imagined you could be. It will do so no matter how out of shape or fat or old or ungraceful you are. Nor does it matter how many times you've tried other exercise regimens only to give up.

If you are already a swimmer, this book will help make you fitter, faster, more efficient, more knowledgeable, and better able to enjoy your sport's special pleasures. It will keep you learning, no matter how long you've been swimming. It will teach you how to improve whether you're twenty-five or seventy-five. And it will show you how to utilize the sport's variety of strokes to stave off the boredom that is so often the downfall of people embarking on a physical fitness program. Follow my advice for working out and you need never be bored again.

HOW THE BOOK IS ORGANIZED

This book is divided into three sections. The first section, "Swim for Your Life," contains five chapters that explain why swimming is universally recognized as the best all-around exercise there is and how swimming can enhance your health, reduce your risk of developing heart disease and a host of other illnesses and ailments, help you not only lose weight but remain fit and trim throughout your life, and, finally, actually help you live a fuller, more satisfying, and longer life.

The second section, "Getting in the Swim," consists of another five chapters that will teach you the basics as well as many of the finer points of swimming efficiently, fluidly, and effortlessly.

The first chapter in this section explains simply and directly the fundamentals of swimming: the shared principles underlying all swimming strokes. The following chapters are devoted to the four major strokes: freestyle (or crawl stroke), backstroke, breaststroke, and butterfly.

Each chapter is organized in this fashion:

- A brief history of the stroke
- Body position
- Arm pull

- Body roll (for freestyle and backstroke)
- Breathing
- The kick
- Putting it all together
- The turn
- The start
- Ten Tips

The final section, "Becoming Fit," has four chapters: one on how swimming can improve your love life; a second that deals specifically with women and swimming and includes topics such as pregnancy, osteoporosis, and self-esteem; and a third that explains why swimming is, quite literally, the sport for a lifetime and includes information on the organizations that promote and sponsor swimming for people of all ages. The book's final chapter talks about training: how to get into shape, different training methods, using swimming paraphernalia, and so on.

The book concludes with eight appendices that provide

- Sample training programs
- Information on where to order everything from swimsuits to prescription goggles and training fins
- An annotated list of magazines, books, and videos that will help you learn more about swimming and keep you up-to-date about developments in the sport
- Directions on how to calculate your body-fat percentage
- A test for determining your life expectancy
- A list of swimming records, from age-group swimming (age nine to ten and under through to ages seventeen and eighteen) through Masters (age twenty-five through one hundred plus)
- A list of addresses and phone numbers for additional information
- Dietary guidelines to help you eat more healthfully

THE ARTWORK

A tremendous amount of thought and effort went into the more than 150 pieces of art in this book—particularly in Chapters 6 through 10. The illustrations have been carefully designed to enhance your learning of the strokes.

Ethan Berry, the illustrator, brings a unique background to this challenge: he is an artist who has won wide acclaim for his innovative and provocative work at exhibits and installations throughout the nation, a teacher of art at Montserrat College of Art and the Massachusetts College of Art for over twenty years, and an outstanding Masters swimmer in his own right.

Ethan was not content to rely on his own expertise in creating the book's illustrations. With me, he analyzed dozens of videotapes of some of the world's top swimmers. Then he did his own observations of collegiate, Masters, and age-group swimmers, photographing and videotaping them underwater. He then used the photos and video freeze-frames as the basis for his drawings.

The result is a unique style that imparts a maximum amount of information without overloading the reader. The style conveys a feeling of the actual motion of each stroke *pattern*. The arrows illustrate not only how the arms and legs should move—the pattern of the strokes—but, through shading, where power should be exerted. By providing a kinesthetic feeling of how your body should be moving through the water, these illustrations not only communicate factual information simply and directly but also transmit a feel for the sensuous nature of swimming.

DO IT!

Now it's time to start reading. *The Complete Book of Swimming* is meant to inspire you. But you'll never get in shape simply by reading. If I've done what I've set out to do, by the time you finish this book, you'll be eager to jump in the nearest pool and take the first stroke in a process that will transform your life.

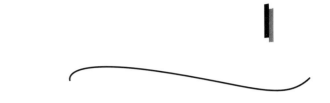

SWIM FOR YOUR LIFE

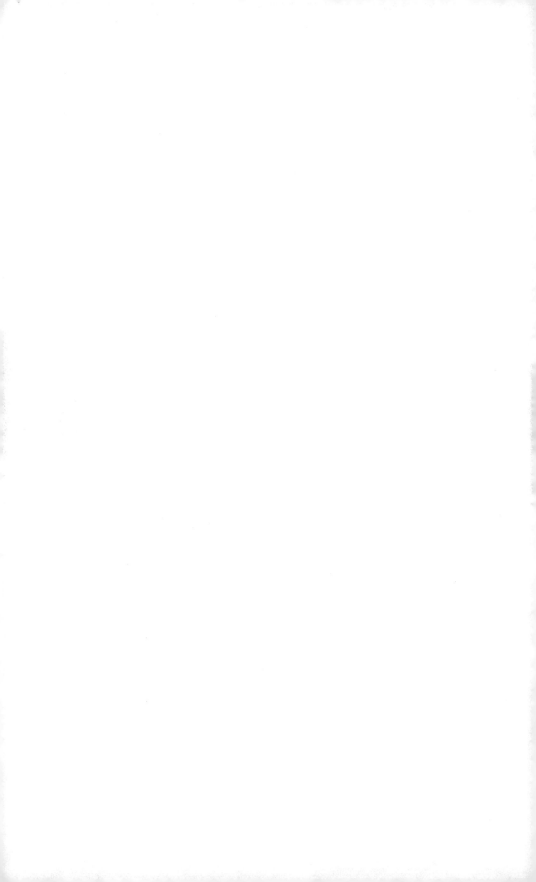

SWIMMING AND HEALTH

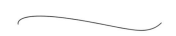

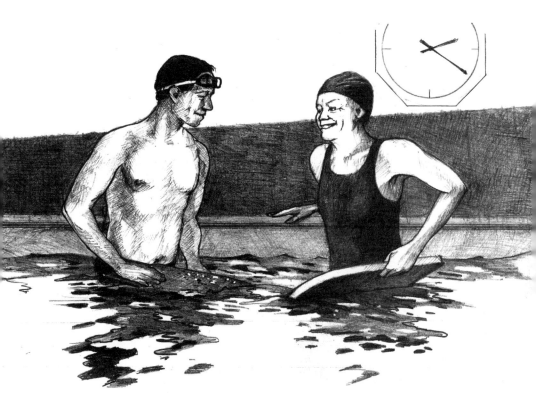

Rest is rust.
—PAUL BRAGG,
ninety-eight-year-old swimmer

Swimming is like taking a daily vacation.
—JUDY COLLINS,
popular singer and swimmer

IF EVERY TIME you take a short flight of stairs you find yourself huffing and puffing, think of Paul Bragg. When you next bend down to tie your shoelaces but discover you can't see them because there's a spare tire where empty space used to be, consider Paul Bragg. If a steady diet of cigarettes has left you hacking and coughing and gasping for air, reflect on the experience of Paul Bragg.

If the headache you get from doing the least bit of housework is so intense that you wish it on Saddam Hussein, think of Nellie Brown. If each Memorial Day you discover that last year's bathing suit seems to have shrunk over the winter, stop a moment and consider Nellie Brown. If you know you should be exercising but don't have the energy or commitment to begin any of the programs you've been considering, reflect on the experience of Nellie Brown before putting it off for another day, week, month, year.

Paul Bragg and Nellie Brown are just two of the many fascinating people you will meet in this book. Some of these people have overcome serious illness or debility. Others are ordinary folks in ordinary health burdened by all those ordinary problems that wear most of us down—career, family, school, parenting, taxes. What they have in common, whatever their backgrounds, are swimming and remarkable good health. Their experiences will help you realize that, yes, the seemingly inevitable progression toward deteriorating health can be slowed and even reversed, even after those first wrinkles and wisps of gray hair have started to appear. It doesn't matter whether you are seventeen or seventy, whether you were a professional athlete in your youth or have never exercised a day in your life, whether those extra fifteen or twenty pounds have been around so long you can't even remember not having them or seem to have jumped onto your figure over the past two weeks. You can swim your way to the same vibrant good health so many regular swimmers enjoy. In the process, you will be adding years to your life—vigorous, healthy, productive years. Best of all, you will enjoy doing it!

When I met Paul Bragg, in 1978, he had already become a living legend on Honolulu's Waikiki Beach. As a child, he had been frail and sickly, and when he contracted polio at the age of fourteen, it appeared he might have to resign himself to a lifetime as an invalid. But young Paul was made of sterner stuff and found a miraculous path that he followed to great health: "constant activity and exercise—swimming, tennis, running, and lots of sunshine." Paul went on to become a wrestler on two U.S. Olympic teams, a practicing osteopath, an expert on nutrition, and the author of over a hundred books on health. At the age of ninety-eight he became the oldest person ever to swim competitively—though there are three centenarians competing today. To stay in shape, he ate a good diet, churned through the warm waters off Waikiki every day, and jogged up to five miles a few times a week. His motto: "Rest is rust."

At first glance, the "unsinkable Nellie Brown," as she was affectionately known to just about everyone in her hometown of Alexandria, Virginia, seemed an unlikely celebrity. But at age eighty-seven, this retired first-grade teacher ("I never made it into second grade") looked to be at least twenty years younger and was in constant demand, besieged by requests for appearances on *Good Morning America,* interviews with local newspapers, an award as Alexandria's Woman of the Year, and speeches at YMCAs and community centers. It was a remarkable schedule, and you may wonder where she found the time to get in her daily one-mile swim. But Nellie was a remarkable woman.

Nellie did not always swim a mile a day. In fact, she didn't even learn to swim until she was sixty-eight. A childhood bout with polio had left her with one leg two inches shorter than the other. By 1961 ravages wrought by childhood sickness, later injuries, and advancing age had produced devastating results. "I could barely walk anymore," she recalled. "I was afraid I'd have to spend the rest of my life in a wheelchair. For the first time in my life, I really felt old. I felt foolish and . . . just plain useless. It was frustrating and depressing." Then her doctor recommended swimming as therapy for her legs, "and that made all the difference in the world," she said with a twinkle. "People told me I'd never learn, that you can't teach an old dog new tricks. But I wanted to learn. I had no intention of being an invalid. I've got too much living to do!"

When I interviewed her, Nellie Brown was not only swimming but teaching swimming classes for Alexandria's mentally retarded and handicapped children. She was in the best health of her life, and she attributed it all to swimming. "I feel great," she explained. "Swimming gives me the exercise I need to keep going." She reported that it was easy to learn to swim, even at an advanced age, and that she intended to keep at it for a long, long time to come.

Admittedly, Paul Bragg and Nellie Brown are extraordinary people who have overcome extraordinary adversity. But they are only two of literally thousands of men and women with equally compelling stories whom I have met over the past twenty-odd years. You will meet many of these people through the pages of this book.

But, more to the point, there are tens and even hundreds of thousands of your fellow Americans—from teenagers and young adults to senior citizens—who have made themselves healthier and enriched their lives through swimming. These are people who only a few years ago were sedentary, overweight, overwrought, or simply overburdened by the stresses of job, family, and taxes. Some were seriously ill. Yet today many of these people have had their lives transformed: they have fewer anxieties, enjoy markedly better health, take pride in their strong and healthy bodies, and find they have more satisfying sex lives and better relationships generally with their spouses and children. Many now delight in a youthful, zestful outlook on life that they once thought they could never recover.

Their elixir is swimming. Over the past few decades, medical experts have come to agree, almost unanimously, that regular exercise is a prime contributor to good health and long life. And of all the forms of exercise Americans have taken up with such gusto since the 1970s—tennis, bicycling, jogging, racquetball, jumping rope, aerobics, whatever—swimming has attracted the most participants. Not only has this thoroughly enjoyable activity become America's most popular participant sport but it is fast gaining recognition as the best form of exercise for most adult Americans, all things considered, especially for those of us who have passed the big 3-0!

Judy Collins surely needs no introduction. For years, her soulful melodies and enchantingly beautiful voice have delighted millions. Seeing her, it is hard to believe that Judy is over fifty. Her skin radiates health and well-being, her body is strong and supple, and she seems relaxed and at peace with herself. Judy continues to give concerts throughout Europe and the United States, but only in recent years has she started to become the kind of singer she wants to be. "I'm beginning to learn what I want to sound like," she explains. "My singing is stronger. I'm adding more humor and making more daring choices in the kind of material I sing." In the last few years she has also begun to spend more time writing—new songs, a book, and an autobiography, *Trust Your Heart,* published in 1987. It is women like Judy Collins who give the over-fifty stage in life such a great image.

But things were different for Judy not long ago. "When I was younger, I drove myself mercilessly, made a lot of demands on my body, and didn't treat myself very well," she confides. What turned things around for her? Swimming. "I've been a workaholic for so long that it's hard for me to take a vacation, and I rarely do. But if I swim,

I get a vacation every day." When Judy took up swimming about ten years ago, she found almost immediately that she was feeling better about herself physically. She stopped smoking and drinking (though she still has a cup of coffee every day), changed her diet, and lost twenty pounds. She tries to swim every day and finds that when she does she's less tense about everything. "Swimming," she says, "has taught me to be good to myself."

"The first thing that my swim coach let me know," reports Dwight Stones, the flamboyant former world high-jump champion, "was that if I planned to swim competitively, I would have to get into condition." He couldn't believe his ears. Here he was—a former world-record holder, two-time Olympic bronze medalist, winner of numerous national championships in the high jump—and he was being told he wasn't in good enough shape to compete in a sport that did not seem to require much training. Today Stones accepts that even an athlete can be brought to a new level of fitness through regular swimming. Along with his running and weight training, he swims an impressive 4,000 yards three times a week at the Belmont Plaza pool in Long Beach, California.

Stones started swimming merely to prepare himself for TV's "Superstars" competition. The venture nearly cost him his amateur status when he decided to ignore an AAU edict and keep the money he had won. But during his subsequent enforced layoff from high-jump competition, Stones kept up his swimming. To his surprise, he found that injuries that had plagued him for years, including a chronic hip problem, began to disappear.

Stones believes that swimming can be beneficial to athletes in all sports. "It's the best form of exercise for me," he notes, "because it's a natural body balancer. In high jumping you use one side of your body more than the other, but swimming counteracts the muscle imbalance this creates." The same is true, he might have added, of other sports that stress the use of only one set of muscles—tennis, racquetball, basketball, even aerobics and jogging. Further, Stones points out, swimming is an excellent recuperative aid and when used as a limbering exercise can actually prevent injury.

Roberta Kresch, a forty-eight-year-old biology teacher in Westfield, New Jersey, feels that swimming has given her a new lease on life. An avid, accomplished skier for twelve years, Roberta was skiing in the Canadian Rockies in February 1976 when she had a bad fall. She was hospitalized for five weeks and confined to bed for an additional two months. "I was in constant, agonizing pain in my back and legs," she recalls. "I was able to walk only with the aid of crutches or a cane much of the time."

Not satisfied with her recovery, Roberta sought out some of the top physicians in New York City to find out if anything could be done. "Eventually," she says, "I met with a doctor in Millburn, New Jersey, who agreed to operate if I were willing to take the chance." The risky eight-hour operation took place in August 1977. Three of Roberta's disks were removed, and her vertebral column was opened up and widened in the entire lumbar region.

After seven weeks in the hospital and four months of recuperation at home, Roberta was ready to resume teaching at Westfield Senior High. Even before her operation, several physicians had recommended swimming, and now, before she returned to her classroom, she returned to the pool. "There's no doubt," she says today, "that my rapid recovery is attributable to my swimming."

Roberta kept right on plowing through the water, improving her stroke and increasing her strength. In 1979 she felt she was ready to enter her first Masters competition. "It was only a small, local meet," she reminisces, "but I almost cried when I won my first ribbon." Two years later, she had won thirteen, along with a silver medal for the 200-yard backstroke at the eastern championships. Today she has won too many ribbons to count.

Roberta works out five or six times a week now. "I never miss," she says. "Six o'clock every morning finds me in the pool. My back will never be 100 percent, but I'm almost never in pain anymore, and I threw my crutches and cane away many years ago."

In addition, the workouts and swim meets opened up a whole new social world to replace the one Roberta lost when she had to give up skiing. "Everyone is so friendly," she offers. "Some of the younger guys help me with my technique. And when I see swimmers thirty and forty years older than I am looking so incredibly good and able to continue their swimming with so little effort, I know I'm going to keep on swimming for the rest of my life."

Herb Kern and Tom Whiteleather are teammates in Fort Lauderdale's crackerjack Gold Coast Masters swim club. Both in their early sixties, each could easily be mistaken for someone a decade younger. Several years back they combined with Dan Malone and Bill Moffit to set a national record in their age-group for the 200-yard freestyle relay.

But before they got into the swim, they were, as Whiteleather puts it, "your typical middle-aged slobs, well on the way to self-destruction."

Kern hadn't exercised in years and was smoking three packs of cigarettes a day when he resolved to break his habit and get into shape. It was not the first time he had tried to stop smoking. "Oh, I had quit a thousand times before," he recalls with a smile. "But every time, sooner or later, I found myself going back to that infernal weed." This time, however, he vowed it would be different.

Kern started jogging, working his way from one to three miles a day. But like so many people over thirty, he found jogging was too hard on his legs and joints. "Besides," he explains, "it was just plain boring." So he decided to try swimming. "I used to swim for the University of Miami," he recalls, "but I must admit I was a little rusty after a twenty-five-year layoff." He persisted, gradually increasing his distance, and soon found his old skills coming back. He also found he was sticking to his vow. "It's amazing," he says, "but I no longer had any urge to light up. Swimming leaves me feeling so relaxed, so good, that smoking just doesn't interest me anymore."

When Tom Whiteleather was a student at Ohio State University, he was national collegiate champion in the 50- and 100-yard freestyle events. But after he graduated he gave up the sport. Twenty years later he found himself much heavier than he wanted to be. He tried a "starvation" diet first, and it worked, at least temporarily. His weight dropped from 223 to 170 pounds in a little over two months. But as so many dieters have found to their chagrin, there's no such thing as a free lunch. "It was insane," he says now. "I wound up sick much of the time. That's when I decided I needed exercise more than dieting. I had always talked about getting back into swimming. Now I knew I had to."

Tom read about Masters swimming in a local newspaper and decided to attend one of the meets. "I went there and saw some guys I had competed against in college. They looked absolutely fantastic! I knew if they could do it, I could do it too."

And he did! Today Tom is an avid Masters swimmer. Although he has not won any individual national championships, he is back down to his collegiate weight and claims to feel better than he has in years.

Mary Beth Hurt has never had any serious health problems and was never a top competitive swimmer. But like Roberta Kresch and Herb Kern, she finds swimming a delightfully invigorating way to stay in shape. Several times a week the slender actress interrupts her hectic schedule and heads for the Paris Health Club on New York's West Ninety-seventh Street, where she swims a mile or more.

In the past few years, Mary Beth has found her career blossoming. Known for her work on the Broadway stage, she has been acclaimed as well for performances on television and in films, for example, in the PBS presentation of John Cheever's *The Five Forty-eight* and in Woody Allen's *Interiors*. With all that emoting, Mary Beth finds swimming "incredibly relaxing. Nothing feels better after a hard day's work," she says, "than to jump in the pool and swim."

At age seventy-seven, Mardie Brown is one of the youngest people I know. Active, thoughtful, funny, and attractive, Mardie has a zest for life equaled by few people her age—or any age. She attributes her youthful enthusiasm and energy to her swimming, an activity she has engaged in since the age of four, and pursued faithfully since 1973. A mother, grandmother, and until recently member of a motorcycle club, the former probation and parole officer lives on a farm in Palermo, Maine, with Donald, eighty-four, her husband of more than fifty years.

Although I've known Mardie for almost twenty years, it was only in 1988, at the World Masters Swimming Championships held in Brisbane, Australia, that we became close friends. One of my favorite recreational activities is scuba diving. Mardie took up the sport in 1981, and I was duly impressed when she told me that she and Don had stopped for several days before the swim meet to dive off Australia's Great Barrier Reef. But the couple also stopped in Hawaii, and I was even more impressed when I saw the photos of her surfing off Waikiki Beach. "The waves were small," she says modestly. "It's not as if I were surfing the Pipeline [on Oahu's North Shore]."

In 1973, at the urging of her doctor, Mardie gave up smoking. But, to her dismay, after breaking her lifelong habit she found her weight and her blood pressure rising. An article she happened across explained how swimming could bring both under control, so, as she recounts, she "marched across the street to the YMCA" and began swimming. Within months, her weight and blood pressure were back to normal.

Two years later, she says, "I began my competitive career." And she's been at it ever since, winning several national and two world titles for women in her age-group. "I don't ever intend to quit," she told me. "I have more energy than I did at forty, I've met some wonderful people, and I'm having too much fun."

• • •

In the past two decades, America has undergone a fitness revolution. In 1961, Herb Elliott, the great Australian middle-distance runner, remarked that our soft, sedentary life-style had turned America into a nation of "mollycoddled milksops." Statistics bore him out. That year a survey found that only 24 percent of American adults exercised regularly. The stereotypical male, notes my good friend T. George Harris, founding editor of *American Health* magazine, was "twenty pounds overweight, used a car to commute any distance over two blocks, and got his exercise by trimming the lawn on a sit-down power mower. His wife was a perfect match: overweight, underexercised, with a vague notion of 'sports' as something her husband watched on television."

By the 1980s the picture had changed dramatically. America had gotten off its collective rear and begun swimming, running, dancing, and bicycling its way to physical fitness. According to a recent study commissioned by Perrier, *Fitness in America,* 59 percent of all Americans eighteen years and over—more than 90 million adults—were participating in some sort of physical activity on a regular basis. We were mollycoddled milksops no longer.

One result of the physical fitness boom has been a remarkable improvement in the nation's health. Americans have never been healthier. According to the U.S. surgeon general, our average life expectancy is now seventy-five years. That's an increase of over five years in just the last two decades. Deaths from heart disease, the country's leading killer, have dropped dramatically—about 40 percent over the past twenty years. And deaths from stroke are down 30 percent.

Of course, factors other than exercise have contributed to this remarkable turnabout. A decrease in the amount of salt, sugar, and fats many Americans consume, closer monitoring of blood pressure, and a steady decline in smoking have been significant. But many physicians and exercise physiologists agree that the quest for physical fitness has been an important factor in the decline of heart disease and several other major illnesses.

Because the Perrier study, conducted by the Louis Harris Polling Company, provides the most comprehensive in-depth reading of the behavior, knowledge, and attitudes of the American public regarding physical fitness and exercise, we will be looking at some of its major findings throughout this book.

Among the questions the study asked a cross-section of adults was the following: "Please tell me which of these activities you personally participated in on a *regular* basis at any time during the past year." The pollsters found ample evidence for the fitness revolution: the total of adult Americans regularly participating in the listed activities came to over 290 million. (Since there were only about 150 million adult Americans when the survey was conducted, it's clear that a lot of people participate in more than one.) Nineteen and a half million people reported that they use their bicycles to pedal their way to fitness. Over 16 million have taken to the roads, dodging irate drivers and territorial dogs, and braving noxious fumes to jog. Another 13.5 million have crowded the nation's tennis courts.

This explosive growth in sports for adults has proven equally healthy for the media: running, tennis, and aerobics "gurus" appear almost daily on TV and radio talk shows to extol the virtues of their sports. Sports medicine experts appear on the same shows to tell us what shoes to wear and how to deal with our shinsplints, stretched Achilles tendons, painful tennis elbow, and pulled hamstrings. Hollywood and made-for-television movies celebrate the mystique of long-distance running. How-to books are churned out at an astonishing rate. Countless newspaper and magazine columns offer advice on getting and staying in shape.

But while sports like jogging, aerobics, and tennis have garnered the lion's share of media attention, the Perrier study confirmed what has been shown in every study of America's fitness habits since 1967: America's most popular sport is *swimming*. Twenty-seven million American adults swim on a regular basis, about as many as the number of joggers and tennis players combined. Away from the glare of the media and the blare of traffic, in more than 220,000 public and private club pools and some 1.2 million residential pools across the nation, in lakes and rivers and reservoirs, in the ocean surf off the east, west, and southern coasts, 27 million Americans are celebrating the fitness revolution by crawl stroking, backstroking, breaststroking, and butterflying their way to better shape.

More recently the media have started to pay a little more attention to this old favorite. Citing its immense popular appeal as well as its myriad health benefits, both the *Los Angeles Times* and *The New York Times* have anointed swimming "the sport of the '90s."

In the next few chapters you will learn why swimming has attracted so many adherents, why medical experts regard it as the ideal form of exercise, and why it is, indeed, the sport of the nineties.

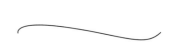

SWIMMING: THE BEST FORM
OF EXERCISE

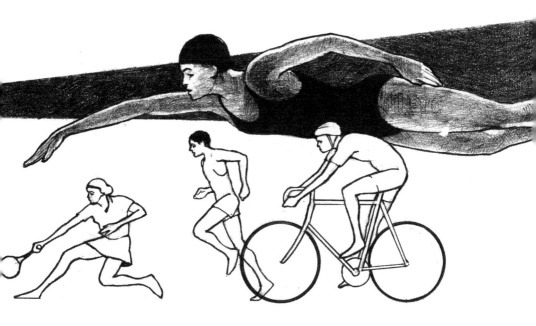

MORE AND MORE people are getting in the swim—to relieve stress, to improve their health, or simply to look and feel better. These people are wise in choosing swimming to reach their goals, for extensive research conducted since the early 1970s has shown that no matter your age or physical condition, no matter how long you have neglected or abused your body, here is an activity that can help get you back on track toward a richer, happier, healthier, and longer life.

THE MOST POPULAR FORM OF EXERCISE

Over the past two decades, as a by-product of a booming national concern with better health as well as with self-improvement and personal growth, and a desire to crowd more gusto into their lives, Americans have become the leaders of a worldwide fitness revolution. Although some experts predicted a rapid peaking and then sure decline in this trend, it has only recently begun to level off. And, for a significant proportion of the population, regular exercise has become a permanent part of their life-style, because the rewards are so gratifying.

How does swimming fit into this new scheme of things? Every poll addressing the question has shown that swimming is far and away America's most popular recreational/athletic activity. Yet we might never guess this from the media coverage of the fitness craze, which seems to focus on virtually every activity *except* swimming.

There are several reasons for this lack of coverage. First, swimming is not economically driven. There are few expensive swimming-related products for companies to market and sell. No $200 designer warm-up suits, no $175 running shoes, no $150 tennis racquets, no $1,000 home gyms. All you really need for swimming is a swimsuit, the less fancy the better, and perhaps goggles and a cap—items that will last a year or more and from which you will never need to graduate to the more advanced model. Because swimming does not create a lucrative market in equipment and attire for potential sponsors, the sport rarely intrudes on the television-controlled consciousness of the American public. Thus, what is an advantage from the point of view of the individual swimmer becomes a disadvantage from the point of view of the sport itself. Only every four years, when the Olympics roll around, is swimming accorded the recognition it deserves. And even this quadrennial moment in the public eye comes about only because American athletes have dominated Olympic swimming competition for over thirty years, as they have no other sport.

Second, an important impetus to the fitness craze is the ever-expanding public consciousness of the health benefits of exercise. Each new study brings out a rush of zealots extolling the virtues of whatever exercise the study found beneficial. But it is hard to do science with people who are in the water. If you are looking to hook people up to scientific apparatus, it is much easier to do so with those on treadmills than with those slicing through water. For convenience, and to protect their expensive equipment, scientists much prefer to conduct their research on out-of-water subjects.

Third, employing the various accepted swimming strokes requires skills not used in everyday life; whereas most people can run reasonably well without instruction, you must learn to swim efficiently. Further, although babies can swim before they can walk, adults tend to perceive the water as a foreign environment and swimming as a means of locomotion unnatural to humans. It is therefore easier for spectators to identify with runners than with swimmers.

Finally, swimmers are simply less visible than joggers. They participate in their activity in pools, lakes, and oceans, generally away from the public eye. But make no mistake about it: invisible as they may be to the nonswimming public, the swimmers are out there, churning up the laps.

All these factors have given rise to and supported the myth that running has become America's foremost nonspectator pastime and therefore must be the ideal form of exercise. Unfortunately, we have learned over the past few years that running may be one of the worst exercise choices for people over thirty. Yes, it is aerobically sound, but, as ever greater numbers of runners are learning to their sorrow and frustration, the human body is simply not built to withstand the constant pounding on hard surfaces running deals it.

THE BEST FORM OF EXERCISE

Experts now recognize that swimming is the best and most complete form of exercise. It provides most of the aerobic benefits that running does, with many of the benefits of resistance training thrown in. Further, unlike running and most other forms of exercise, swimming works all the muscles of the body. Possibly most important, it does not put the strain on connective tissues that running, jogging, aerobics, and some weight-training regimens do.

It seems that more and more people are taking to the water to stay in shape—former senator and presidential candidate Paul Tsongas, supermodel Kim Alexis, writer Stephen King, television anchorwoman Paula Zahn, businessman Vidal Sassoon, designer Donna Karan, even Pope John Paul II, who gets in a workout at his Castel Gandolfo pool whenever he can.

And many are returning to the water after a decade or more on dry land. Take Pat Richard, for example. Married for twenty-six years, the mother of three grown sons, a nurse with her own practice monitoring high-risk obstetrical patients, Pat had not swum since the early sixties, when she was a member of the Michigan State University varsity squad. In 1991, at age forty-six, she took stock. "I had gotten so overweight it was ridiculous," she recalls. "As a nurse, I realized what that meant, so I decided to do something about it." She went on a low-fat diet and started swimming again. A year later, she had lost over forty pounds, "with a few more to go." She had also regained her competitive spirit and finds that she not only enjoys her workouts but also savors the return to competition Masters meets afford her.

But swimming's strongest recommendations come from highly successful competitive athletes in other sports, people who know well the strengths and limitations of the human body but who would be expected to be partial to the sport that provided them their success. A surprising number of such champions, past and present, now rely on swimming to keep them in shape: Parry O'Brien, the former world-record holder in the shot put, who competes for a southern California Masters squad; Yuri Vlasov, the 1960 Olympic heavyweight weight lifting champion, who swims backstroke for the Kiev Masters in Ukraine; Dwight Stones, the former U.S. record holder in the high jump, whom you met in the last chapter; and NBA "mighty-mite" Muggsy Bogues, who stays in shape by swimming when he isn't playing basketball, to name just a few. Countless other athletes have used swimming to rehabilitate from injury: Nancy Kerrigan, Bo Jackson, Joan Benoit Samuelson, and Larry Bird come immediately to mind. Even racehorses are swimming to stay in shape as they recover from injuries. It never ceases to amaze me how many former runners are now swimmers. I don't know how many times I have heard people say, "I used to run to stay in shape, but now I swim." As our population grows and ages, the number of people making this switch will increase.

To reap the benefits of swimming, you do not have to be a household name. At age forty-seven development economist Carl House began to suffer lower back pain. It was excruciating, and nothing seemed to help. Desperate, House went to a specialist who told him that exercise, especially swimming, might help a little but that basically he would simply have to learn to live with the chronic pain.

House had never exercised as an adult, but he was willing to grab at any straw. If exercise could help, even a little, it was worth a shot. So he began running. "It was boring as hell and I hated it," he recalls. "What's more, it didn't help my back at all. In fact, it made things worse." So he quit. He tried biking next. About the same result. Then one day he read about Masters swimming in a local newspaper. The next day he simply showed up at the pool. He was hooked immediately. "Within three months my pain was completely gone," he reports. Six years later he's still swimming, and he is still pain free. "As long as I swim four times a week, about an hour and a quarter a day, I have no problem with my back." At first barely able to complete one lap, House has come along surprisingly well, even sneaking occasionally into the national top ten rankings in the 200-meter butterfly. "But you have to remember," he qualifies, modestly, "that that's an event no one likes to swim."

Ever-growing numbers of people are taking the plunge, drawn to swimming for a variety of reasons nearly as wide as the number of swimmers joining in. Virtually all report immediate therapeutic benefits, but there are also joys that keep them at it, and this book will discuss both.

As mentioned in the last chapter, all exercise provides at least some benefit for those who do it regularly. Then why is it that exercise physiologists and fitness experts agree almost unanimously that one form of exercise—swimming—is the best?

Much of the remainder of this book is concerned with the many ways to answer that question. For now, I will focus mainly on the fitness benefits swimming confers. Later chapters will discuss the health and psychological benefits that come with regular swimming.

SWIMMING FOR FITNESS

As previously noted, swimming provides most of the aerobic benefits running does. Tests have shown that swimmers can get their heart rates up almost as high as comparably fit runners'. What's more important, however, is that the sport is virtually injury free. Because water provides so much natural buoyancy, exercise in water is easy on the joints and tendons. You can work out as aggressively as you like without concern that you will be disabled by aching feet, blisters, shinsplints, tennis elbow, or runner's knee. Even more assuring, you can have confidence that your zeal for the sport is not condemning you to a future plagued by a variety of knee, leg, hip, or back ailments. In fact, if you have developed any of these problems from your other activities, swimming may help make them better.

Not only does swimming provide aerobic benefits but because it takes place in water, a medium in which you must push against resistance to propel yourself forward, it confers many of the benefits of resistance exercises like Nautilus workouts and weight lifting.

SWIMMING: THE SPORT FOR LIFE

The advantages of swimming over other forms of exercise are myriad. Heading up the list may be that swimming is fun. As will be discussed in Chapters 6 and 14, there is an almost infinite variety of ways to exercise as you swim. You can kick, using only your legs; pull, using only your arms; use any of the four competitive strokes; and employ any of a variety of training aids. You can use an assortment of drills or focus on techniques that will strengthen particular parts of your body. But there is no swimming activity that will cause you pain (Gain, No Pain! is the swimmers' motto), and most will give a special refreshing and sensual experience that only hydrotherapy—a sort of return to our origins—can provide.

Another important benefit is that swimming does not leave you hostage to the weather. Although you can not swim outdoors throughout the year in all parts of the country, you can always find an indoor pool. Especially pleasurable in summertime, when you are most eager to be more active, swimming comes with its own body-cooling apparatus. In fact, a high percentage of the strain on your heart during out-of-water exercise is brought about by the body's need to have blood pumped close to the surface so that it can be cooled. This is especially so, for example, if you are running outdoors on a hot, humid day, when evaporation of perspiration cannot do the whole cooling job. But the pool provides its own heat sink, as engineers would put it, absorbing all the heat you can produce as fast as you can produce it, leaving the heart to concentrate on responding to muscle demands for energy.

You can vary the distance you swim and the amount of rest you give yourself. You can develop skill at all four competitive strokes. By timing your swims, you can keep an accurate record of your progress in the various strokes.

Compare this bountiful variety with the boredom of running. Basically, there is only one way to run: put one foot in front of the other. If you do it slowly, you're walking; do it a little faster, and you're jogging; go faster still, you're running. That's about it. Of course, you can change your distance and the ups and downs of the terrain, if your neighborhood provides such variety, but basically running affords only one way of exercising, and it works your legs primarily. In contrast, swimming exercises the entire body.

Consider these other benefits of swimming:

- It provides the best overall fitness and does so with minimal assault on body parts, even on formerly unused muscles and joints. Here is an exercise for a lifetime. You can start swimming at age 8, 38, or 108 and continue to reap the benefits as long as you live.
- It helps you develop and maintain an ideal body, one that not only looks good but is strong, flexible, supple, better able to resist disease, and quicker to recover from illness or injury.
- It will help you control your weight and, more important, the percentage of your body that is fat.
- It will decrease stress, increase alertness, improve mental functioning, even enhance self-esteem.
- Research shows that it will improve your love life (see Chapter 11). You will find yourself making love more often and enjoying it more, no matter what your age.
- Physiologically, it will allow you to turn back the hands of time. Part of the reason you will derive all these benefits is that swimming will transform your body into that of a much younger person. And it will keep you young! As long as you swim, your body will display the physical attributes of a person many years your junior.
- The changes your body undergoes will help you resist the ravages of disease, such as diabetes, asthma, arthritis, heart disease, possibly some forms of cancer, and many other major and minor diseases. And if you do fall ill, the widespread benefits swimming provides your general health will improve both your odds and speed of recovery.
- Finally, I am sure you will be happy to learn that epidemiological evidence seems to confirm that swimmers live longer, although just how much longer is still being debated by experts. What is *not* debated is that the *quality* of your life will improve dramatically.

In the next three chapters, you will see how swimming can help bring about all these changes for you and how it can help you live a longer, fuller life.

3

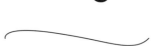

GETTING TO THE HEART
OF THE MATTER

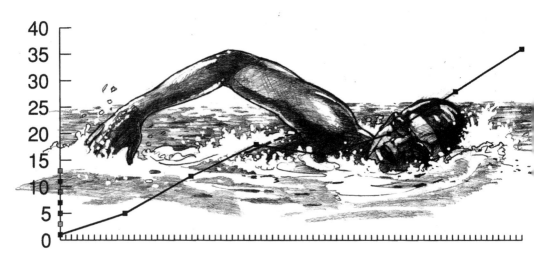

It was about nine-thirty on a cold February night in 1981 when Arnie Spector first felt the pain in his right arm. He was working late in his pharmacy on the corner of Essex and Chestnut streets, in Lynn, Mass-achusetts, a business he had owned since 1960.

At first he ignored it. After all, a fifty-year-old man should expect a few aches and pains every now and then. But the pain in his biceps grew more intense, then excruciating. Fearing the worst, he phoned for a relative to drive him to a nearby hospital.

While waiting in the emergency room, Arnie felt pain in his chest, and his feet grew colder than they had ever been. "Please hurry," he told the nurse. "I think I'm having a heart attack." Feeling very sleepy, he tried his best to stay awake. "I felt that if I fell asleep, I'd never wake up."

But he did lose consciousness, and did wake up, in a hospital bed the next morning, where he learned that he had suffered a massive heart attack. His heart had stopped beating for a minute and a half, and an emergency medical crew had had to defibrillate him. That explained the scabs on his chest. Shortly thereafter, Arnie underwent quadruple bypass surgery at New England Medical Center in Boston. Two of his coronary arteries had been totally clogged, a third obstructed 70 percent, and a fourth 40 percent.

SICK AT HEART

Arnie Spector was one of the lucky ones, for heart disease is a treacherous assassin. Silent for years, this killer often strikes with scant warning. Cardiovascular illness, which accounts for half of the deaths recorded in the United States each year, affects all of us: men, women, blacks, whites, the elderly, even the young; nearly a quarter of fatal heart attack victims are below the age of sixty-five. As a comparison, cancer, although more feared, claims only a third as many victims as heart disease.

Over two thirds of deaths attributable to cardiovascular disease are occasioned by heart attacks or strokes. Heart attacks, which take about 520,000 lives annually, occur when the coronary arteries, which supply oxygen-bearing blood to the heart, become clogged and the oxygen-deprived heart muscle is damaged. If too much tissue is affected, the heart becomes so weakened it can no longer pump effectively. But even mild damage can disrupt the electrical impulses that govern the heart's rhythmic beating, and this can lead to sudden death. Stroke, which claims another 150,000 lives each year, can also be caused by obstructed blood flow, this time to the brain, or by the blowout of a blood vessel supplying the brain.

All is not doom and gloom, however. The situation has improved radically over the past two decades. The incidence of fatal heart attacks has fallen by 25 percent, while the incidence of strokes has plummeted 40 percent. The reasons for this turnabout are clear: the fitness boom, which has brought home the importance of exercise in maintaining good health, a sharp decline in the number of Americans who smoke, an improvement in the diet of a significant portion of the population, and better diagnostic evaluation before a coronary event, including an aggressive campaign waged by the American Heart Association to detect and treat high blood pressure.

So the situation is improving. Still, it could be much better. Consider this: over 1.5 million Americans are stricken with heart attacks each year, more than one third of them fatal; heart failure afflicts an additional 2 million people, reducing the quality of their lives and limiting their activities; and millions more endure angina (chest pain or discomfort caused by narrowed coronary arteries) that causes them to live in fear as well as pain.

Medical experts agree that most of this suffering could be avoided if we all endeavored to adopt life-style changes that we already know reduce the odds of contracting heart disease. The first important step is to get into a regular program of exercise, which can eliminate, reduce, or help compensate for almost every major risk factor for heart disease. And, as we have seen, the exercise program that offers the highest benefit-to-risk ratio is swimming. So dig out your old bathing suit and get ready to take the plunge.

But first, to assure that there will be no backsliding of resolve, let's examine the causes of cardiovascular illness and look at the ways swimming can improve your chances of avoiding this sneak thief of life.

RISKY BUSINESS

The causes of heart disease are well-known. One factor we have no control over is heredity, the luck of the draw in the genes we received from our parents. But many other causative agents are almost synonymous with modern urban living: stress, smoking, a diet high in saturated fat, and a sedentary life-style.

The box on page 23 lists the leading cardiovascular risk factors, according to the American Heart Association. If you have any two of these factors, you should be concerned about the increased risk of suffering heart disease. If you have more than two, you should actively strive to eliminate all those you can, for these factors have a sort of multiplier effect: the more you have, the more dangerous each of them is.

Let's explore some of the most important risk factors.

MAJOR CARDIOVASCULAR RISK FACTORS

Genetic Factors
• Male sex
• Family history (parent or sibling) of heart attack under age fifty-five

Life-style Factors
• Lack of exercise
• High blood pressure
• High blood cholesterol
• Smoking
• Obesity

HIGH BLOOD PRESSURE

Having our blood pressure taken is a ritual with which we are all familiar. Most of us know our blood pressure—120/80, 135/95, or whatever. But what do the numbers actually mean? Blood pressure is simply the force exerted by the bloodstream against the walls of the arteries. Traditionally, it is expressed as a ratio, a larger number over a smaller one, for example, 120 over 80, usually written as 120/80, although the ratio between the two is irrelevant. What blood pressure of 120/80 means is this: the pressure when the heart contracts to pump blood to the arteries can drive a column of mercury up a tube to a height of 120 millimeters, known as the *systolic,* or pumping pressure. And when the heart relaxes between beats, the pressure exerted can support a column of mercury only 80 millimeters high, called the *diastolic,* or resting pressure.

Blood pressure is measured with an instrument called a sphygmomanometer, which is Greek for "pulse-pressure measurer." Usually a nurse wraps an inflatable cuff around your upper arm. Squeezing a rubber bulb, she pumps air into the cuff, which cuts off the blood flow to your lower arm. She then opens a valve and gradually releases the air. As she does, she listens with a stethoscope placed on an artery just below the cuff for a thumping sound that signals that the blood has started to flow again. The level of the mercury when she hears the first thump is your systolic pressure.

As the air is released and the cuff loosens its grip, the sound softens, eventually disappearing, signaling that your blood flow is no longer impeded, even in the heart's resting stage. The mercury level at the instant the thumping sound disappears is your diastolic pressure.

Generally speaking, the lower your blood pressure the better off you are. Readings between 110/75 and 140/90 are considered normal, but research has shown that people who live to advanced ages almost always have low blood pressure.

One of the myths about blood pressure is that it rises inevitably as we age. There seems little truth to this notion, especially when it comes to the more critical measurement, the diastolic pressure. But whether or not blood pressure tends to rise in older folks, such rises should not be treated as benign. Studies have found that older people with blood pressures of 140/90 or below live longer and have fewer strokes, heart attacks, and instances of heart failure than those whose pressures are even slightly higher.

The Silent Killer

High blood pressure is often called a silent killer: silent because even people with extremely high readings may experience no symptom of the disease; and killer because hypertension is one of the leading precipitators of heart attack, congestive heart failure, stroke, and kidney disease.

About one third of adult Americans—some 60 million people—are hypertensive to some degree. Even if you suffer from mild hypertension only, which begins as you cross 140/90, your risk of contracting heart disease is considerably greater than if your reading is below 140/90. Moderate high blood pressure—readings between 145/95 and 160/115—results in even greater risk. If your blood pressure measures 160/115 or over, you have severe hypertension and are shortening your life every day you leave your blood pressure at that level.

Controlling Hypertension

Fortunately, in most cases, hypertension can be controlled. A good first step? Swim.

Large clinical studies have shown that regular aerobic exercise combined with meditation or relaxation (such as Dr. Herbert Benson's famous "relaxation response") is very effective in lowering blood pressure for most people with high blood pressure. And no aerobic exercise is more effective in inducing a relaxed state than swimming.

My own experience provides a good example. I suffer from what doctors call *essential hypertension,* a tendency toward high blood pressure in the absence of any of the other factors doctors often find in hypertensive patients—obesity or high body fat, a lifetime of high cholesterol readings, an inactive life-style. When I was twenty-eight, before I began swimming again, my blood pressure consistently measured about 140/96—a high reading for a young man and one that signaled danger for the future. Because it involves no correlating factors, many doctors find essential hypertension the most intractable to treatment other than drug therapy. Yet within months after I began swimming, my blood pressure had declined to 130/90. Today, twenty-two years later, my blood pressure is a very healthy 116/74.

Because most antihypertensive drugs produce unpleasant side effects in many people, the first step the doctor will recommend for most people with high blood pressure is losing weight or, more precisely, lowering body fat percentage. The belief is that less fat in the diet will lead to less fat in the blood, which in turn will lead to less plaque formation on the inside walls of the arteries. As Chapter 4 will show, swimming is an effective way to reduce body fat. At one time it was thought that salt consumption was a major cause of hypertension and that reducing it would lower blood pressure. But researchers now believe that for many people who do not eat a high-salt diet, further reducing salt is not likely to bring about lower blood pressure.

So if you want to keep your blood pressure down, here is the two-pronged prescription. Swim, and set aside some time to relax each day. True, it takes a bit of self-discipline. But this is your life we are talking about, and these changes will make your life more pleasurable as well as longer. The alternative, drug therapy, may seem easier, but it is not very attractive over the long haul: a lifelong dependency on chemicals, most of which cause drowsiness, dry mouth, fatigue, skin disorders, or impotence in many people.

HIGH BLOOD CHOLESTEROL

Another major risk factor for heart disease is high serum cholesterol or, simply put, an excessive amount of cholesterol in the bloodstream. But what exactly is cholesterol? And what constitutes "excessive"?

Cholesterol is a waxy lipid, or fat, that is produced by the body and found in the cell membranes, nerve linings, and blood. Serum cholesterol is measured in milligrams per deciliter of blood; if your cholesterol level is 220, you have 220 milligrams of the fatty substance for every tenth of a liter of blood.

Less than half the cholesterol in your body comes from the foods you eat. The rest is manufactured in your liver and other body organs. After it is synthesized, the cholesterol is released into the bloodstream, where it is carried to different destinations.

Like high blood pressure, high blood cholesterol can be a silent killer, causing your body injury while presenting no symptoms. So it is important to have your cholesterol measured at least every two years. According to the National Institutes of Health, your blood cholesterol should not exceed 200. Readings of 200 to 240 are considered borderline. A reading above 240 is categorized as high and considered a significant cardiac risk factor (see Table 3.1).

TABLE 3.1
Cholesterol Levels

Health Status	*Total Cholesterol*
Desirable	170–200
Borderline	200–240
Risky	over 240

Just how significant a factor cholesterol is depends on your other risk factors. Let's say, for example, that your cholesterol level is 240. If you are a fifty-year-old man who smokes a pack of cigarettes a day, is obese (27 percent body fat or above), rarely exercises, has a blood pressure of 140/95, and whose father died of a heart attack at age fifty-nine, you are in big trouble.

If, however, your blood cholesterol is 240 but you are a trim, non-smoking, fifty-year-old woman, with normal blood pressure and healthy, elderly parents, your risk of having a heart attack is much lower. Still, you would be in an even better position if that 240 were reduced, for it is no longer deniable that lowering your cholesterol reduces your chance of having a heart attack. The Japanese are an impressive illustration of the strong influence of cholesterol in bringing about heart attacks. In Japan, the average blood cholesterol is very low, and heart attack rates are correspondingly low. This is true even though smoking is common and blood pressure tends to be higher than among Americans. But ethnic Japanese who live in America and eat the high-fat American diet have higher cholesterol levels and more heart attacks than their relatives eating the Japanese diet.

HDL and LDL: "Good" and "Bad" Cholesterol

Actually, we have learned recently that the cholesterol issue is a bit more complicated than knowing your total blood cholesterol. There are several types of lipoproteins (transporters of cholesterol), the most important of which are HDL (high-density lipoprotein) and LDL (low-density lipoprotein). They act in very different ways, and with very different consequences for your health.

It turns out that LDL delivers cholesterol to the walls of the arteries, where it is deposited as plaque. Over time these fatty deposits accumulate, narrowing the arteries. The result is heart disease. However, HDL does just the opposite. It strips the cholesterol from arterial walls and carries it back to the liver, where it is converted to bile and then eliminated. So HDL actually reduces the total amount of cholesterol in the body. Generally speaking, the more HDL you have, the better off you are: 45 milligrams per deciliter is about average. Levels of HDL under 35 are considered risky, while figures of 55 and above provide greater protection against heart disease.

One way to think of the heart's health is as a battle waged between the good guys, HDL, and the bad guys, LDL. When a person develops heart disease, the contest has been won by LDL. So, if you want to know how the battle is going in your own body, you should be most interested in the amounts of HDL and LDL rather than total cholesterol.

What seems most important is the amount of HDL relative to total cholesterol. This is sometimes expressed as the percentage of total cholesterol that is HDL, but more often it is put the other way, as the ratio of total cholesterol to HDL. In the first way of measuring HDL, the higher the number the better for you; in the second, the lower the ratio, the better. Table 3.2 shows a range of values and their associated levels of risk.

Let's say your total cholesterol is 200 and your HDL is 44. That would give you a ratio of 4.5. This ratio means you have an average risk of developing heart disease. Another example: imagine that your total cholesterol is a desirable 180, but your HDL is only 30. This gives you a ratio of 6.0, which means that your risk is about double the aver-

TABLE 3.2
HDL and Total Cholesterol

Ratio Total/HDL	Percentage HDL in Total	Risk
8.0	12.5%	Very High
7.0	14.3	
6.0	16.7	High
5.5	18.2	
5.0	20.0	
4.5	22.2	Average
4.0	25.0	
3.5	28.6	
3.3	30.3	Low
3.0	33.3	
2.5	40.0	Very Low

age. If with the same total cholesterol your HDL were 60, then the ratio would be 3.0 and you would have about half the average risk.

Shifting the Odds in Your Favor

There are two ways to change the ratio in your favor: lowering LDL or raising HDL. The best strategy, I believe, is a dual approach. Most doctors will tell you that it is easier to reduce LDL, by changing what you eat: cut down on saturated fats and increase the amount of dietary fiber you take in. The best way to reduce saturated fats is to limit the amount of red meat and dairy products you eat and replace highly saturated tropical plant oils (such as coconut and palm oil) with less saturated vegetable oils.

As for the amount of fiber we should be consuming, let's look at the diet we humans evolved eating. A fascinating study of the diet of prehistoric people, originally published in *The New England Journal of Medicine,* indicates that they ate about 100 grams of fiber a day. Nutritionists, apparently resigned to modern reality, recommend that we eat at least 25 grams of fiber a day. But the average American diet falls far short even of this modest goal, containing only about 10 to 12 grams.

Vegetables such as carrots, broccoli, artichokes, peas, radishes, and collard greens and fruits such as apples, berries, figs, pears, and nectarines are particularly rich in dietary fiber. By the way, fiber has an added bonus: it protects against colon cancer.

The other way to shift the ratio in your favor is to increase your level of HDL. And this is much more easily done than most doctors believe. The key is contained in one eight-letter word: exercise.

Studies have shown that you must exercise for at least twenty minutes, three days a week, to get minimal results. But to raise your HDL significantly, all it takes is a little more: a total of only two to five hours a week, spread out over five or more days. We know that swimmers begin to raise HDL levels about six weeks into this kind of regimen.

Not long ago I discovered just how effective swimming can be in boosting HDL. In late 1990 I came down with a mysterious liver ailment after spending two weeks in the Amazon. The illness kept me bedridden for almost six months. At the end of that time, blood tests showed that my total cholesterol was 227 and my HDL was 49. That gave me a ratio of 4.6, meaning my risk of developing heart disease was just slightly above average. After recovering I began training again, swimming about five to seven hours a week.

Within a year my total cholesterol had improved only modestly, down to 209. But my HDL level had almost doubled, to 90. This changed my total cholesterol-to-HDL ratio to 2.3, which my doctor informed me was off the chart on the safe side.

OTHER MAJOR RISK FACTORS

The American Heart Association reports the major life-style cardiac risk factors as lack of exercise, smoking, and obesity. Not far behind are two institutions as American as apple pie: a diet high in fat, especially saturated fat, and our fast-paced, stressed-out way of life. Fortunately, swimming, by itself, can ameliorate all these factors.

Lack of Exercise

Exercise does much more than improve the total cholesterol to HDL ratio. For instance, it builds heart and lung capacity and improves circulation. Yet, more than two decades into the fitness revolution, and after hundreds of scientific studies proving the many health benefits of physical fitness, an estimated 60 percent of American adults still get no exercise. Citing this fact, the American Heart Association in 1992 added inactivity to its list of major risk factors for heart disease. An AHA committee headed by Dr. Gerald F. Fletcher noted that a sedentary way of life was as big a risk factor for heart disease as high cholesterol, high blood pressure, or smoking.

According to Ralph S. Paffenberger, a professor of epidemiology at Stanford Medical School and one of the pioneers in studying the health benefits of exercise, if every American exercised, deaths from heart attacks and strokes might drop an additional 25 to 30 percent, and deaths from all causes might decline by as much as 15 percent. "That's equivalent to what you'd get if you abolished smoking," Paffenberger says.

Paffenberger was the author of a seminal study that first clinched the argument for exercise. In it he followed 17,000 Harvard alumni, ages thirty-five to seventy-four, for twenty years. People who made a lifetime habit of regular exercise (for example, swimming at least three times a week) had about half as many heart attacks as those who were sedentary. Even smokers, obese people, and those with high blood pressure or family histories of heart disease benefited from exercise. Another study, of 6,000 San Francisco longshoremen over twenty-two years, produced the same results.

Smoking

Americans are finally getting the message about tobacco: in terms of the number of people affected, it is the deadliest drug around. Since 1965 the percentage of people who smoke has declined steadily; by 1993 only about one in four Americans were still puffing away.

Nevertheless, cigarette smoking remains one of the AHA's top-ranking coronary risk culprits. Aside from being by far the most important cause of lung cancer and a major factor in other forms of cancer, it also affects the heart; smoking is implicated in about one fourth of deaths from all causes. How does it do all this damage? By speeding up the heart rate, raising blood pressure, constricting blood vessels, and depressing HDL levels. Smokers are twice as likely as nonsmokers to have a heart attack and three times as likely to die from heart disease. The AHA estimates that more than 150,000 deaths from heart disease alone could be avoided each year in the United States if people gave up smoking.

While there have been no conclusive scientifically controlled studies to test whether regular swimming will cause you to stop smoking, two studies I conducted thirteen years apart suggest that almost all smokers who begin swimming for health and fitness reasons give up the nasty weed. Those few who do not quit altogether significantly reduce the number of cigarettes they smoke each day. These studies are detailed in Chapter 5.

Obesity

Related to high blood pressure, high cholesterol, and lack of exercise is obesity. In plain English, being too fat. Obesity is a major cardiac risk factor in itself. But as well, people who are fat are more likely to have high blood pressure, a high cholesterol count, and a sedentary life-style.

Fortunately, there is a painless cure for obesity: *swim.* As the next chapter will show, contrary to what some experts contend, swimming is one of the best ways to lose weight, especially when combined with a prudent diet. Far more important, it is an ideal way to decrease body fat.

Let's say you can swim a mile in forty minutes—the equivalent of running the same distance in ten minutes. That will burn about 415 calories—more if you swim a stroke other than freestyle. If you swim your mile four times a week, you will lose about a pound each week, most of it fat. So not only will you be losing weight but much of the weight you lose will be fat.

Take, for example, a 180-pound man with 25 percent body fat. He is lugging around 45 pounds of fat on his frame. Although that is about average for a thirty-five-year-old American male, it is well over the 19 percent that signals the onset of cardiovascular risk. And he is only 2 percent away from being classified as morbidly obese.

Five months after beginning a program of swimming a mile a day, four or five times a week, our typical American male will have dropped to a svelte 160 pounds and, no doubt, will be out purchasing a new wardrobe. More significant, he will have reduced his body fat to about 18.7 percent of his total body weight, or approximately 30 pounds. That's enough to get him below the level of risk for developing cardio-vascular disease. Still, he has a way to go before reaching the "ideal" 15 percent body fat level that medical experts say indicates physical fitness. Another six to eight weeks of swimming should do the trick.

Or consider a woman weighing 135 pounds with 33 percent body fat. Again, although she is about average for a thirty-five-year-old American female, she's already well beyond the 24 percent figure that puts a woman at risk for developing heart disease. And she is only a single percentage point from the medical classification of morbid obesity.

Half a year after beginning a swimming program of just one mile a day, four or five days a week, our model American female will have dropped her weight to about 115 pounds. With fat constituting most of the weight loss, her body fat percentage will be down to 24—significantly lower than the average thirty-five- or even twenty-five-year-old and within striking distance of the "ideal" 22 percent level that defines physical fitness for women. More important, she will have eliminated the risk that comes with being obese.

There is nothing unusual about these examples. I have seen such transformations happen hundreds, perhaps thousands, of times. And at Masters swim meets, I see all around me men and women in their fifties, sixties, and older with the bodies of twenty- and twenty-five-year-olds. They look the way the human animal is supposed to look: trim, well-muscled, flexible, healthy, and strong. What they have done is simply kept a promise to themselves to do the best form of exercise there is—swimming—on a regular basis. The payoff—a healthy heart, an attractive body, boundless energy, a renewed enthusiasm for life—more than justifies the time commitment. And if they can do it, so can you.

Modern Life

Some of the standard components of life in modern industrial society also constitute significant risk factors for heart disease. Among these are stress and a diet high in saturated fat. Once again, these factors are often seen in combination with other risk factors—for instance, hypertension and high cholesterol—which magnify their negative effects.

Rhythmic, aerobic exercise has been discovered to be an effective means for reducing stress and so has helped many Americans deal with their lives in a more healthy way. But it remains true that no exercise is better for reducing stress than swimming.

Much has been written about "runner's high," the endorphin-induced state of relaxation that often accompanies distance running. Actually, the name is a misnomer, for the state can be induced by many activities, among them swimming. Not only does swimming provide the same high and the same stress-reducing benefits as running or biking but it does so in an environment, water, that is especially soothing to the body and psyche. When I finish a swim, no matter how tough or tiring, I always feel a sense of inner peace and relaxation.

As for diet, swimming cannot affect what you eat directly. You can fill your body with high-fat junk food whether you work out or not. But once most people commit themselves to improving their health through exercise, they also begin to experience a taste for a healthier diet. Chapter 4 will explain what constitutes a healthier diet and how swimming and diet can work hand in hand to reward you with optimal health throughout your life.

SWIM FOR YOUR LIFE

I hope you agree at this point that swimming can literally save your life. Here is a summary of what extensive scientific research conducted over the past thirty years has shown swimming can do to help you eliminate the chances of cardiovascular disease:

- Lower your blood pressure
- Lower your total cholesterol
- Increase your HDL, the "good" cholesterol
- Help you stop smoking
- Improve your ability to dissolve blood clots (we haven't discussed this one yet, but we will)
- Lower your heart rate

In doing all this, it may well prevent that heart attack or stroke you could be heading for.

Table 3.3 (see page 34) shows how my heart's health has been affected since I began swimming again.

Once again, there is nothing extraordinary or magical about what I have achieved. Thousands, perhaps tens of thousands, of other people have turned their hearts' health around in exactly the same way. And all we have done to achieve this result is made swimming a given in our lives. From this commitment, everything else follows.

TABLE 3.3
Effects of Swimming on Author's Health

Variable	At Age 28	At Age 50
Weight	188 lbs.	180 lbs.
% body fat	17.6%	9.8%
Blood pressure	140/96	116/74
Total cholesterol	229	209
HDL cholesterol	unknown	90
Chol:HDL ratio	unknown	2.3
Heart rate	64	42

HOW MUCH IS ENOUGH?

"Okay," you say. "I buy what you say, but I'm a busy person. I've got a career, a family, other obligations. Just *how much* do I need to swim to keep my heart healthy?" The answer, say experts, is surprisingly little.

According to the AHA, a regular program of swimming—a minimum of thirty minutes at least three times a week—will improve the condition of heart, arteries, and lungs while lowering blood pressure, decreasing total cholesterol, and raising HDL. It will also lower your percent of body fat and help you lose weight. Four or five sessions each week will provide even better results. The American College of Sports Medicine suggests you swim fifteen to sixty minutes a day, three to five days a week.

A recent study published in the magazine *Circulation* demonstrated that only four thirty-minute sessions a week—two hours a week—reduced blood pressure by an average of six points for the systolic and ten points for the diastolic for a group of middle-aged, out-of-shape men with mild hypertension. And it only took ten weeks.

A study published in *The New England Journal of Medicine* found that people who are physically unfit have more than three times the risk of dying of a heart attack as people who are fit, regardless of their cholesterol levels, age, or whether they are smokers. How much do you need to swim to reduce your risk of heart attack threefold? "About 30 to 40 minutes, three to four times a week," according to the study's lead author, Dr. Lars-Goran Ekelund, associate professor of medicine at the University of North Carolina at Chapel Hill.

Two additional studies, conducted at the University of Washington, demonstrated that exercise such as swimming four times a week for forty-five minutes results in an increase of over 40 percent of the body's production of tissue plasminogen activator, or TPA, the substance that dissolves blood clots that can block coronary arteries narrowed by atherosclerosis and precipitate a heart attack. Tissue plasminogen activator is a potent clot buster that is given in artificial form to thousands of heart attack victims each year. Moderate exercise, such as swimming, eliminates the need to take this drug.

Another recent study, this one conducted at the University of Massachusetts Medical School under the direction of Dr. Ann Ward, found that moderate exercise combined with a modest reduction in fatty foods produced major cardiovascular benefits in only four months. Ward's subjects, overweight, sedentary, middle-aged men, dropped their total blood cholesterol by twenty-three points while increasing their HDL six points.

The list of such studies goes on and on. But Dr. Manuel Sanguily of New York, one of the top Masters swimmers in the world and an expert on the effects of exercise on cardiovascular health, sums it up this way: "If you're one of the 60 million Americans who are at risk for a heart attack, the very best thing you can do for yourself is to start swimming."

HOW HARD SHOULD YOU SWIM?

There is no way around it. If you want cardiovascular benefits from any exercise, you are going to have to make your heart work. But how hard? If you are over thirty-five, be sure to consult your doctor before starting any fitness program. The same holds if you are under thirty-five and have any major risk factors for heart disease, such as high blood pressure. But once you have gotten the go-ahead, you have to determine how much you want to exercise your heart and lungs.

To come to some intelligent guidelines that will work for you, you will need to do a few calculations. The first is *heart rate,* simply the number of times your heart is beating in a minute. Place your finger where you can feel your pulse in the hollow at the upper inside area of your wrist or at the side of your neck and count the beats for five seconds. Then multiply that number by 12. The answer will be your heart rate. If you do this when you haven't been exercising, the number is your resting heart rate (RHR).

Next you have to compute your maximum heart rate (MHR), the most times a minute a heart your age should beat. You can do this by subtracting your age from 220. Thus, if you are 40, your MHR is about 180.

The next number you will have to know is your *training range,* the range within which you want to keep your heart rate while exercising so that it is high enough to do your heart some good but not so high that it creates a risk for you. To calculate your training range, multiply your MHR first by .60, which will give you the lower threshold of your training range, and then by .80, to establish a safe upper limit. For a forty-year-old, the training range is between 108 to 144 beats per minute. Or you can just consult Table 3.4.

TABLE 3.4
Training Range for Cardiovascular Benefits by Age

Age	*Beats per Minute*
25	117–156
30	114–152
35	111–148
40	108–144
45	105–140
50	102–136
55	99–132
60	96–128
65	93–124
70	90–120
75	87–116
80	84–112
85	81–108
90	78–104

Table 3.4, based on AHA recommendations, is easily understood and simple to use. But it is only a rough approximation. If you would like a more precise estimate of your training range, there is a more complicated formula that yields a more personal value. Its advantage is that it takes into account improvements in your aerobic fitness level as you continue training. Here's how it works:

First figure your maximum heart rate (MHR) by subtracting your age from 220.

Then find your resting heart rate (RHR), preferably just before you get out of bed in the morning.

Now, calculate your target heart rate using these two formulas:

0.6 (MHR − RHR) + RHR
0.8 (MHR − RHR) + RHR

If you are thirty-five years old and have a resting heart rate of 55, it would work out this way:

0.6 (185 − 55) + 55 = 0.6 × 130 + 55 = 133 minimum rate
0.8 (185 − 55) + 55 = 0.8 × 130 + 55 = 159 maximum rate

So, because your heart is now in good shape, as indicated by your low RHR, 55, your heart rate while swimming should be a little higher than the range in the table.

IT'S NEVER TOO LATE TO START

Of course, the ideal time to begin swimming is when you are young. A lifetime of swimming will yield a lifetime of benefits. But research has shown that it is never too late to begin, even if you already have heart disease. My good friend Dr. Dean Ornish, of the University of California Medical School at San Francisco, has demonstrated conclusively that moderate exercise combined with a low-fat diet and meditation can actually reverse severe hardening of the arteries. Other studies have produced similar evidence attesting to the benefits of exercise for people with cardiovascular illness. In fact, properly prescribed swimming can help even if you have had a heart attack. Of course, you should get good medical advice before you begin.

SWIMMING AFTER A HEART ATTACK

European specialists have long prescribed swimming for their heart disease patients, but only recently has the practice caught on in the United States. Research conducted by Thomas G. Manfredi and his colleagues at the University of Rhode Island Human Performance Laboratory and the Cardiac Rehabilitation Program bears witness to the value of swimming and water exercise in the rehabilitation of cardiac patients. A series of studies found that swimming provides all the cardiovascular benefits that land-based exercises do. And swimming has several major advantages: the energy cost of swimming was similar to that of treadmill and arm exercises, but blood pressure was lower. And swimmers were far less likely than patients who engaged in land-based exercises to suffer heart arrhythmias while exercising. Most important, swimming uses a greater muscle mass than treadmill or arm exercises. Also, a swimming pool is conducive to supportive rather than competitive group interaction, as evidenced by the number of cultures that employ communal bathing as a regular unwinding activity. This improves the chances that the exerciser will stay with the program, which can mean the difference between life and death.

Remember Arnie Spector, the Lynn, Massachusetts, pharmacist? After his heart attack in 1981, Arnie was in such bad condition that he was unable even to take a stress test. But he had no intention of sliding into permanent invalidism. After his surgery, on the advice of his cardiologist, Arnie began swimming. At first he didn't get very far. The first time in the water he was only able to manage two or three strokes! But he kept plugging away. Two weeks later he swam the length of the pool—twenty-five yards. Within four months he was swimming a mile, in a very respectable forty minutes. He has been a regular swimmer ever since.

Now age sixty-three, Arnie swims a mile three days a week and a half mile three other days. He supplements his swimming by training on a stairclimber for twenty minutes three days a week. And on pleasant evenings he takes a leisurely two-mile walk with his wife, Sandy. He also made some other life-style changes: he quit smoking (he'd been a light smoker), broke the twelve- to fourteen-cup-a-day coffee habit he had started in the navy, and began eating a low-fat, low-sodium diet.

The results of all these changes have been dramatic. At age sixty-three, Arnie Spector is far healthier than he was at fifty—or forty! His blood pressure is down to 128/86, his heart rate is down to sixty, his cholesterol is down to 190, his cholesterol-to-HDL ratio is an excellent 3.8, and his body fat percentage is an "ideal" 15 percent. Not only is he alive but he is fully alive—healthy, happy, and active. And it all started with those first few strokes he took in a pool when he thought he might never again be able to do anything strenuous.

Chapter 5 will explain how swimming can add years and enjoyment to your own life. But first let's look at swimming and weight.

4

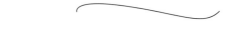

SWIM AND BE TRIM

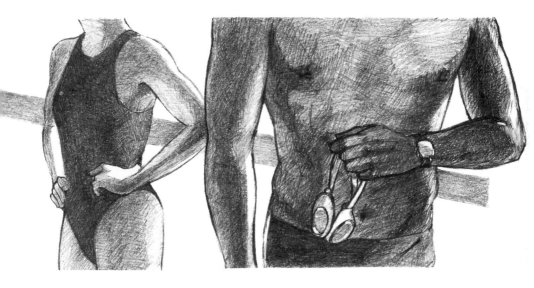

ONE OF THE major reasons people say they swim is that it makes them look and feel more youthful. The vast majority of Masters swimmers certainly appear much younger than nonswimmers their age.

After being around swimmers for a while, you come to accept as the norm this youthful appearance, as well as the youthful attitude that seems to go with it. It is only when suddenly confronted with the larger world that you are reminded just how unusual swimmers are. I recall how shocked I was several years ago when I traveled to Washington, DC, for a meeting of the American Sociological Association right after attending the U.S. national Masters swimming championships. Having just been with almost 2,000 extraordinarily youthful and fit men and women between the ages of twenty-five and eighty-seven, I was shocked to see what the real world looked like. Many of the sociologists were smoking, quite a few were noticeably fat and out of shape, almost all took elevators to the second or third floor of their hotels and cabs between hotels only a few blocks apart; many munched on the doughnuts the meeting organizers provided as "snacks" at the back of each lecture room.

THE LOOK

Americans have long viewed the swimmer's body as a cultural ideal. A recent Valentine's Day article in *The Boston Globe* on dating services (both straight and gay) reported that over a quarter of men and women placing personal ads described themselves as having "a swimmer's body."

This cultural ideal has existed for at least hundreds of years, as Michelangelo's *David* testifies. Often cited as representing the epitome of masculine beauty, this statue does not have the gaunt, almost emaciated look of a distance runner. Nor does it have the bulky appearance of a bodybuilder. *David* looks like a swimmer, freshly emerged from a workout. He has a strong, V-shaped torso; a well-defined body with long, smooth, supple muscles; and low body fat. In short, he looks remarkably much more like Mark Spitz or Matt Biondi than Arnold Schwarzenegger.

For women too the swimmer's body defines the cultural ideal. Most women want strong bodies, but they also want to retain a natural feminine build, not the haggard look of a distance runner. Nor do most consider the bulky, power-lifter look an ideal feminine form. Most women would rather look like 1992 Olympic hero Summer Sanders, Academy Award–winning actress Mary Steenburgen, or fifty-plus singer Judy Collins, projecting confidence, supple strength, and radiant good health.

SWIMMING AND WEIGHT LOSS

By now you are aware that swimming is the best, most complete form of exercise there is, that it provides all the cardiovascular benefits of running while exercising all the muscles of the body, and that it offers protection against a host of deadly diseases. But you may not be convinced that swimming is also an excellent way to lose weight. The reason is that many of the experts are themselves confused and do not stress swimming as the excellent weight-reduction exercise it can be.

Take, for example, Covert Bailey, author of *The New Fit or Fat.* In a recent article in *Men's Health* magazine, Bailey extols the benefits of swimming but writes that swimmers carry more body fat than runners or cyclists. He concludes, "If you're overweight, I don't recommend it as your only exercise." He goes on to suggest that overweight people start with swimming before moving "on to exercises that burn more fat."

The reason such experts are confused and their conclusions misleading has to do with the way calorie-burning capabilities of different sports are compared. Studies by University of California exercise physiologist Steven Gregg, Educational Testing Service statistician Howard Wainer, and others indicate that one mile of swimming is about equivalent to four miles of running. This 4-to-1 rule of thumb is supported by a comparison of the world records for men and women in the 400-meter freestyle and the one-mile (about 1,600 meters) run. The records are almost identical.

Think of it this way: if you work out for an hour, you might be able to run about eight miles or swim two. But the energy expended, and the calories burned, will be approximately the same.

I did say approximately, for it is true that because of the buoyancy of water and the swimmer's horizontal position swimming burns slightly fewer calories than running. But the difference is very small, and the benefits of swimming—including the fact that it is virtually injury free and therefore more likely to be continued without interruption—far outweigh this tiny difference in leading to complete a successful weight-loss program.

Bailey is not the only exercise guru to sell swimming short. An article by runner Hal Higdon in *American Health* presents a chart comparing the benefits of thirteen forms of exercise. Again, swimming is acknowledged as "great" for building aerobic endurance and upper-body strength, improving flexibility, and reducing stress, but it is rated as only "fair" for weight control. The chart states that you will burn 320 calories per half hour at a speed of 50 yards per minute and 150 per half hour at 20 yards per minute.

The problem is the swimming speeds Higdon has chosen as his

examples. These are extremely slow paces, resulting in thirty-five-
and eighty-eight-minute miles. Using the 4-to-1 rule, they translate to
running a mile in about nine minutes at the faster pace and twenty-
two minutes at the slower. The first is the equivalent of a moderate
jog. The second is slower than walking!

If you compare calories burned in equivalent running and swimming efforts, here is what you get:

| | Calories per 30 minutes | |
Pace for One Mile	Running	Swimming
6-min. run = 24-min. swim	450	440
10-min. run = 40-min. swim	355	310

These results are for the crawl stroke, the most efficient of all swimming styles. If you swim at the same pace using one of the other
strokes—backstroke, breaststroke, or butterfly—you will actually
burn *more* calories.

REDUCING BODY FAT

So swimming is an excellent way to lose weight. But simply losing
weight does not mean getting fit. You can be thin and still be
unhealthy. The key is reducing *body fat*. Here swimming's credentials
are even more impressive, for, contrary to Bailey's contention,
Olympic swimmers have close to the lowest body-fat percentages of
any athletes: about 6 percent for men and 12 percent for women.

But what about ordinary folk like you and me? Medical experts
agree that to be fit, a man should have 15 percent body fat or less; a
woman 22 percent or less. In general, women have a higher percentage of body fat than men because women's breasts are composed of
fatty tissue and women have more internal fat to protect their reproductive organs.

If you are above these levels, you must consider yourself overweight even though you may be within normal limits on an insurance
company chart. According to the most recent health statistics, at age
thirty-five the average American male carries 25 percent of his weight
in fat, the average female 33 percent. These figures are perilously
close to those that place your health in serious jeopardy.

Without exercise, people lose muscle and add fat as they grow older. Their weight may stay the same, but by middle age the average American is carrying far too much fat. Excessive levels of body fat are strongly correlated with heart disease, diabetes, cancer, and many other diseases.

People who exercise regularly add body fat much more slowly as they age. The typical man in an exercise program carries 16 percent of his body weight in fat at age twenty-five and 23 percent at age fifty-five. For women, the figures are 19 percent at age twenty-five and 29 percent thirty years later.

As mentioned, numerous studies have shown that regular swimming results in significant weight loss. More important, it leads to a decrease in body fat. In one study, overweight middle-aged men lost twelve to fifteen pounds of body fat during just twelve weeks of swim training. In another, overweight women lost fifteen to twenty pounds after swimming for ten weeks. Masters swimmers who train a minimum of forty-five minutes a day, three or more times a week, fare even better.

Forty-six-year-old Bill Purdin was horrified when he weighed in at 194 pounds, more than 30 pounds above his college weight. A body-fat analysis showed that at 22 percent he was lugging around almost 43 pounds of fat. The busy Boston-area advertising executive had tried working out over the years but had never stuck to a program. His imminent encroachment on 200 pounds must have provided special motivation, for this time he did. As a result of training six hours a week, Bill's weight dropped to 164 in less than six months. More important, his body fat percentage dropped to just over 16 percent. His goal is to reach 12 percent and stay there.

My own experience is similar. In 1971 I was a twenty-eight-year-old hotshot, several years into a promising publishing career and probably a bit more active than most guys my age. I had been a competitive swimmer in college and had continued to work out on and off while in graduate school. Although I no longer exercised in any sort of program, I did go for a bike ride once or twice a week and tried to squeeze in an occasional game of touch football or a set or two of tennis. I even got into the pool every now and then. On top of that, as a single father I was kept hopping by my then three-year-old son, Russell.

But clearly I was on the road of ever-decreasing activity that ultimately would lead to serious health problems. I already weighed in at 188 pounds, 10 pounds above my competitive weight in college. And my waist had expanded five inches, to a nice round girth of thirty-six inches. My body fat was 17.6 percent, not terrible but well above the 15.0 percent that defines fitness for a man and less than 2.0 percent from the point at which coronary risk begins.

In December 1971 I began swimming again, and I have been doing it ever since. Now, at the age of fifty, I am in far better shape than I was twenty-two years ago. My weight is back down to the 180 pounds I weighed as a college freshman, my waist is a trim 32 1/4 inches, and my body fat is 9.8 percent. (See Table 4.1 for a more detailed comparison.)

TABLE 4.1
Effects of Swimming on Author's Weight and Body Fat

Variable	At Age 28	At Age 50
Weight	188 lbs.	180 lbs.
Chest	44 in.	44 in.
Waist	36 in.	32 1/4 in.
Lean body weight	154.9 lbs.	162.4 lbs.
Body fat	33.1 lbs.	17.6 lbs.
% body fat	17.6%	9.8%

I have *lost* over seventeen pounds of fat while *gaining* seven pounds of muscle. And I have never been healthier.

There is nothing unique about my experience. In 1991–92, I tested the body fat of over 700 Masters swimmers from throughout the United States and several other countries. The results are shown in Table 4.2.

TABLE 4.2
Body Fat of Masters Swimmers by Age

| Age | Percent Body Fat | |
	Women	Men
25–34	17.6%	10.1%
35–44	17.7	13.6
45–54	19.3	14.3
55–64	20.4	15.6
65–74	19.9	15.7
75–84	21.6	17.4

These dramatic figures demonstrate that losing muscle mass and increasing fat are not inevitable parts of the aging process. In fact, it seems crystal clear that if you swim regularly, you can remain fit and trim, with little increase in body fat.

Table 4.3 illustrates this point by comparing Masters swimmers with people in an exercise program and with sedentary individuals to illustrate how body fat changes with age.

TABLE 4.3
Changes in Body Fat with Age

Age	Sedentary		Exercising		Masters Swimmers	
	Men	*Women*	*Men*	*Women*	*Men*	*Women*
25	23%	29%	16%	21%	10%	17%
35	25%	33%	18%	23%	13%	17%
45	28%	35%	21%	25%	14%	19%
55+	30%	39%	23%	29%	15%	20%

Figures for sedentary individuals and exercisers adapted from Jeffrey Fischer, *The Chromium Program* (HarperCollins, 1990).

Measuring Body Fat

There are several ways to determine how much body fat you have. The original method, and theoretically the most accurate, is called *hydrostatic weighing,* or water weighing. Here you are weighed while you hold your breath under water. Then you are weighed again as you duck your head under water and exhale all the air in your lungs.

The *skin caliper* test is another common method of measuring body fat. A caliper gathers up and measures the thickness of your fat and skin at specific spots on your body, such as your triceps.

A third method, called *electrical impedance,* is based on the fact that muscle contains more water than fat and thus is a better conductor of electricity. Sensor pads connected to a monitor are placed on your ankle and wrist; then a small current is sent through the sensors. The time it takes the electrical impulse to travel the length of your body reveals how much fat and lean tissue you have.

All these techniques require special equipment and some expertise in its use. But not to worry. According to Jack H. Wilmore, an exercise physiologist at the University of Texas, you can estimate your body-fat percentage fairly accurately using only a scale, a tape measure, and the charts in Figure 4.1. Here's how:

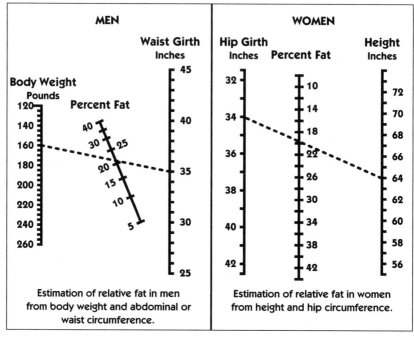

Figure 4.1. Body-Fat Estimation Charts for Men and Women

Men: Weigh yourself, then measure your waist at the belly button. Using a straightedge, line up the two figures on the chart. Your body-fat percentage is where the straightedge crosses the percent body-fat line.

Women: Measure your hips at their widest point. Using a straightedge, draw a line connecting your hip girth with your height. Read your body-fat percentage where the line crosses the percent body-fat line.

A highly accurate method for calculating your body fat involves only slightly more effort. The only tools you need are a scale, a tape measure, and the ability to perform a simple arithmetic calculation.

Body-Fat Calculation for Women

1. Measure your hips at their widest point and your waist at your belly button.
2. Measure your height without shoes.

3. Record these measurements on the work sheet on page 48.
4. Find each of these measurements in the table in Appendix D and record the constants on the work sheet.
5. Add Constants A and B, then subtract Constant C from this sum. Round to the nearest whole number. The figure is your percentage body fat.

Let's say that you are 5 feet 6 inches tall. Your hips are 36 inches, and your waist is 27 inches. Here is how to calculate your body fat:

Hips: 36 inches   Constant A = 41.86
Waist: 27 inches   Constant B = 19.20
Height: 66 inches   Constant C = 40.23
Add Constants A and B:

$$\begin{array}{r} 41.86 \\ +19.20 \\ \hline 61.06 \end{array}$$

Now subtract Constant C:

$$\begin{array}{r} 61.06 \\ -40.23 \\ \hline 20.83 \end{array}$$

Round out to the nearest whole number, and you get 21 percent.

Some things to keep in mind: Take all your measurements on bare skin, making sure the tape is snug but not too tight. The best procedure is to take each measurement three times, then use the average. When taking your waist measurement, be sure you measure at the belly button and not at the narrowest point.

I have found this simple procedure to be remarkably accurate and a good way to keep a record of your progress as you get into shape. However, it is important to keep in mind that the procedure was developed using averages based on the measurements of thousands of women. My experience is that it tends to overestimate slightly the body-fat percentage of women in excellent shape and women with smaller than average breasts. It also underestimates somewhat the body-fat percentage of women with larger than average breasts.

Your body composition is an important measure of your physical fitness. How do you compare with other women? Table 4.4 lists the body-fat percentages for different reference groups. This list will help put your own body-fat percentage in perspective. It will also allow you to measure your progress as you get into shape.

WORK SHEET FOR
WOMEN TO CALCULATE BODY-FAT PERCENTAGE

Hip measurement: _____ (for Constant A)
Waist measurement: _____ (for Constant B)
Height: _____ (for Constant C)

Using Appendix D, look up each of the measurements in the appropriate column. Enter these constants here:

Constant A = _____
Constant B = _____
Constant C = _____

To determine your approximate body-fat percentage, add Constant A and Constant B. Then subtract Constant C:

Constant A: _____
plus Constant B: +_____
Subtotal: _____
Minus Constant C: −_____
% Body Fat: _____

TABLE 4.4
Women's Body-Fat Percentages

Reference Group	Body Fat
Lowest female measured	6%
Average anorexic patient	10
Medically unsafe for most females	11
Gymnasts	14
Swimmers	14
Racquetball players	15
Distance runners	15
Cyclists	15
Masters swimmers, age 25–44	17
Aerobic dance instructors	17
Cross-country skiers	18
Masters swimmers, age 45–54	19
Average 25-year-old in exercise program	19
Masters swimmers, age 55–74	20
Tennis players, alpine skiers	20
Hurdlers, basketball players, volleyball players	21
Masters swimmers, age 75–84	21
"Ideal" fit female	22
Upper limit for professional athletes	22
Average 35-year-old in exercise program	23
Maximum percent before coronary risk factors begin	**24**
Average 45-year-old in exercise program	25
U.S. military's "desired" percent, all ages	26
Military's maximum allowable for 17- to 20-year-olds	28
Average American female at age 25	29
Average 55-year-old in exercise program	29
Military's maximum allowable for 21- to 27-year-olds	30
Average 65-year-old in exercise program	31
Military's maximum allowable for 28- to 39-year-olds	32
Average American female at age 35	33
Classified as morbidly obese	**34**
Military's maximum allowable for 40 years and up	35
Average American female at age 45	35
Average American female at age 55 and up	39

Adapted from Barry Sears, *Biosyn Technical Manual,* 1991, Appendix F.

Body-Fat Calculation for Men

The formula for calculating men's body fat is even simpler than that for women.

1. Measure your waist at your belly button.
2. Measure your wrist where it bends, at the space between your hand and wrist bone.
3. Record these measurements on the work sheet on page 51.
4. Subtract your wrist measurement from your waist measurement and find the resulting value in the table in Appendix D.
5. Find your weight on the left-hand side of the table. Move to the right. Then move down from your waist-minus-wrist figure. At the point where these two intersect, simply read your body-fat percentage.

Let's say that your waist measures 34 inches, your wrist is 7 inches, and you weigh 165 pounds. Here is how to calculate your body fat:

Waist: 34 inches
Wrist: 7 inches

Subtract your wrist measurement from your waist measurement:

$$\begin{array}{r} 34 \text{ inches} \\ - \ 7 \text{ inches} \\ \hline 27 \text{ inches} \end{array}$$

Use Appendix D to find your weight: 165 pounds. Where 165 pounds intersects with 27 inches you will find your body-fat percentage: 16 percent.

Be sure to take your measurements on bare skin, keeping the tape snug but not too tight. Take each measurement three times, using the average. Remember to measure your waist at the belly button, not the narrowest point.

As with women, a man's body composition is one of the most significant indicators of his physical fitness. How do you measure up against other men? Table 4.5 lists the body-fat percentages for different reference groups. This list will help put your own body-fat percentage in perspective and allow you to measure your progress as you swim yourself into condition. Note that the athletic groups listed are world-class or professional.

WORK SHEET FOR
MEN TO CALCULATE BODY-FAT PERCENTAGE

Waist measurement: _____ inches
Wrist measurement: _____ inches
Subtract your wrist measurement from your waist measurement:

Waist: _____
minus Wrist: – _____
Subtotal: _____

Using Appendix D, find your weight in the left-hand column. Then find your waist minus wrist number. Your body-fat percentage is where the two columns intersect.

% Body Fat: _____

TABLE 4.5
Men's Body-Fat Percentages

Reference Group	Body Fat
Lowest male measured	3%
Gymnasts, amateur wrestlers	4
Medically unsafe for most males	5
Swimmers, top bodybuilders	6
Basketball centers	7
Cross-country skiers	8
Cyclists	9
Racquetball players	9
Masters swimmers, age 25–34	10
Basketball forwards, soccer players	10
Distance runners, football defensive backs	11
Basketball guards, football linebackers	12
Football offensive backs	13
Masters swimmers, age 35–44	13
Football quarterbacks	14
Masters swimmers, age 45–54	14
"Ideal" fit male	15
Masters swimmers, age 55–74	15
Upper limit for professional athletes	15
Average 25-year-old in exercise program	16
Power lifters, shot putters, discus throwers	17
Masters swimmers, age 75–84	17
Average 35-year-old in exercise program	18
Maximum percent before coronary risk factors begin	19
U.S. military's "desired" percent, all ages	20
Average 45-year-old in exercise program	21
Military's maximum allowable for 21- to 27-year-olds	22
Average 55-year-old (or older) in exercise program	23
Average American male at age 25	23
Military's maximum allowable for 28- to 39-year-olds	24
Average American male at age 35	25
Military's maximum allowable for 40 years and up	26
Classified as morbidly obese	27
Average American male at age 45	28
Average American male at 55 years and up	30

Adapted from Barry Sears, *Biosyn Technical Manual,* 1991, Appendix F.

SWIMMING AND DIET

One of the things I used to tell people when they asked me why I swim, is that swimming allows me to eat anything I want. And I *love* to eat. I have heard many athletes express similar sentiments.

In a way it was true. I made sure to get all the basic nutrients in my diet, but on top of that I piled on the high-carbohydrate foods I loved, particularly frozen yogurt. Sure enough, as long as I was working out, I could eat just about anything and never put on weight. But as I learned several years ago, I was fooling myself, and in the process cheating myself of a valuable training tool and a key to long-term health.

For years nutritionists have told us that it is important to eat a balanced diet, one high in carbohydrates and low in both protein and fat, and one containing the basic vitamins and minerals and a high level of fiber. But in recent years a new discipline has emerged that offers a powerful and compelling challenge to the conventional wisdom about the ideal diet.

Dietary Endocrinology

Dietary endocrinology, a new area of nutrition, studies our bodies' hormonal responses to the foods we eat. One of the leaders in this field is Barry Sears, a former research instructor at the Boston University School of Medicine and the Massachusetts Institute of Technology, and now president of Surfactant Technologies, Inc.

Although dietary endocrinology originally was developed for the treatment of cardiovascular patients, it appears to be applicable both to the enhancement of athletic performance and to the maintenance of ideal levels of body fat. Since 1989 research in this area has been conducted with the Stanford University men's and women's swim teams, and dietary endocrinology played an important role in the impressive success of the Stanford swimmers who participated in the 1992 Olympics.

New Attitudes about the High-Carbohydrate Diet

Contrary to sports nutrition gospel, it appears that high-carbohydrate diets may limit athletic performance. This statement is based on thirty years of endocrinological studies which indicate that the food you eat generates a powerful hormonal response. According to this new theory, you have a choice: either you control these biochemical responses or they control you. Athletes, particularly endurance athletes, often believe that their bodies do not obey the laws of biochemistry and endocrinology that govern everybody else. As I used to do, they treat their stomachs like blast furnaces; they believe that because they are *athletes* they can digest anything. Nothing could be further from the truth.

Several basic biochemical facts govern athletic performance. First and foremost, the primary source of muscle energy is fatty acids—that is, fats. The problem is that muscle cells contain very limited amounts of fat. Fatty acids must be released from the fat in your body into the bloodstream to be used as an energy source by the muscle cells. If the muscles cannot access fatty acids, they are forced to use a secondary and inferior source for energy: carbohydrates. Although the muscle cells contain much of the body's stored carbohydrates, only the carbohydrates in the liver can be mobilized to maintain the blood-sugar levels your brain needs to function. The task becomes to mobilize the stored carbohydrates from the liver into the bloodstream at levels the brain can access.

An athlete's body has a virtually unlimited supply of stored fat, but it has limited supplies of stored carbohydrates. For example, a world-class marathon runner or a long-distance swimmer can store twenty to forty times more energy as fat in his or her body than as carbohydrate, so carbo loading makes absolutely no sense at all. What we should be discussing is how best to utilize the fat in our bodies.

It is important to note that the brain can use only carbohydrates as an energy source. As long as the muscles can access fatty acids and the brain has its carbohydrates, the body works smoothly during exercise. The trouble begins when the muscles and brain start to compete for carbohydrates. This is the worst possible dilemma for an athlete, because if the brain is deprived of its carbohydrate supply, the athlete will simply lose concentration.

According to Sears, the problem with nutrition in general, and sports nutrition in particular, is that the conventional wisdom has people looking at the trees and ignoring the forest. Nutrition, he points out, is far more complex than counting the calories you eat or calculating how much fat or carbohydrates are in a serving. "Every time you put a piece of food in your mouth," he points out, "you trigger a hormonal response. This response ultimately dictates how our bodies perform."

With this background, we can look at the effects that high-carbohydrate diets have on hormonal response. Initially there is a rise in blood sugar, which causes the secretion of the hormone insulin. As insulin levels increase in the bloodstream, blood-sugar levels begin to fall. Once blood sugar drops below a critical threshold, the brain begins to demand more of it. This starts the cycle over again, and it accounts for the constant hunger and carbo cravings experienced by many athletes, as well as people on high-carbohydrate weight-loss diets.

Several additional facts must be explained. First, the rate of the rise in blood sugar determines insulin levels in the bloodstream. However, not all carbohydrates have the same effect on insulin secretion. In fact, some complex carbohydrates actually increase insulin levels faster than simple sugars. The faster that insulin rises, the more rapidly blood-sugar levels drop. For example, pasta increases insulin levels much faster than a Snickers candy bar. This is why many people, including athletes, become hungry only two to three hours after eating a high-carbohydrate meal.

Second, the human body has a limited capacity to store carbohydrates as glycogen. Once the glycogen pools are full, the rest of the carbohydrates are stored as fat. So high levels of insulin, which are a direct consequence of a high-carbohydrate diet, lead in a roundabout way to an increase in body fat.

Third, elevated insulin prevents the release of free fatty acids from the fat stores. The end result is that a high-carbohydrate diet actually cuts off the primary energy source for your muscles.

The Benefits of Balancing Hormones

Just as carbohydrates affect insulin, protein affects other hormonal responses. In particular, protein in the diet drives up the blood levels of the hormone glucagon. It is the dynamic balance between insulin and glucagon that ultimately determines an athlete's endurance.

Glucagon has the opposite physiological effect of insulin. For example, whereas insulin prevents the release of fatty acids from your fat stores, glucagon mobilizes these fatty acids. Likewise, glucagon mobilizes carbohydrates from the liver to maintain blood-sugar levels while insulin lowers blood sugar. So it is important to keep a favorable ratio between insulin and glucagon in order to maintain the flow of energy to your muscle cells. The key point to remember is that the glucagon-to-insulin ratio is determined totally by the food you put in your mouth.

There are a number of immediate and profound benefits for anyone who follows a glucagon-favorable diet, but athletes in particular can gain by these advantages:

- Hunger is eliminated because blood-sugar levels are maintained for up to six hours.
- Muscular endurance is increased because fatty acids are being released from your fat stores.
- You stay more mentally alert since blood-sugar levels are stabilized.
- Finally, your body fat decreases because you are utilizing stored fat.

The Ideal Diet

How can you establish a balanced, glucagon-favorable diet? The key is the ratio of carbohydrates to proteins that you eat. This determines the ratio of insulin to glucagon in your bloodstream.

The typical athlete's diet contains 60 to 70 percent carbohydrates, 15 percent protein, and 15 to 25 percent fat. In addition, the carbohydrates often have a high glycemic index, causing blood sugar to rise rapidly. High-glycemic carbohydrates include pasta, bread, and starches. This type of diet is guaranteed to promote high insulin levels and ultimately limit your performance.

The diet of the typical American is even worse: 50 percent carbohydrate, 13 percent protein, and 37 percent fat. This is a tailor-made prescription for developing heart disease, diabetes, and several forms of cancer.

Research has shown that a favorable glucagon balance can be achieved with a diet consisting of 40 percent carbohydrates, 30 percent protein, and 30 percent fat. What is most important is maintaining the 4-to-3 ratio between carbohydrates and protein. It is interesting that recent research by anthropologists indicates that this 4-to-3-to-3 ratio closely approximates the diet eaten by our prehistoric ancestors.

Thirty percent fat is the level recommended by the American Heart Association. For good health, your diet must include at least some fat, but this poses no health risk because most people, as a result of well-established diet preferences, find it difficult to get fat levels much below 30 percent. However, if you are one of the few who can get your fat intake below 30 percent, you can still maintain the essential 4-to-3 carbohydrate-to-protein ratio. For example, with a diet containing only 22 percent fat, you can have a 4-to-3-to-2 ratio between carbohydrates, proteins, and fats, yielding the same 4-to-3 ratio in carbohydrate-to-protein intake.

To further complicate things, you must try to maintain the 4-to-3 ratio at every meal, and you must also eat about a third of the vitamins and minerals you need at every meal. At one time medical authorities believed vitamins' only role in health was preventing or curing diseases specifically caused by vitamin deficiencies. But recent studies have shown many vitamins to be useful in protecting overall health. Among these are vitamin C, and the antioxidants, vitamin E and vitamin A, especially in the form of beta carotene.

Some may protest that this diet appears to be just what they have long been told is not conducive to weight loss. But you *will* lose weight, because using your stored body fat as a primary source of energy means that you will not have to put as many calories in your mouth to maintain your energy level. In fact, people on a glucagon-favorable diet eat only about half the total calories of a typical American diet because of better appetite control as well as the diet's ability to provide better access to stored fat.

Once you calculate the number of grams of protein and carbohydrates you will need in a glucagon-favorable diet, it quickly becomes apparent that this is a low-calorie, low-fat, protein-adequate, and high-nutrient diet. It is precisely this kind of diet that geneticist Roy Walford has shown experimentally can lead to a significant increase in life expectancy.

Why are scientists only now beginning to understand the powerful hormonal effects of diet? The reason is that there is a very narrow target zone of protein to carbohydrate that generates the favorable glucagon-to-insulin ratio. If an athlete eats too much carbohydrate (relative to protein), excess insulin is released. If he eats too much protein and not enough carbohydrate, he will develop a physiological state known as ketosis. Ketosis is actually far worse for an athlete than excess insulin production because it inhibits the release of glucagon and promotes the loss of muscle mass.

Therefore, it is essential to eat just the right balance of protein and carbohydrate at every meal—not an easy task. Appendix H provides examples of meals with the proper protein-to-carbohydrate balance.

How do you know if you are in the target zone? Your lack of appetite. If your blood-sugar levels are stabilized, your brain will be satisfied and not send out any hunger signals for four to six hours. If you are out of the target zone, you will constantly be hungry. It's as simple as that.

THE FOUNTAIN OF YOUTH
DISCOVERED:
SWIMMING AND LONGEVITY

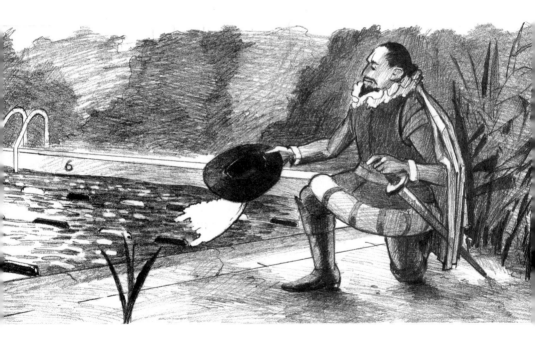

IN 1513 THE SPANISH explorer Juan Ponce de León braved the unknown perils of the swampy Everglades and the fierce Carib and Seminole Indians in his search for the mythical Fountain of Youth. Although he is remembered today for his accidental "discovery" of Florida, Ponce never did find the legendary source of eternal youth. He died in 1521 at the unremarkable age of sixty-one, reportedly looking every bit his age.

In 1989 Lynda Myers, a thirty-nine-year-old business executive, homemaker, and mother of two teenagers, found the real Fountain of Youth less than a mile from her home in a Washington, DC, suburb: she started swimming five days a week during her lunch hour. Today, Lynda is happier and healthier than she ever remembers being. What's more, according to recent scientific studies and data gathered by life-insurance companies, Lynda has added over thirty years to her life expectancy! Later in this chapter I will explain how she accomplished this. More important, I will show you how you can do the same.

THE ENIGMA OF LONGEVITY

Ever since the dawn of civilization, human beings have attempted to probe the mystery of longevity. Why, we have wanted to know, do some of us die young while others live well beyond our biblical allotment of three score and ten years? Today, although much research remains to be done, scientists are beginning to unravel the mysteries of long life. Biologists such as Roy Walford have learned, for example, that we have a genetic capability to live for at least 100, and possibly 120 years. Why, then, do almost half of us fall 50 years short of our genetic potential? There are two basic answers: our heredity and our life-styles.

If your parents and grandparents lived to be eighty, ninety, or more, the chances are that, barring accidents, you too will live to about their ages. If your parents or grandparents died of heart disease, stroke, cancer, diabetes, or other such illnesses in their forties or fifties, you are more at risk than most people of dying young from one of these diseases.

Though there is not much you can do yet about your heredity, you must understand that heredity creates propensities only, not predestinations. But you *can* do something about the way you live, and the way you live, regardless of your genetic endowment, can add many healthy years to your life.

Scientists have learned that we are killing ourselves prematurely by how we live. First of all, we eat too much; more than 60 million adult Americans are classified as obese. And much of what we eat—excess fat, sugar, and salt—contributes to our demise. Add in environmental pollution, smoking, sedentary but stressful jobs, too much driving, and not enough exercise, and you have an accurate portrait of an all-too-typical American: fat, frustrated, unhappy, and unhealthy. The only question remaining for most of us is whether we will die young of a heart attack, stroke, lung cancer, or some other deadly disease.

SWIMMING AND LONGEVITY

"Four years ago," Lynda Myers told me, "the pathetic portrait you've painted described me to a T. Outwardly, I'm sure I seemed the epitome of the successful woman: I was moving up rapidly in my profession, and I had a 'good marriage' with two kids who were popular, did well in school, and never gave me any grief. As we used to say in the eighties, it seemed like I had it all. But inside," she admitted, "I was seething with anger and frustration, and I didn't know why.

"I had been smoking two packs a day for eighteen years and had put on a good twenty pounds since my college days. Whenever I looked in the mirror, I couldn't believe that the frown-lined, frumpy image that stared back was really me. I knew, of course, that smoking was bad for me. But whenever I tried to stop, I put on even more weight. I didn't want to blimp out."

Lynda recalls that she was constantly yelling at her kids at the slightest provocation. "And my sex life with Bob can best be described as almost nonexistent—once a month at most. Even that was quick and unsatisfying. We were both too tired, and we just seemed to be going through the motions. The spark was gone."

Like so many people, Lynda tried jogging for a while, but all she got for her efforts were shinsplints, sore legs, and a pulled Achilles tendon. "And that wasn't the worst of it," she reports. "I hated breathing in all those exhaust fumes and having dogs nipping at my heels. But most of all, it was boring. Just plain B-O-R-I-N-G."

Lynda's boss had been in the Masters swimming program for a few months, and when he suggested she join up she wasn't very enthusiastic. But he definitely seemed more relaxed than he had been and looked much trimmer, so she figured, "Why not give it a try? What've I got to lose?"

Lynda found that it wasn't all that easy at first. "I had learned to swim as a kid," she told me, "but my first time back in the pool I barely made two laps. There I was, huffing and puffing and feeling sorry for myself. Then this sweet old lady who had been swimming next to me stopped to give me some encouragement. She told me to stick with it, that she hadn't been able to swim a stroke when she'd started two years before. Then she went back to finish her mile. Later I found out she was eighty-three! Eighty-three, for Chrissakes! I figured, if she can do it, so could I."

Now Lynda tries to swim at least a mile a day—more if she is feeling really good. She has learned to swim all the strokes, even butterfly. "And I'm even thinking about competing in some Masters meets," she says with a laugh. "I'll never be mistaken for a potential Olympic champion," she goes on. "I'm no Summer Sanders. I'm not even one of the fastest swimmers my age on our team. But it doesn't matter. The people are fantastic—friendly, supportive, always willing to help me with my technique. The atmosphere's just great."

Lynda claims that swimming has made her a new woman. She hasn't lit a cigarette, or even wanted to, in over four years. It didn't happen all at once, but after a while she just stopped smoking. Even she isn't sure why: she just knows that she gradually lost the desire to draw carbonized tar particles into her lungs.

"Swimming has also firmed me up," she says. "I'm back down to my college weight, and for the first time in years I feel proud of the way I look. I've even gone out and bought a two-piece for the beach this summer. Bob started noticing the difference in me after a few weeks. Our sex life has been reborn; it's exciting, and I think we are closer now than we've ever been. He even began swimming with me last year, so now it's something we share. You've got to know Bob to realize how radical a change this is. Before he started swimming, his idea of exercise was to plunk himself down in front of the boob tube for the afternoon, six-pack in hand."

Lynda Myers is delighted with the ways swimming has enhanced her life, but it has done even more than all this: it has lengthened her life.

THE LIFE-EXPECTANCY TEST

Diana S. Woodruff has devised a life-expectancy test based on statistical data and medical studies that has been modified slightly to accommodate the most up-to-date scientific studies. The test consists of thirty-two items in four broad categories: heredity and family, education and occupation, life-style, and health:

I. *Heredity and Family*
   1. Longevity of grandparents
   2. Longevity of parents
   3. Cardiovascular disease of close relatives
   4. Other hereditable diseases of close relatives
   5. Childbearing
   6. Mother's age at your birth
   7. Birth order
   8. Intelligence

II. *Education and Occupation*
   9. Years of education
   10. Occupational level
   11. Family income
   12. Activity on the job
   13. Age and work

III. *Life-style*
   14. Urban vs. rural living
   15. Marital status
   16. Living status if single
   17. Life changes
   18. Friendship
   19. Aggressive personality
   20. Flexible personality
   21. Risk-taking personality
   22. Depressive personality
   23. Happy personality

IV. *Health*
   24. Percent body fat
   25. Dietary habits
   26. Smoking
   27. Drinking
   28. Exercise
   29. Sleep
   30. Sexual activity
   31. Regular physical examinations
   32. Health status

You probably have noticed that only one of the thirty-two items on the test is directly concerned with exercise. This factor by itself can add up to three years to your life. If that was all swimming could do, it would be pretty spectacular. Who, after all, would not like to live an extra three healthy, vigorous years? But, as will be shown, a regular program of swimming can affect many other aspects of your life as well: from your weight and percent body fat to your blood pressure and smoking habits; from your susceptibility to disease to your personality and even your sex life. It can change the way you feel and the way you feel about yourself. These changes are reflected in ten additional items on the life-expectancy test, totaling thirty to fifty years.

As my editor reminded me, however, it is important to keep in mind that nothing will make you immortal, not even swimming. Some years ago the hype surrounding running seemed to imply that you could live forever if only you ran long enough and consistently enough. This hype came to an abrupt end in 1984, when running guru Jim Fixx tragically died of a heart attack at the early age of fifty-two while out for a jog on a country road.

Many people concluded that all Fixx's running did not avail him a bit. Or worse still, that his running caused his early death. In fact, the likelihood is that exercise helped Fixx live longer than he would have otherwise. Fixx was the unfortunate recipient of bad genes: his father had died in his mid-forties of a heart attack. And before taking up running in early middle age, Fixx himself had lived a life designed to lead to an early death: he smoked heavily, weighed over 200 pounds, and exercised only sporadically.

I'm not saying I'm superstitious, but Jim Fixx's editor is now my editor, so when he implored me not to claim any benefits for swimming that are not firmly grounded in scientific fact, I took what he said seriously.

Swimming will not—repeat, *not*—make you immortal. But it can add many dynamic, robust years to your life.

The benefits swimming can confer are now well-established by scientific research. Aside from the three years that it can add directly to your life, swimming can favorably affect almost every aspect of your life not determined by your genes. The life-expectancy test illustrates how this can happen.

Here is how the test works:

Begin by finding your life expectancy from an actuarial table. This figure shows how many years the "average" American of your age, sex, and race can expect to live. The most recent actuarial table, produced by the U.S. Department of Health and Human Services, appears in Appendix C.

Then, by keeping a running score based on your personal attributes, you will end up with a personalized life expectancy. Of course there is no guarantee that you actually will live the precise number of years predicted by the test. These figures are based on a large pool of people and only predict what is *likely* to happen to the majority of people in your age, sex, and racial category.

Here is how it worked for Lynda Myers (see Table 5.1).

TABLE 5.1
How Swimming Affected Lynda Myers's Life Expectancy

	Before (age 39)	*After* (age 43)
Average Life Expectancy (from actuarial table)	80.1	80.4
PART I. Heredity and Family		
1. Longevity of grandparents	+1.0	+1.0
2. Longevity of parents	—	—
3. Cardiovascular disease of close relatives	−2.0	−2.0
4. Other hereditable diseases of close relatives	−2.0	−2.0
5. Childbearing	—	—
6. Mother's age at Lynda's birth	—	—
7. Birth order	—	—
8. Intelligence	═	═
	−3.0	−3.0
PART II. Education and Occupation		
9. Years of education	+3.0	+3.0
10. Occupational level	+1.0	+1.0
11. Family income	+1.0	+1.0
12. Activity on the job	−2.0	−2.0
13. Age and work	═	═
	+3.0	+3.0
PART III. Life-style		
14. Urban vs. rural living	−1.0	−1.0
15. Marital status	+1.0	+1.0
16. Living status if single	—	—
17. Life changes	—	—
18. Friendship	—	+1.0
19. Aggressive personality	−4.0	−2.0
20. Flexible personality	—	+1.0
21. Risk-taking personality	—	—

	Before *(age 39)*	*After* *(age 43)*
22. Depressive personality	−2.0	—
23. Happy personality	—	+2.0
	−6.0	+2.0
PART IV. Health		
24. Percent body fat	−3.0	—
25. Dietary habits	—	—
26. Smoking	−7.0	—
27. Drinking	+3.0	+3.0
28. Exercise	—	+3.0
29. Sleep	−2.0	—
30. Sexual activity	—	+2.0
31. Regular physical examinations	+2.0	+2.0
32. Health status	−5.0	—
	−12.0	+10.0
Total years gained or lost	−18.0	+12.0
LYNDA'S PERSONALIZED LIFE EXPECTANCY	62.1	92.4

Part I. Heredity and Family (items 1-8).
Part I is not affected by swimming. Lynda's heredity loses her three years. Although she had two grandparents who lived beyond the age of seventy (item 1), her father died of a heart attack at age fifty-nine (items 2 and 3), and a grandmother died of breast cancer (item 4).

Part II. Education and Occupation (items 9-13).
The items in this part of the test also are not affected by swimming, but here Lynda picks up three years. Her educational background (item 9), occupational level (item 10), and family income (item 11) all work in her favor, although her sedentary job works against her.

All in all, the factors Lynda could not change are a wash: they don't affect her life expectancy at all.

Part III. Life-style (items 14-23).
Changes in Lynda's life-style that she identifies as resulting from her swimming account for a shift of eight years, from −6 to +2. Her new activity, she feels, has led to new friendships (item 18) and has made her a less aggressive, more flexible, happier person (items 19, 20, 22, and 23).

Part IV. Health (items 24–32).

Here is where Lynda's swimming makes the biggest difference. Before she began swimming, Lynda could have expected to lose eighteen years from her life because of the destructive way she was treating her body. Four years later there was a dramatic change. Lynda had gained twelve years over the average life expectancy.

How? She lost the excess weight she had been carrying around for years and reduced her body-fat percentage from 33 to 28 percent (item 24); she quit smoking (item 26); she was exercising daily (item 28); she slept better (item 29); she increased her sexual activity (item 30); she saw her blood pressure drop to normal and her chronic colds disappear almost completely (item 32). She looked better, felt better, and lived better. Her daily sessions in the pool had added thirty years to her life expectancy—literally, the gift of life. Lynda sums up her attitude this way: "I know that with every stroke I take, I'm adding to my life. As a plus, I'm making that life more worth living."

Lynda Myers is only one of tens of thousands of people whose lives have been both enriched and lengthened by swimming. I am another.

CHANGES SWIMMING HAS MADE IN MY LIFE

I first learned of the Masters swimming program in December 1971, when I was twenty-eight. At the time, I was divorced, living in Connecticut with my three-year-old son, and working as the publisher of a small educational publishing firm. I had had chronic back problems for the previous four years—debilitating periods every six months or so, during which it hurt just to turn my head. Even so, I felt I was in reasonably good shape for a guy my age. I didn't smoke, and I drank only occasionally. Once a week or so, I played a game of touch football at lunchtime or managed to get in a brief jog, a regimen I thought made me a pretty active fellow for my age.

But I was playing a perilous game of self-delusion. A physical examination revealed that my weight had crept up, as had my cholesterol. My blood pressure, marginally high, was still waving a red flag of danger that I was ignoring. Moreover, the emotional and physical pressures of trying to be both father and mother to a young child while advancing in a highly competitive profession with a difficult boss were taking their toll. I often found myself feeling anxious, harried, worried, and depressed.

Had I taken the life-expectancy test then, I would have discovered I could expect to live to the age of 60.1, barely enough time to see my son into manhood. Even less than poor Ponce de León.

Today my life has changed dramatically. At the age of fifty, I am physically much younger than I was at twenty-eight. In fact, it may be that at fifty I can look forward to more years of life—healthy, vigorous, productive life—than I could have at twenty-eight!

How did I bring this about? In December 1971, after my physical exam, I decided to try to do something about the state of my health. I began swimming, and I have been swimming ever since, about two miles a day, five days a week. Results: as pointed out in Chapters 3 and 4, since resuming swimming I have improved my health by many measures. My weight is down to 180, about the same weight I carried as a competitive swimmer in college. My body fat has decreased from over 17 to less than 10 percent. My blood pressure has dropped to an excellent 116/74. My overall blood cholesterol has dropped to 209. More significantly, my HDL level is 90. My resting pulse rate, which was 64 twenty-two years previously, is now a strong 42. What is more, I have not had a single back problem since I started swimming again.

My son, Russell, graduated from the University of California at Santa Barbara in 1991 and is now studying to be a chiropractor. Raising him was one of the great pleasures of my life, an incredibly rewarding experience. As a result, there is a bond of love and respect between us that can never be severed.

I am still working hard—as a writer, lecturer, magazine editor, and university professor. But these days I feel relaxed, happy, and in control of my life. Recently I remarried, and Donna has added an extra dimension of happiness to my life. I find it significant that I met my wife-to-be at a swim meet.

Just how much difference swimming has made to me is revealed by the life-expectancy test. I can now expect to live to the ripe old age of 92, an increase of over thirty years.

HOW LONG WILL *YOU* LIVE?

All right, you may be thinking. It's interesting to read how people like Lynda and Phil have increased their likelihood of living to ripe old ages. But what I'd really like to know is, How long am *I* going to live? And what can I do to increase *my* life expectancy? Fair enough.

There is no way anyone can tell you with absolute certainty how long you will live. But the results of Diana Woodruff's life-expectancy test should be taken seriously. Based on the best scientific evidence now available, it points out those aspects of your life-style that may shorten or lengthen your life.

TAKING THE LIFE-EXPECTANCY TEST

Begin by finding your life expectancy from the actuarial table in Appendix C. Enter this figure on the score sheet on page 77.

This figure is your average life expectancy and is based on your age, sex, and race. Now, by keeping a running score based on your personal attributes, you will end up with a personalized life expectancy. Add and subtract years according to how you answer the questions in the work sheet beginning on page 70.

After you have filled in this work sheet, transfer your scores to the score sheet on page 77 and tally up your personal life expectancy.

How did you measure up? If you are like most Americans, the results probably are pretty depressing. Chances are that unless you change your way of living, you will not see eighty or ninety.

Fortunately, there is something you can do: *swim.* Whether you are twenty-five or sixty-five, male or female, ten pounds or one hundred pounds overweight, a former Olympic swimmer or a total non-swimmer, whether you are one of the millions who have tried jogging and found it just wasn't for you or have never exercised before, this enjoyable, refreshing, ideal form of exercise can add years to your life—vigorous, productive, fulfilling years.

HUMAN GROWTH HORMONE: HOW SWIMMING LITERALLY MAKES YOU YOUNGER

According to the life-expectancy test, a regular program of swimming can add up to three years directly to your life expectancy. Not a bad start! But *indirectly,* its effects can be much greater.

Chapter 3 showed how swimming can lower your blood pressure and increase the amount of "good" cholesterol (HDL) in your blood, decreasing substantially your risk of dying of stroke or heart attack.

LIFE-EXPECTANCY TEST
WORK SHEET

PART I. Heredity and Family

1. *Longevity of grandparents*
    Have any of your grandparents lived to age eighty or beyond? If so, *add one year for each grandparent living beyond that age.* Add one-half year for each grandparent surviving beyond the age of seventy.   _____

2. *Longevity of parents*
    If your mother lived beyond the age of eighty, *add four years.* Add two years if your father lived beyond eighty. You benefit more if your mother lived a long time than if your father did.

    _____

3. *Cardiovascular disease of close relatives*
    If any parent, grandparent, sister, or brother died of a heart attack, stroke, or arteriosclerosis before the age of fifty, *subtract four years for each incidence.* If any of those close relatives died of the above before age sixty, *subtract two years for each incidence.*   _____

4. *Other hereditable diseases of close relatives*
    Have any of your parents, grandparents, sisters, or brothers died before the age of sixty of diabetes mellitus or peptic ulcer? *Subtract three years for each incidence.* If any of these close relatives died before sixty of stomach cancer, *subtract two years.* Women whose close female relatives have died before sixty of breast cancer and men whose close male relatives have died of prostate cancer before sixty should also *subtract two years.* Finally, if any close relatives have died before the age of sixty of any cause except accidents or homicide, *subtract one year for each incidence.*   _____

5. *Childbearing*
    Women who have never had children are more likely to be in poor health, and they are also at a greater risk for breast cancer. Therefore, if you can't or don't plan to have children, or if you are over forty and have never had children, *subtract one-half year.* Women who have a large number of children tax their

bodies. If you've had or plan to have over seven children, *subtract one year.* _____

6. *Mother's age at your birth*
    Was your mother over the age of thirty-five or under the age of eighteen when you were born? If so, *subtract one year.*

    _____

7. *Birth order*
    Are you the firstborn in your family? If so, *add one year.*

    _____

8. *Intelligence*
    How intelligent are you? If your intelligence is superior, that is, if your IQ is over 130 or you feel you are smarter than almost everyone you know, *add two years.* _____

PART II. Education and Occupation

9. *Years of education*
    How much education have you had? *Add or subtract the number of years shown in Table A.* _____

TABLE A.
Education and Life Expectancy

Level of Education	Years of Life
Four or more years of college	+3.0
One to three years of college	+2.0
Four years of high school	+1.0
One to three years of high school	0.0
Elementary school (eight years)	−0.5
Less than eighth grade	−2.0

---

10. *Occupational level*
    If you are working, what is the socioeconomic level of your occupation? If you do not work, what is your spouse's occupation? If you are retired, what is your former occupation? If you are a student, what is your parents' occupational level? *Add or subtract the number of years shown in Table B.* _____

Occupation and Life Expectancy

Occupational level	Years of Life
Class I —Professional	+1.5
Class II —Technical, administrative, managerial, and agricultural	+1.0
Class III—Proprietors, clerical, sales, and skilled workers	0.0
Class IV—Semiskilled workers	−0.5
Class V —Laborers	−4.0

11. *Family income*
    If your family income is above average for your education and occupation, *add one year.* If it's below average for your education and occupation, *subtract one year.* _____

12. *Activity on the job*
    If your job involves a lot of physical activity, *add two years.* On the other hand, if you sit all day on the job, *subtract two years.*

    _____

13. *Age and work*
    If you are over the age of sixty and still on the job, *add two years.* If you are over the age of sixty-five and have not retired, *add three years.* _____

PART III. Life-style

14. *Urban vs. rural living*
    If you live in an urban area and have lived in or near a city for most of your life, *subtract one year.* If you have spent most of your life in a rural area, *add one year.* _____

15. *Marital status*
    If you are married and living with your spouse, *add one year.*
    A. *Formerly married men.* If you are a separated or divorced man living alone, *subtract nine years.* If you are a widowed man living alone, *subtract seven years.* If as a separated, divorced, or widowed man you live with other people, such as a partner or family members, *subtract only half the*

years given above. Living with others is beneficial for formerly married men.

B. *Formerly married women.* If you are separated or divorced, *subtract four years.* Widowed women should subtract *three and a half years.* The loss of a spouse through divorce or death is not as life-shortening to a woman, and she lives about as long whether she lives alone or with a family, unless she is the head of the household. Divorced or widowed women who live with family as the head of their household should *subtract only two years.* _____

16. *Living status if single*
    If you are a woman who has never married, *subtract one year for each unmarried decade past the age of twenty-five.* If you live with a family or friends as a male single person, you should also *subtract one year for each unmarried decade past the age of twenty-five.* However, if you are a man who has never married and are living alone, *subtract two years for each unmarried decade past the age of twenty-five.* _____

17. *Life changes*
    Are you always changing things in your life—your job, your residence, your friends and/or spouse, your appearance? If so, *subtract two years.* Too much change is stressful. _____

18. *Friendship*
    Do you generally like people and have at least two close friends in whom you can confide almost all the details of your life? If so, *add one year.* _____

19. *Aggressive personality*
    Do you always feel that you are under time pressure? Are you aggressive and sometimes hostile, paying little attention to the feelings of others? *Subtract two to five years depending on how well you fit this description.* The more pressured, aggressive, and hostile you are, the greater your risk for heart disease.

    _____

20. *Flexible personality*
    Are you a calm, reasonable, relaxed person? Are you easygoing and adaptable, taking life pretty much as it comes? *Depending*

upon the degree to which you fit this description, *add one to three years.* If you are rigid, dogmatic, and set in your ways, *subtract two years.* _____

21. *Risk-taking personality*
     Do you take a lot of risks, including driving without seat belts, exceeding the speed limit, and taking any dare that is made? Do you live in a high-crime neighborhood? If you are vulnerable to accidents and homicide in this way, *subtract two years.* If you use seat belts regularly, drive infrequently, and generally avoid risks and dangerous parts of town, *add one year.* _____

22. *Depressive personality*
     Have you been depressed, tense, worried, or guilty for more than a year or two? If so, *subtract one to three years depending upon how seriously you are affected by these feelings.*

     _____

23. *Happy personality*
     Are you basically happy and content, and have you had a lot of fun in life? If so, *add two years.* Happy people live longer than unhappy people. _____

PART IV. Health

24. *Percent body fat*
     Is your body-fat percentage too high? Obesity places an added

---

TABLE C.
Body-Fat Percentage and Life Expectancy

% Body Fat Women	Men	Years of Life
under 11%	under 5%	−4.0
12–20	6–13	+4.0
21–24	14–17	+2.0
25–27	18–20	+1.0
28–30	21–24	0.0
31–33	25–26	−3.0
over 34	over 27	−6.0

strain on your heart and can shorten your life; if you are morbidly obese, your susceptibility to a host of diseases rises rapidly. If your body-fat percentage is too *low,* you may be suffering from anorexia; extremely low levels of body fat can also shorten your life. Calculate your body-fat percentage using the formula presented in Chapter 4. Then *add or subtract the number of years shown in Table C.* _____

25. *Dietary habits*
Do you prefer vegetables, fruits, low-fat meats, and simple foods to foods high in fat and sugar, and do you *always* stop eating before you feel really full? (What constitutes a healthy diet is explained in detail in Chapter 4.) If your honest answer to both questions is *yes, add one year.* _____

26. *Smoking*
How much do you smoke? If you smoke two or more packs a day, *subtract twelve years.* If you smoke between one and two packs a day, *subtract seven years.* If you smoke less than a pack a day, *subtract two years.* If you do not smoke or have quit smoking, congratulations. You subtract no years at all! _____

27. *Drinking*
If you are a moderate drinker, that is, if you never drink to the point of intoxication and have one or two drinks per day, *add three years.* If you are a light drinker, that is, you have an occasional drink but do not drink almost every day, *add one and one half years.* If you are an abstainer who never uses alcohol in any form, do not add or subtract any years. Finally, if you are a heavy drinker or an alcoholic, *subtract eight years.* (Heavy drinkers are those who drink more than three ounces of whiskey or drink other intoxicating beverages excessively almost every day. They drink to the point of intoxication.) _____

28. *Exercise*
How much do you exercise? If you swim (or do another aerobic exercise) on at least three nonconsecutive days a week, for a minimum of twenty to thirty minutes, at about 80 percent of your maximum attainable heart rate (see Chapter 3), *add three years.* Exercising on weekends does not count. _____

29. *Sleep*
If you generally fall asleep right away and get six to eight hours of sleep per night, you are average and should neither add nor subtract any years. However, if you sleep excessively (ten or more hours per night), or if you sleep very little (five or less hours per night), you probably have problems. *Subtract two years.*

        _____

30. *Sexual activity*
If you enjoy regular sexual activity, having intimate sexual relations once or twice a week, *add two years.*

        _____

31. *Regular physical examinations*
Do you have an annual physical examination by your physician, which includes a breast exam and Pap smear for women, and a proctoscopic examination every other year for men? If so, *add two years.*

        _____

32. *Health status*
Are you generally in poor health? Do you have a chronic health problem (for example, high blood pressure, heart disease, cancer, diabetes, ulcers), or are you frequently ill? If so, *subtract five years.*

        _____

1. Adapted from Diana S. Woodruff, *Can You Live to Be 100?* (New York: Chatham Square Press, 1987), pp. 3–22. Reprinted by permission.

LIFE-EXPECTANCY TEST SCORE SHEET

Your Average Life Expectancy (from actuarial table)   _____

PART I. Heredity and Family
  1.   Longevity of grandparents   _____
  2.   Longevity of parents   _____
  3.   Cardiovascular disease of close relatives   _____
  4.   Other hereditable diseases of close relatives   _____
  5.   Childbearing   _____
  6.   Mother's age at birth   _____
  7.   Birth order   _____
  8.   Intelligence   _____

PART II. Education and Occupation
  9.   Years of education   _____
 10.   Occupational level   _____
 11.   Family income   _____
 12.   Activity on the job   _____
 13.   Age and work   _____

PART III. Life-style
 14.   Urban vs. rural living   _____
 15.   Marital status   _____
 16.   Living status if single   _____
 17.   Life changes   _____
 18.   Friendship   _____
 19.   Aggressive personality   _____
 20.   Flexible personality   _____
 21.   Risk-taking personality   _____
 22.   Depressive personality   _____
 23.   Happy personality   _____

PART IV. Health
 24.   Percent body fat   _____
 25.   Dietary habits   _____
 26.   Smoking   _____
 27.   Drinking   _____
 28.   Exercise   _____
 29.   Sleep   _____
 30.   Sexual activity   _____
 31.   Regular physical examinations   _____
 32.   Health status   _____

Total years gained or lost   _____

YOUR PERSONALIZED LIFE EXPECTANCY   _____

Chapter 4 outlined how swimming can make you trimmer and keep you trimmer, eliminating the risk factors that accompany obesity. Later chapters will examine some of the *psychological* effects of swimming: how it will improve your self-image and outlook, factors that affect your longevity. In addition to all this, recent research demonstrates how swimming can retard and even reverse some of the "normal" processes of aging.

In 1990 the world was startled by reports of the youth-conferring effects of human growth hormone (hGH). Human growth hormone, as its name implies, is important in the growth process of young people. During childhood and adolescence, the hormone, which is produced by the pituitary gland, stimulates development of the muscles, bones, kidneys, liver, and immune system and prods fatty tissue to shrink. After adolescence, secretion of hGH begins to decline; by age fifty it has decreased significantly, and ultimately it stops altogether in some people.

For years scientists have speculated that at least some of the changes attributed to normal aging result from hGH deficiency. If so, giving hGH to older people might slow or reverse bodily changes associated with aging. Daniel Rudman, a professor of medicine at the Medical College of Wisconsin, decided to test this theory. What he discovered started a mass media avalanche.

In his 1990 report, Rudman described what happened when twelve men, aged sixty-one to eighty-one, gave themselves hGH injections three times a week for six months. Their lean body mass increased by almost 9 percent, their fatty tissue decreased by over 14 percent, and their skin thickened by 7 percent. These changes, Rudman declared, amounted to washing away the effects of ten to twenty years of living. A larger study published in 1991 reported similar results; it also found that the liver, spleen, and muscles from ten areas had increased in volume by 8, 23, and 11 percent respectively.

Unfortunately, what Rudman did *not* report is that injecting hGH can result in a wide range of adverse side effects, from swollen joints and enlarged breasts in men to an elevation in insulin or blood sugar (which can lead to diabetes). In addition, once normal individuals begin receiving hGH injections, their bodies stop producing the hormone naturally; it takes months after the injections stop for the pituitary gland to begin secreting hGH again. Finally—and most significant of all—it is not necessary to inject this seemingly magic potion at all: *it is produced naturally by the body when you exercise!* And *without* the adverse side effects.

It is thus no wonder people who swim regularly report feeling stronger, sexier, more vital, younger. Aside from all the other positive changes, the release of hGH triggered by their swimming *actually turns back the clock.*

FORESTALLING THE AGING PROCESS

As we get older, our bodies change. It seems to take us longer to recover from anything: an injury, a cold, or a workout. We have aches and pains where we never had them before, and we often find that once easy physical tasks are now difficult or impossible. For most Americans, aging is synonymous with inexorable physical decline. But how much do we decline with age? Can exercise forestall the ravages of the aging process?

The One-Percent Rule

For years, gerontologists had an ironclad rule of thumb: after age twenty-five, there was about a 1 percent decline per year in a host of physical attributes, from maximum oxygen uptake ($VO_{2\,max}$) to strength and speed. Thus, a person could expect to decline about 25 percent between ages twenty-five and fifty. Numerous studies of the general population bore out this conclusion.

With the advent of Masters sports in the early 1970s, however, people began seriously questioning the one-percent rule. How much of the decline, they asked, was caused by aging itself, and how much by a sedentary life-style?

A long-term study I am conducting and a smaller study by Jane A. Moore, M.D., provide good news: almost all the decline may be the result of a sedentary, unhealthy life-style. The guiding principle is "use it or lose it," and most Americans simply do not exercise enough. If you live like a couch potato, you will come to resemble one. But if you exercise regularly, you can retain most of the strength and vitality of youth. This view is supported by anthropological studies of more physically vigorous peoples, such as the Abkhazians, among whom men and women remain robust and energetic well into old age.

Earlier studies on the effects of exercise were less encouraging. They seemed to suggest that training had only a slight impact on the one-percent-decline-per-year rule. But these studies either followed moderate exercisers over relatively short periods of time or looked at different people at one point in time. Meanwhile, anecdotal evidence suggesting that there were "exceptions" to the rule began to accumulate.

By the 1990s middle-aged superstars became almost a cliché in a number of sports. At age forty-three, Nolan Ryan was crowned the major league strike-out king; tennis ace Jimmy Connors at age thirty-nine battled his way into the semifinals of the U.S. Open; forty-something George Foreman and Larry Holmes found themselves once again among the world's top-rated heavyweight boxers; and near-forty-year-old Robert Parish, the seven-foot center of the Boston Celtics, enjoyed one of his finest seasons in the NBA. What does it all mean?

Masters Swimming: A Living Laboratory

For scientists studying the aging process, Masters swimming provides a natural laboratory with tens of thousands of subjects. For the first time ever, we can follow the changes that occur in conditioned athletes over time. Moreover, swimming is an ideal sport to study because in it performance can be measured precisely, to the hundredth of a second.

That is exactly what I have done. Instead of comparing the performances of different people at one point in time, I have studied the same individuals over a long period. This is known as a *longitudinal study*. Such studies are now possible because Masters swimming is over twenty years old, and we have data going back to 1971. Ultimately, I plan to follow the same people over a lifetime—perhaps fifty years or more.

How the Study Was Done
Because there were relatively few Masters swimmers in the early 1970s, I began this study using performances from 1975. Looking at six representative events—the 100- and 500-yard freestyle, 100-yard backstroke, 100-yard breaststroke, 100-yard butterfly, and 200-yard individual medley—I picked out the *third*-best time in the nation.

Swimmers were assigned to appropriate "age cohorts." Cohort A, for example, consisted of people who were in the twenty-five to twenty-nine age-group in 1975. They were born between 1946 and 1950. Cohort B was composed of those in the thirty to thirty-four age-group in 1975, and so on, all the way to Cohort H, men and women who were aged seventy to seventy-four in 1975.

The study then compared the third-best times of each cohort in each of the six events every five years. For example, Cohort A was twenty-five to twenty-nine in 1975, thirty to thirty-four in 1980, thirty-five to thirty-nine in 1985, and forty to forty-four in 1990. In the 100 free, this cohort produced the following times: 49.04 in 1975, 49.14 in 1980, 50.34 in 1985, and 49.82 in 1990. Thus I was able to measure how performances changed over fifteen years and four age ranges.

What Was Learned

The results obtained were in startling contrast to studies conducted with sedentary people. I believe the evidence is overwhelming that most of the decline associated with aging is caused by inactivity rather than the aging process itself. Folks who swim regularly can perform physically at levels typical of much younger individuals in the general population.

Here are the highlights:

- The one-percent-per-year-after-age-twenty-five rule applies only to a sedentary population. The decline among Masters swimmers is a small fraction of one percent. Figure 5.1 illustrates how the physical abilities of Masters swimmers change with age.

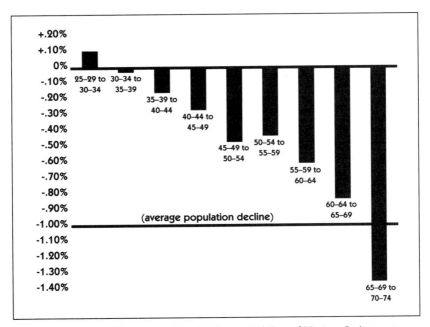

Figure 5.1. Percent Change per Year in Physical Ability of Masters Swimmers

- For people who swim regularly, physical decline begins not at age twenty-five, but in the mid-thirties. Men are actually *faster* in their early thirties than in their late twenties.
- The change that occurs with age is not linear. The rate of decline increases gradually as we grow older. Decline for regular swimmers begins, almost imperceptibly, in the mid-thirties. At that time it is 0.04 percent per year—one twenty-fifth the rate among the sedentary. In the early forties, the rate of decline is 0.13 percent per year—about one eighth the rate among nonswimmers. As Figure 5.2 illustrates, these differences are cumulative.

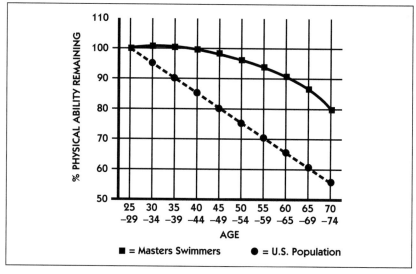

Figure 5.2. Cumulative Change in Physical Ability with Age Among Masters Swimmers

- People who remain healthy and swim regularly can expect to be about as strong and agile at forty as they were at twenty-five. Sure, it takes commitment and self-discipline to maintain a consistent training program over many years. There is no question that it is harder to be physically fit at forty than at twenty-five. But the people who are so are not genetic freaks. They represent what all of us can achieve if we take the time and make the effort to maintain our bodies.
- Swimmers do not decline at the one-percent-per-year rate until they reach their early seventies. This is a dramatic finding. What it means is that if you live a sedentary life-style, you will lose 25 percent of your physical capacity by your fiftieth birthday. By age sev-

enty-five, you will be half the person you were at twenty-five. In contrast, if you swim regularly the decline is only 3.5 percent by age fifty and 19.1 percent at seventy-five. For example, my study suggests that a seventy-year-old swimmer will have the strength and vitality of a normal forty-five-year-old. (See Figure 5.2.)

But the results away from the pool are far more significant than those *in* it. People who are physically fit are happier, healthier, and far more productive than those who are not.

Looking Ahead

I believe that the next few decades will witness a revolution in our understanding of the aging process. This study represents only a modest first step in learning how swimming affects the physical changes we normally associate with aging. I intend to continue the study over the course of my lifetime.

As dramatic as my results to date may be, however, I suspect that they understate what is theoretically possible. After all, most Masters swimmers have family and job responsibilities. They are unable to train more than an hour—or, at most, two hours—a day. Were they able to put in the time and mileage that top collegiate swimmers do, they probably could swim even faster.

But there is more to life than swimming. Most of us are happy to live in the real world of family, community, and career. What I find most heartening about the results of this study is that with a commitment to swim only an hour or so a day, a person can remain strong and vital until well into old age.

SWIMMING AND SMOKING

Smoking is the single most important factor leading to disease and premature death in North America. An estimated 550,000 people die each year in the United States as a direct result of smoking. Indeed, according to a 1992 study published in the journal *Lancet,* smoking causes fully one fifth of all deaths in the developed world. It is also entirely controllable: although nicotine is highly addictive, ultimately a person can quit and thereby add years to his or her life.

Fortunately, smoking is one of the factors that seems to be most affected by swimming. If you look back at the life-expectancy test (item 26), you will see that smoking can be the single greatest factor in shortening your life: if you smoke two or more packs of cigarettes a day, you are likely to live twelve years less than if you didn't smoke; if you smoke "only" a pack or so a day, you can figure on dying seven years early.

According to the Centers for Disease Control, educational programs to reduce smoking have yielded good news. Since 1980 the proportion of the adult population that smokes has declined from 36 to 26 percent. Still, that leaves well over 40 million people puffing away.

The Perrier study found no significant differences in smoking habits between those who exercise and those who don't. However, two studies I conducted indicate that swimming and smoking do not mix. Most Masters swimmers never smoked, and of those who did, most dropped the habit entirely.

At the 1991 National Masters Swimming Championships in Elizabethtown, Kentucky, I asked a sample of 162 competitors—83 men and 79 women—about their smoking habits. On average, the men in my survey had been swimming in the Masters program for about six years, the women a bit under five. About 27 percent of the men and 25 percent of the women indicated they had smoked before they began swimming—slightly below what was then the national average. By 1991 smoking among this group had disappeared almost entirely: only 5 percent of the women and barely *1 percent* of the men (only one individual) reported that they were still smoking.

TABLE 5.2

The Effects of Swimming on Smoking

| | Men | | Women | |
	Before	*After*	*Before*	*After*
Nonsmokers	73.5%	98.8%	74.7%	94.9%
Smokers	26.5	1.2	25.3	5.1
Of those who smoke:				
1 pack or more/day	4.8	0.0	3.8	0.0
1 pack/day	12.0	0.0	8.9	1.3
1/2–1 pack/day	6.0	1.2	7.6	1.3
<1/2 pack/day	3.6	0.0	5.1	2.5

What is more, those few who did still smoke were smoking less. The results of this study are summarized in Table 5.2.

All things considered, Masters swimming appears to be bad news for the tobacco companies.

Exactly how swimming works to reduce smoking is not known: it may be physiological, psychological, or a combination of the two. However, it does seem to work, as Lynda Myers found out. This should be welcome news for the millions of smokers who have struggled in vain to break their habit. One forty-two-year-old stockbroker, a former college football player, summed up the experience of many swimmers: "I didn't particularly try to stop smoking when I started swimming. I hurt my knee in college, and for me swimming was just a way to help keep my weight down without putting stress on my knee. But after a few months, I just didn't seem to need to smoke anymore. I'd find myself reaching in my pocket for a pack out of habit and then catch myself and think, Hey, what am I doing this for? Why should I destroy my lungs? That was that. No withdrawal pains—nothing. Oh, sure, every once in a while I still feel an urge to take a puff, but now it's something I can control. I feel a whole lot better now that I've stopped smoking. Hey, if swimming helped me to lick this thing, that's just great. It's one more thing it's got going for it."

GIVING YOURSELF THE GIFT OF LIFE

Swimming makes sense—for you, for me, for just about everyone. Study after scientific study documents its beneficial effects on the body and the mind. Not only is swimming the best form of exercise, but it is a sensual and highly enjoyable activity as well. By the time you finish this book, I hope you will be convinced to get in the swim. To help you see how much swimming can mean to your health, three score sheets for the life-expectancy test are included in Appendix C, in addition to the one on page 77. Take the test and fill in a score sheet before you begin your swimming program. Be honest with yourself: this is serious business. Then take the test after just six months of swimming, and again after one year. This way you will be able to chart for yourself the extraordinary benefits you'll be deriving—how swimming will be your gift of life.

The Fountain of Youth exists. And unlike the unfortunate Juan

Ponce de León, you won't have to voyage halfway around the world to find it. It exists right in your own community—at the local pool, in a nearby lake, in the ocean. You won't need to brave the unknown dangers of uncharted lands. All you will need is a swimsuit, goggles, and a little motivation. Swimming will add years to your life—and life to your years.

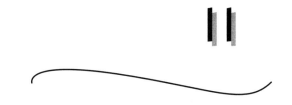

GETTING IN THE SWIM

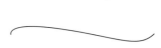

6

HOW TO BEGIN SWIMMING: DIFFERENT STROKES FOR DIFFERENT FOLKS

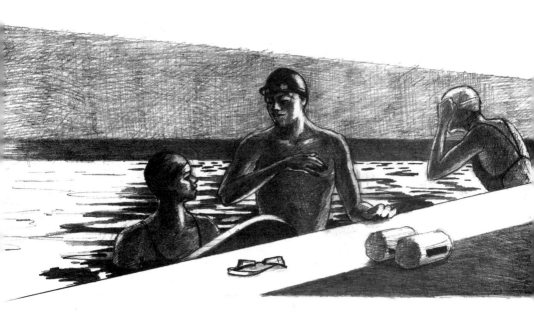

NOW THAT YOU are convinced of the benefits of swimming, what comes next is to learn the strokes and start. I can't guarantee that you will ever be another Mark Spitz or Summer Sanders. I *can* guarantee, though, that in the process of becoming a more proficient swimmer, you will enjoy yourself thoroughly.

THE BARE ESSENTIALS

Before you take your first stroke, you will need to get outfitted. Fortunately, that will be easy. Swimming is an inexpensive sport. In fact, you can easily equip yourself for a year or longer for less than fifty dollars. You do not need expensive shoes, tights, or other paraphernalia. The only equipment you *really* need is a swimsuit (and even that can be optional at times).

Swimsuits

Nowadays, racing suits are made of two basic materials: nylon and Lycra. (Actually, "Lycra" suits contain only about 23 percent Lycra.) The nylon suits are sturdier and last longer, but they absorb more water. The Lycra suits mold themselves to your body's contours and do not absorb water. Because they reduce resistance, Lycra suits allow you to swim faster, but they tend to lose their elastic quality with frequent use. So most swimmers prefer to use nylon suits in practice and Lycra suits in competition. (Among the avant-garde, the latest and "fastest" swimsuit material is paper. That's right, *paper*. As you might expect, paper suits tend not to last very long.)

Your swimsuit should fit snugly to minimize resistance. Men's sizes are based on waist measurement. During workouts, I wear a size 32 nylon suit, the same as my waist size. But when I don my Lycra suit for a meet, I squeeze into a size 30.

For women, choosing the proper size is a bit more problematic. Women's sizes are based on bust measurement. If your bust is 34 inches, you will probably wear a size 34 nylon suit and a 32 Lycra. But your best fit may differ depending on your shape. And, as with other items of clothing, swimsuit sizes vary by manufacturer. A friend of mine, one of the top female swimmers in the country, advises: "Start with your bust size, but then try on different sizes to see which one fits you best. Find a size you can squeeze into, but make sure it's not too short or too tight." You should just be able to squeeze yourself into your suit.

Several manufacturers produce high-quality racing suits: Speedo, TYR, The Finals, Hind, Arena, the Victor, Ocean Pool, and Jantzen, among others. Men's nylon suits run about ten to fifteen dollars; Lycra ones cost thirteen to twenty-four dollars, depending on style and manufacturer. Women's nylon suits range from about fifteen to twenty-five dollars; Lycra suits go for twenty-five to fifty-five dollars, again depending on style and manufacturer. Children's and youths' swimsuits cost a little less. You can buy a racing suit at most sporting goods stores. But you often can get discounts from some of the larger mail-order suppliers. Appendix B lists several of the leading mail-order houses along with their 800 numbers.

Many swimmers wear two or more suits when training. This practice has a dual purpose: (1) It increases the resistance or *drag,* so that when you take the extra suits off your body feels much lighter; and (2) it allows you to continue using worn-out suits, which if worn alone might create a scandal.

Goggles

I would add goggles to the very short list of swimming essentials. In my opinion, this piece of equipment ranks as the second greatest invention of the twentieth century—right after the microwave oven! Like many Masters swimmers, I remember well what my son likes to call "the olden days"—before the 1970s—when goggles were worn only by airplane pilots and steelworkers. Many were the evenings I would come home from practice, my eyes painful and red from chlorine, unable to do my homework.

All that is changed now. These days virtually all swimmers wear goggles. Not only do they protect your eyes but they allow you to see clearly underwater. You make fewer blown turns, and you can check out your stroke as you swim. You can also observe that heavenly body in the lane next to you as she (or he) swims by.

There are hundreds of styles of goggles made by many of the companies that manufacture swimsuits: Speedo, Arena, Competitor, TYR, Leader, The Finals, Hind, Barracuda, and Speed. They come in a variety of shapes and sizes, and feature different-colored lenses and gaskets, adjustable nosepieces, antifog coatings, UV protection . . . just about anything you could imagine. There are goggles designed to rest on the bony structure of the eye socket, goggles designed especially for women, and even custom-made prescription goggles.

Prices for goggles range from less than four to over thirty dollars. The goggles I use cost about eleven dollars.

A good pair of goggles fits comfortably and snugly and does not come off on starts or turns. I wear contact lenses. When I swim, I keep my lenses on under my goggles—even when I do racing dives in meets. I have not lost a lens while swimming in over ten years.

The best style of goggles for you is the one that fits the contours of *your* face. Test several varieties before making a decision. Other swimmers will let you try their goggles on and offer advice on which styles they have found best.

Other Equipment

Although it definitely does not qualify as an essential, like many swimmers, I like to wear a *swim cap*. Caps are cheap ($1.50 to $3.00 apiece), and they help protect your hair. Just massage a little cream rinse into your hair before putting on your cap, and you're ready to go. I also find that swim caps are decorative and fun to trade or give as presents. Many swimmers who are prone to the sniffles also wear nose clips ($1.50 to $2.50 each).

That just about covers it: a swimsuit, goggles, cap, and maybe some nose clips. There is other equipment you may want to use in your workouts—kick boards and pull buoys, for example. But these items are usually supplied by the pool at which you swim. Chapter 14 will discuss training equipment and how it should be used.

GETTING WET

A good part of the enjoyment of swimming comes from the variety it offers. I try to swim at least five days a week, and I rarely repeat the same workout. Sometimes I concentrate on freestyle; at other times I stress one of the other strokes. Sometimes I work mostly on my sprinting, at other times on distance. In some workouts I emphasize my legs by using a kick board or swim fins; in others I work mainly on my arms, placing a pull buoy between my legs to maintain my body position and keep myself from kicking. And so on. There are literally thousands of variations!

In this section I will concentrate on the four major strokes: freestyle (or crawl stroke), backstroke, breaststroke, and butterfly. You may want to try to perfect your technique in all of them. Or you may find that you enjoy doing one or two of the strokes more than the others. As the immortal Sly and the Family Stone so melodiously put it: "Different strokes for different folks."

By now you should feel reasonably comfortable in the water. If you are over thirty-five, you have gotten a medical checkup and an enthusiastic "okay" from your doctor. So the next step is simply to start swimming. Swimming is one of those things you have to learn by *doing.* This book can provide you with the motivation to swim, and it can give you some useful information about how to do the strokes and how to train. But the only way you will ever become a good swimmer is by practicing.

Some people like to learn by trial and error. That's fine. If you are one of those folks, just get in the water and start stroking. You probably won't be very efficient at first, but you'll improve. Your goggles will help you see where you're going and allow you to observe the techniques of other swimmers underwater. When you see a particularly good swimmer, ask him or her to give you some pointers. Most people will be flattered you asked and delighted to help.

Or you may prefer formal instruction. No problem. Swimming has become so popular in recent years that virtually every YMCA and community center in the country has classes for people of all ages and abilities—from infant to senior adult and from rank beginner to accomplished swimmer. It should be easy to find a class suitable for you no matter where you live.

A good way to supplement lessons is through videos. In recent years, a number of high-quality videos have been produced for swimmers at every ability level. Appendix G reviews some of the top videos currently available, lists their prices, and provides information about how you may purchase them.

Whether you learn on your own or from an instructor, the important thing is to proceed at your own pace, mastering each skill at every step. Don't try to learn everything at once. Concentrate on one thing at a time—your body position, breathing, arm stroke, kick, whatever. Pretty soon you will be slicing confidently through the water.

BASIC PRINCIPLES OF SWIMMING

Part of the charm of swimming is the constant variety it offers. But since all four strokes involve propelling oneself through water as efficiently as possible, it is not surprising that they share basic elements. Dr. James E. "Doc" Counsilman—perhaps the world's foremost authority on swimming technique—outlines five principles that all swimming strokes have in common. It is important to keep these in mind as you learn to swim better and faster.

1. Streamline Your Body

In order to move through the water more efficiently, you should try to create as little drag as possible. To do this you must keep your body in a flat, or horizontal position. If you are swimming freestyle or back-stroke, for example, and you lift your head too high to breathe, your hips and legs will drop, and you will be moving at an angle, creating unnecessary resistance (see Figure 6.1). For the same reason, you must avoid excessive rolling from side to side, or wiggling your hips or legs back and forth. The less drag you create, the less energy you will need to propel yourself forward. I like to try to feel the water flowing around me. One swimmer I know likes to think of herself as a smooth, sleek dolphin gliding effortlessly through the water.

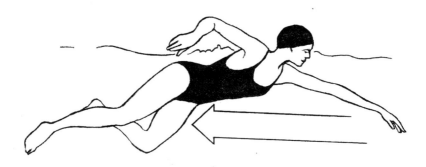

Figure 6.1. Dropping your hips and legs creates unnecessary resistance.

2. Obey Newton's Law

Sir Isaac Newton's third law of motion states that for every action there is an equal and opposite reaction. In swimming, this means that in order to move forward, you have to push water backward. Many swimmers believe this means that if they push directly back in a straight line they will move forward most economically. However, this is not the case.

Why? Doc Counsilman explains by comparing swimming with running: a runner pushes against the ground almost directly backward and, as a result, is pushed almost directly forward. This happens because the ground does not move when he pushes against it. When a swimmer pushes her hand against water, however, the water naturally moves in the direction the hand pushes it. If she continues to push backward in a straight line, the swimmer is pushing water that is already moving backward. Thus, she receives almost no additional propulsion. To solve this problem, she must move her hands in an elliptical pattern to find still water to push against. This is true for *every* swimming stroke. Figure 6.2 illustrates the elliptical pull patterns of the four strokes. The following four chapters will go into these stroke techniques in some detail.

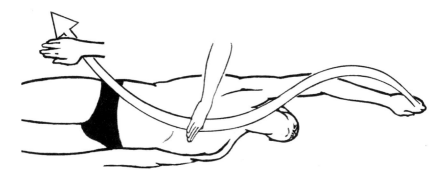

Figure 6.2. Elliptical Pull Patterns of the Four Major Strokes
A. The freestyle pull pattern seen from underneath

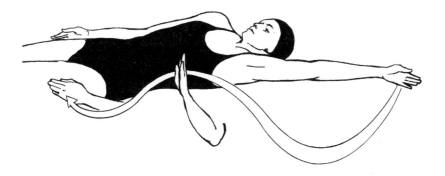

B. The backstroke pull pattern seen from the side

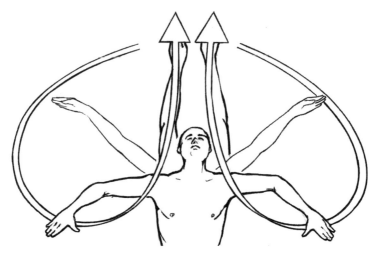

C. The breaststroke pull pattern seen from underneath

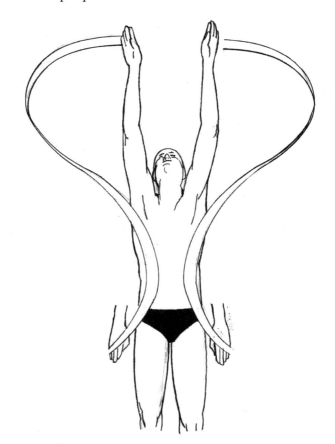

D. The butterfly pull pattern seen from underneath

3. *Use the Proper Pull*

When learning to swim, one of the most important things to concentrate on is using the most effective pull. Most beginning swimmers either drop their elbows or use a straight-arm pull.

The dropped-elbow pull is the least efficient type. As Figure 6.3 indicates, a swimmer using this pull has very little leverage and exerts force backward only at the middle of the stroke. At the beginning, most of the force is applied downward, whereas at the end, most of the force is applied upward. The result is that the swimmer expends a lot of energy for very little forward propulsion.

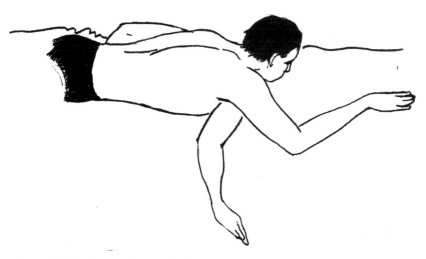

Figure 6.3. The Dropped-Elbow Pull

The straight-arm pull (see Figure 6.4) is a little better. But the same mechanical problems are present: most of the force is exerted downward or upward, rather than backward. This tends to make the swimmer bob up and down, and in the process creates additional drag.

The most effective pull for any of the four strokes is illustrated in Figure 6.5. It begins with the elbow only slightly bent. The elbow increases its bend until it is in a vertical position, directly below the swimmer. As the stroke continues backward, the amount of bend in the elbow decreases steadily until the end, when the elbow is almost straight (except in breaststroke). Notice that the elbow is carried in a high position throughout the pull. As the elbow begins to bend at the start of the pull, the upper arm rotates inward. In this type of pull, the downward and upward forces are minimized and the backward push is maximized. Thus, the swimmer is propelled smoothly through the water.

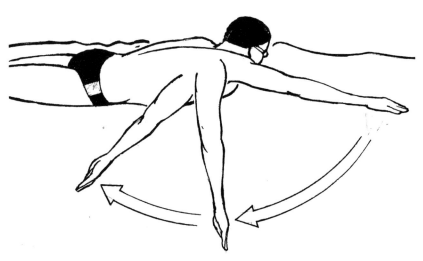

Figure 6.4. The Straight-Arm Pull

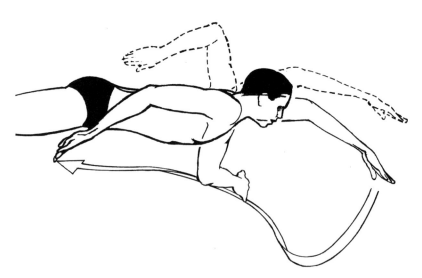

Figure 6.5. The Correct Pull

4. Position Your Hands Efficiently

There are two things to keep in mind about the position of your hands while swimming: how they enter the water and how you hold them during the pull.

Your hands should enter the water by knifing cleanly through it. If you slap the water, air bubbles will form around your hands, decreasing the efficiency of your pull. Likewise, as your hands leave the water they should be as streamlined as possible so they do not exert an upward force, which will push you down.

How should you hold your hands and fingers while swimming? When I first learned to swim, I was taught to cup my hands during the pull. But research by Counsilman using a wind tunnel has demonstrated that this is one of the *least* effective ways of holding your hands while swimming. Why? Because it decreases the hands' surface area and thus reduces the efficiency of the pull. The best way to hold your hands is flat, with the fingers firm but relaxed and spread slightly apart.

5. Apply Propulsion Evenly

When swimming you must try to move forward at as even a pace as possible. This has been termed the continuity of movement principle. If you are continually stopping or slowing down, you will spend much of your energy trying to overcome inertia each time you start up again.

The cost of overcoming inertia can be considerable. Think of how much energy a weight lifter has to use to lift a heavy barbell off his shoulders—and how little he needs once the weight is in motion. Or consider how much force is needed to push your car after it has run out of gas. Once you have gotten the car moving, however, much less force is needed to keep it moving to the next gas station.

The same principle applies to swimming. And it explains why freestyle is the fastest stroke: because in it there is a constant application of propulsive force.

So keep this principle in mind as you swim—apply force evenly. You will find that doing so will make your swimming much more efficient, and much easier.

You are now ready to tackle the four major swimming strokes, which are described in detail in Chapters 7 through 10. As you learn them, remember to put to use the five basic principles:

1. Streamline your body.
2. Obey Newton's law.
3. Use the proper pull.
4. Position your hands efficiently.
5. Apply propulsion evenly.

Don't expect to perfect all the strokes in a week or a month—or even a year. It will take time. But you will find that you are improving noticeably as you master each technique, come to execute it almost automatically, and move on to the next skill. You will feel more comfortable and less tired, and you will have a sense of flowing with the water instead of struggling against it.

My teammate and good friend Abe Olanoff is eighty-eight, has been swimming more than seventy years, and is always asking me to watch his stroke or his turns and suggest ways he can improve. I have been swimming for over thirty-five years, and I'm *still* learning. Indeed, that is part of the fun and part of the challenge! As my son so indelicately put it not long ago: "You're living proof, Dad, that you *can* teach an old dog new tricks." Old dog or young, it's a great feeling to know that there is always more to learn, that you can still improve, still swim better and faster, whether you are thirty, forty, or even eighty.

And now, let's get started.

7

THE FREESTYLE

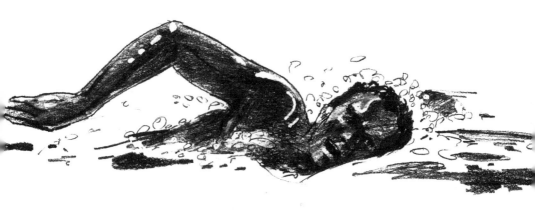

THE FREESTYLE, OR crawl, is both the fastest and the most efficient swimming technique. When it was introduced more than a hundred years ago, many thought the stroke too exhausting to be used for any distance longer than short sprints. But today it is used exclusively for all distance events, including English Channel swims and marathon races. Swum properly, the freestyle uses less energy than any other stroke.

Technically, the name for the fastest of all strokes is the *front crawl*. *Freestyle* literally means you can swim any stroke, or any combination of strokes, you like: backstroke, breaststroke, butterfly, even sidestroke or elementary backstroke. Even in a race. But in modern swimming *freestyle* has come to be synonymous with the *crawl*. Throughout the remainder of this chapter—indeed, throughout this book—I use the two terms interchangeably.

Not only is the freestyle fast and efficient but most people find it the *easiest* stroke to learn. It is no surprise to discover, then, that it is far and away the most popular stroke.

In fact, even if you wind up specializing in one of the other strokes, you will probably find yourself swimming more laps of crawl stroke than of anything else in your workouts. The crawl stroke is the best way to maximize your yardage and squeeze a quality workout into a limited time. So it is important not only that you master the mechanics of this stroke but also that you learn to swim it smoothly and fluently.

A BRIEF HISTORY

The freestyle has roots that go back thousands of years. An ancient Egyptian wall relief clearly shows soldiers of Ramses II using an over-arm stroke to pursue their Hittite enemies across the Orontes River more than 3,200 years ago.

The crawl stroke itself seems to have been invented independently in several tropical areas of the world at least several hundred years ago. In the late eighteenth century, the great explorer Captain James Cook described the inhabitants of the Solomons, and a number of other Melanesian and Polynesian islands, as swimming a type of crawl. More than two centuries earlier, Portuguese explorers of coastal Brazil, near modern-day Rio de Janeiro, noted that the local Indians also swam with an overhand stroke.

It seems that wherever conditions were appropriate, people learned to swim. The islands of the South Pacific, with their warm, calm waters, provided *ideal* conditions. Not only was swimming fun and a respite from the tropical sun but it also had its rewards: fish and shellfish for food, shells for decoration and exchange. Over time, it seems, the islanders became more and more proficient, eventually developing a form of crawl stroke.

It was Australians, however, who first adopted and then refined the technique they observed among their island neighbors. Probably the most sports-minded people in the world, the Aussies have always been particularly fond of swimming. In 1893 a young man named Harry Wickham introduced the crawl in Australia. It seems that Wickham had learned the stroke while visiting the island of Rubiana. He taught it to his twelve-year-old brother, Alick, who caught the eye of George Farmer, a local swim coach. The story goes that Farmer, astounded by the boy's speed and his unorthodox technique, exclaimed, "Look at that bloke crawling on the water!" The name stuck, and the modern era of swimming was born.

In 1902 two Australian brothers, Syd and Charles Cavill, popularized the stroke in Europe. The following year they came to the United States, where the stroke was dubbed the Australian crawl. By the time they arrived, European and American swimmers were already familiar with another overhand stroke, the trudgeon. Named after an Englishman who learned the technique in South Africa in the 1880s, the trudgeon combined an overarm recovery with a wide scissor kick. Even today I occasionally see older people swimming laps using the trudgeon.

The Cavills' Australian crawl featured a two-beat flutter kick: two kicks for each arm cycle. American swimmers promptly improved on it, substituting a faster four-beat kick. Since then the stroke has become progressively faster and its stars well known. The first swimmer to gain world renown was Hawaiian Duke Kahanamoku, a three-time Olympic champion, who is also credited with popularizing the sport of surfing. The sport has seen many superstars: Johnny Weissmuller, the first man to break a minute for 100 meters, who parlayed his swimming success into a Hollywood film career as Tarzan; Mark Spitz, who won an unprecedented seven gold medals in seven events at the Munich Olympics in 1972, setting world records in every one; Russia's Vladimir Salnikov, regarded by many as the greatest distance swimmer of all time and the first man to swim 1,500 meters in under fifteen minutes; and, more recently, America's Matt Biondi, world-record holder in the 100-meter freestyle, swimming's glamour event.

Unlike many other sports, swimming has always had its share of female superstars. These include Gertrude Ederle, an Olympic champion who in 1926 became the first woman to swim the English Channel; Australia's Dawn Fraser, who held the world record in the 100-meter freestyle from 1956 until 1971; Penny Dean, an American whose record for swimming the English Channel is faster than the fastest men's time; and America's sweetheart, Janet Evans, whose world-record times are nothing short of astounding.

BODY POSITION

The key to swimming an efficient freestyle—as for all the strokes—is maintaining the correct body position. That means *streamlining*. If your body is streamlined, you will feel yourself gliding, almost effortlessly, through the water. If it is not, you will feel as if you are struggling against the water, and the drag you create will slow you down and tire you out.

Your kick can help you maintain a streamlined body position by keeping your hips and legs from sinking. Kick steadily, with only a slight bend at the knees, and do not let your feet go any deeper than about twelve to sixteen inches below the surface of the water. The position of your head is especially important, because it affects the rest of your body. If you hold your head too high, your hips and legs will sag. If you pull your head to one side when you breathe, your hips will swing the other way. All these things will force your body out of alignment and create drag.

The ideal body position for the crawl stroke is simple: you should be horizontal, with your body stretched out in a straight line. Your face should be in the water (except when you breathe, of course), with the water at about your hairline. Look forward and slightly downward. That's it. That's all you need to remember.

ARM PULL

In the freestyle, the arms stroke alternately—first one arm, then the other—recovering over the water, while the legs maintain a streamlined body position and provide additional propulsion with a constant "flutter" kick. As explained in Chapter 6, to swim well you must remember Newton's third law: for every action there is an equal and opposite reaction. When you swim the crawl, you move forward by pushing your body past your hands. If you are having trouble visualizing this, think about what you do when you use crutches: you plant the crutches on the ground and then swing your body past them.

In the crawl stroke, your arms furnish about 80 percent of your propulsion—more than in any other stroke. So using your arms as efficiently as possible is very important. The best way to do this is an elongated S-pattern arm pull, illustrated in Figure 7.1. This technique

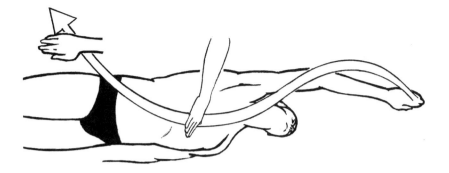

Figure 7.1. The S-Pattern of the Freestyle Arm Pull

gives you a better "grip" on the water because with it you are always pushing against still water rather than water that is already in motion.

The freestyle arm stroke consists of five phases:

1. Entry
2. Catch
3. Pull
4. Follow-through
5. Recovery

As you learn the stroke, try to keep two principles in mind: (1) always *keep your elbows high,* and (2) *accelerate your hand speed* until you have completed the follow-through. If you remember these principles, you will avoid the two most common errors people make when doing the crawl.

One more thing: in the next few pages, I have broken the crawl down into its constituent phases. But remember, when you put it all together, the stroke is one continuous, fluid motion. Okay? Now, let's get started.

The Entry

Your arm enters the water directly in front of your shoulder, with your elbow bent so it is higher than your hand. Enter at about a thirty-degree angle and as "quietly" as you can; try to avoid slapping the water.

Your fingertips enter first, thumb down, and your palm is tilted out slightly. Then slide your arm forward and slightly downward, until it is fully extended. Think of your fingers making a hole in the water. Then let your hand, wrist, elbow, and shoulder slip through the hole.

The Catch

The catch is made as soon as you have completely extended your elbow. As you begin to flex your elbow, turn your wrist downward so that your fingertips point toward the bottom of the pool. Try letting your hands scull out slightly before you begin the pull. Although doing this is not necessary, some people find that it improves their pull.

The Pull

Start the pull as soon as you have made the catch. As you begin the pull, you will feel yourself grabbing an armful of water with your hand, forearm, and upper arm, almost as if you are reaching around a very large barrel. Then—always remembering to keep your elbow high—move your hand backward in an S-pattern, past your shoulders and then under your body. Be careful not to let the pull cross your body's centerline, as this will disturb your body position. As your hand passes beneath your shoulders, your elbow achieves its maximum bend—about ninety degrees.

The Follow-through

Throughout the pull, you have been accelerating your hand speed. Now, in the follow-through, continuing that acceleration, push your hand back past your hips. Push hard! As you straighten and extend your arm to finish the stroke, your palm will be facing your feet. This will allow your hand to exit the water most easily.

The Recovery

The final phase of the arm stroke, the recovery, is a smooth, rounded movement in which the stroke continues into the air. It begins as your elbow leaves the water, followed by your shoulder and then your hand. Your elbow should remain higher than your hand throughout the recovery, and your hand should be just over the surface of the water. Think of your elbow reaching for the sky as your shoulder comes out of the water.

Your arm should remain completely relaxed throughout the recovery. Allow momentum to carry it forward. As you complete the recovery, your hand enters the water again at about a thirty-degree angle, fingertips first, thumb down, palm tilted out. You are now ready for your next stroke.

Figures 7.2 and 7.3 illustrate the phases of the freestyle arm pull as seen from the side (7.2) and head-on (7.3).

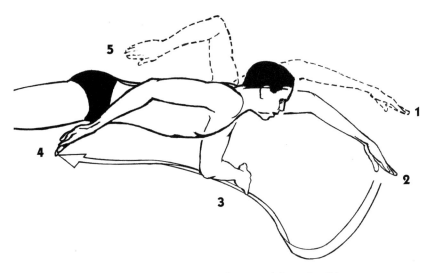

Figure 7.2. Phases of the Freestyle Arm Pull, Viewed from the Side

BODY ROLL

An essential part of swimming the crawl stroke efficiently is the body roll. In fact, if you do the stroke correctly, you will actually spend more time on your sides than in a flat position. Steve Winwood is right on when he sings: "You've got to roll with it, baby."

The roll is a natural motion caused by the rotating of the arm stroke. Don't fight it! It reduces drag, allows you to put the large muscles of your back and shoulders to their best use, and helps you get

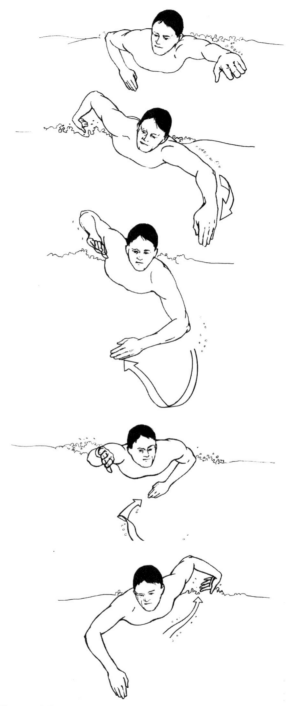

Figure 7.3. Phases of the Freestyle Arm Pull, Viewed Head-on

more distance with every stroke. It also makes your recovery more relaxed and lets you breathe without twisting your head as much.

When your right arm enters the water, let your body, especially your hips, roll about forty-five degrees to the right. Then, when you stroke with your left arm, roll about forty-five degrees to the left. You will probably find that you roll even more when you breathe. That's fine. Although it is possible to roll too much, a more common error is to roll too little. So relax and let yourself roll naturally with the stroke.

A new theory of how power can be maximized in the freestyle argues that swimmers need to roll even more than forty-five degrees. Using frame-by-frame underwater video and computer analysis, Bob Pritchard, director of Somax Posture and Sports in Corte Madera, California, analyzed the strokes of world-class, collegiate, and beginning swimmers. He found that the very best swimmers rotate their hips up to *sixty* degrees and that the hip movement *precedes* the arm stroke. Thus, just as with baseball players and golfers, more power is generated from the hips than from the shoulders and arms.

Matt Biondi, the world record holder for 100 meters, has his hand enter the water at a very shallow angle and lets it glide for an unusually long period of time. He rolls his hips sixty degrees, then begins to rotate them back before he starts the in sweep of his arm stroke.

In contrast, good college swimmers rotate their hips during the out sweep of the arm stroke, making only partial use of the powerful hip muscles. Poor swimmers rotate their hips long after an arm enters the water and is ending the out sweep. They make no use whatsoever of their hip muscles, essentially just dragging them through the water.

BREATHING

For novice swimmers, breathing can be the most anxiety-provoking aspect of swimming the freestyle. Some people twist their heads from side to side with every stroke, causing their bodies to wiggle. Others lift their heads straight up, which makes their lower bodies sink. Still others, perhaps fearful of catching a mouthful of water, hold their breath as long as they can before gasping for air. All of these will lead quickly to exhaustion.

Turning your head to inhale is a simple, easy motion that should be coordinated with the roll of your body. As your body rolls toward your breathing side, turn your head gently and take a deep breath. By inhaling when you roll, you won't need to lift your head out of the water. In fact, you will actually be breathing *below* the water surface. This is because your forward momentum creates a bow wave extending from your head to your neck, giving you a little air pocket in which to inhale (see Figure 7.4).

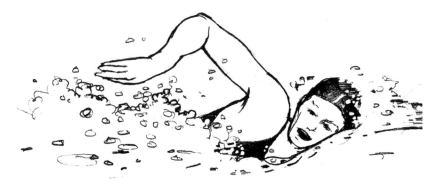

Figure 7.4. Inhaling in the Bow Wave

After you inhale, return your face into the water and exhale slowly as your body rolls toward the other side. Be sure to exhale *completely* before turning your head to inhale again.

Probably the most common error swimmers make is early inhalation. If you turn your head to inhale before your opposite arm has entered the water, you are breathing too early (see Figure 7.5). Early breathing gives you an up-and-down rhythm, making you feel that you are swimming faster. Actually, it pushes your lower body deeper

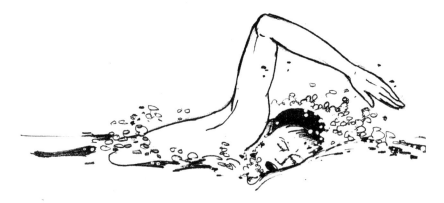

Figure 7.5. The Error of Early Breathing

in the water, increasing drag and thus slowing you down. More important, early breathing can stress your shoulders, possibly leading to injury.

If you experience shoulder pain or tire easily when swimming the crawl, you may be breathing too early. Fortunately, the problem is easy to fix. *Simply make sure you see your opposite hand as it enters the water before turning to inhale.* When you practice, concentrate on perfecting this timing. It may feel awkward at first, but eventually it will become second nature.

You can inhale to the right side, the left side, or both sides, whichever you prefer. I was taught to inhale to one side, my left. Nowadays, most coaches prefer bilateral breathing: inhaling alternately from both sides. Janet Evans, for example, usually breathes every *third* stroke, first to one side then the other. Alternate breathing balances your stroke. So it is worth learning, even though adult swimmers may find it a bit difficult at first.

One of the questions novice swimmers often ask is How often should I breathe? The answer is, It depends—on your lung capacity, your physical condition, and the distance you are swimming. If you are doing a 50-yard sprint, an anaerobic event, you probably do not need to breathe more than three or four times—and maybe not at all. In a 100-yard race, you may only need to breathe every fourth or fifth stroke. Then again, you may need to breathe more often. If your body is crying out for oxygen, *you need to breathe*! Do *not* hold your breath! Doing so will tire you out very quickly.

For distances longer than 100 yards, you will definitely need to breathe much more frequently—probably every second or third stroke. The key is to establish and maintain a rhythm: stroke, stroke/ breathe, stroke, stroke/breathe; or stroke, stroke, stroke/breathe; stroke, stroke, stroke/breathe. Once you are in shape and breathing rhythmically, you will be able to swim long distances without tiring.

THE KICK

The leg action that accompanies the crawl stroke is called the *flutter kick*. The kick contributes only about 20 percent of the total propulsion in the freestyle—less than in any other stroke. But it is essential in maintaining body position and preventing excess wiggling of the hips.

To do the flutter kick, move your legs up and down alternately in a steady, strong, consistent rhythm. The power for the kick comes from your hips, not your lower legs. As you kick downward, bend your knee slightly and keep your ankle loose. On the upbeat, hold your knee relatively straight and raise your foot until your heel breaks the water surface.

Do not bring your feet far out of the water: doing so may make a big splash, but it contributes nothing to your propulsion. And don't kick too deep: your feet should go only about twelve to sixteen inches below the surface. Try to make the water "boil" around your feet.

Practice your flutter kick by using a kick board. Hold the board in front of you, hands about two thirds of the way to the front, and simply kick. Although you may find it tiring at first, you will progress quickly if you keep at it. Kicking is an excellent exercise for firming the thighs and hips, and it will also increase your ankle flexibility.

There are several kicking patterns you can use. The most popular are the *six-beat kick* and the *two-beat kick*. In the six-beat kick, you kick six times for each complete arm cycle (that is, three beats for each arm stroke). The two-beat kick consists of two beats per arm cycle.

Generally speaking, sprinters use the six-beat kick, which has the advantage of generating more power but the disadvantage of using more energy. Distance swimmers tend to use some variation of the two-beat kick. It really doesn't matter very much *which* kick you use. Simply choose the pattern that feels most comfortable and natural to you.

PUTTING IT ALL TOGETHER

By now you have mastered each of the skills that constitute the crawl stroke—the streamlined body position, the bent-arm **S**-shaped arm pull, the body roll, the correct breathing technique, and the flutter kick. Now it is time to put it all together (see Figure 7.6). Janet Evans and Matt Biondi: look out!

These are the essentials of the crawl stroke. But, if you want to swim a smooth, powerful freestyle, you need more than good stroke mechanics. You need to develop both a "feel" for the water and a sense of momentum.

Freestyle, former Olympic champion Rowdy Gaines points out, is very much a "feel" stroke. As you practice the basics, he advises, sensitize yourself to the feel of the water on your fingertips, your hands,

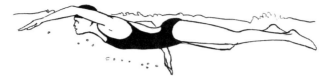

Figure 7.6. The Freestyle: Putting It All Together
A. One arm enters the water as the other begins the recovery with a bent elbow. The legs kick up and down in a steady flutter kick throughout the stroke.

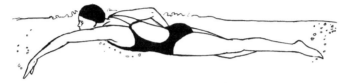

B. After the catch is made, the S-pattern arm pull begins. Note that the elbow is held high and the body has begun to roll.

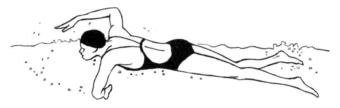

C. As the body rolls, the pulling arm passes under the chest and the elbow reaches its maximum bend, about ninety degrees. The other arm prepares to enter the water, directly in front of the shoulder.

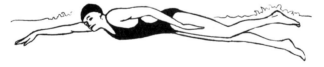

D. As the swimmer completes the pull with the follow-through, she begins to rotate her head to the recovering side to inhale.

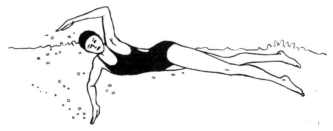

E. As the swimmer inhales, her body achieves its maximum roll. Her other hand enters the water to begin the next stroke.

your arms, your torso, your legs, your feet. *"Learn to feel the water,"* Rowdy counsels. "Don't fight against it. Become one with the water."

You should also learn to maintain constant momentum. This is the best way to overcome resistance. As you swim, imagine yourself moving forward at a constant speed on an invisible conveyor belt. Canadian Olympic coach Cecil Colwin explains: "Momentum never starts, ends, nor is interrupted. The entire freestyle action should be fluent, continuous, and free-flowing."

THE FLIP TURN

The flip turn is, by far, the fastest way to do a freestyle turn. In my experience, almost everyone loves doing it. I have taught the turn to hundreds of people—from children as young as five to adults as old as eighty-six. It seems that as soon as people learn the crawl stroke, they want to learn how to flip.

What you are trying to accomplish with the flip turn is reversing the direction of your body in the shortest time, without losing speed and while using the least amount of energy possible. The sequence of drawings in Figure 7.7 illustrates the phases of the flip turn.

As you approach the wall, stop the recovery of one arm and hold it at your thigh. Take the final stroke with the other arm. Then hold both arms at your sides, palms facing down.

Begin the somersault by ducking your head and shoulders. At the same time, press down with your palms. Add a dolphin kick to help raise your hips and rotate your body. (The dolphin kick is described in detail in Chapter 10.)

With your body in a pike position and your hands still pushing down, complete the somersault by bringing your legs over the water. Move your hands toward your head to reduce resistance and prepare for a streamlined push off the wall.

Whip your legs directly overhead. Then plant your feet on the wall. Now, as you bring your arms forward, push off the wall with your legs. With the thrust off the wall, extend your arms, keeping your head squeezed between your upper arms, and streamline your body. Finally, as you push off, twist your body so that you "corkscrew" through the water and end up on your stomach before taking your first stroke. The time you spend on the wall should be very little—half a second or less.

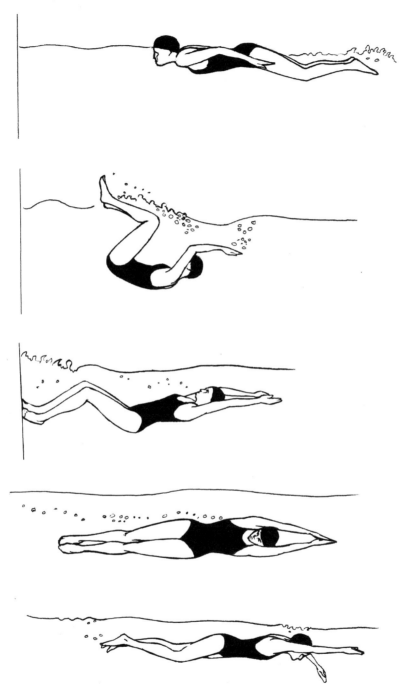

Figure 7.7. The Freestyle Flip Turn

As soon as you feel yourself slowing down, begin flutter-kicking with a small, fast kick. Then let your head break the surface and begin stroking. When you practice your turns, remember to explode off the wall, assume a streamlined position, and kick hard. You should be able to glide four or five yards, or even farther, before you begin stroking.

THE START

You won't need to learn how to execute a start unless you choose to swim in competition. So if you are swimming solely to improve your health and fitness, you may want to skip this section.

A word of caution: as you practice your starts, *make sure you dive into deep water—at least seven feet.* Beginners often dive too deep. To avoid injury it is important to give yourself plenty of room for error.

Fast starts are an important part of competitive swimming. A good start can give you an advantage of one or two feet over your competition before the first stroke is taken, sometimes providing the margin of victory in a tight race.

In freestyle, as in breaststroke and butterfly, the start is made out of the water from a starting block. (The backstroke start, explained in Chapter 8, is made *in* the water.) There are a number of starting techniques. Here I will concentrate on the most widely used: the *grab start* (see Figure 7.8).

After mounting the block, curl your toes over the front edge, placing your feet at about hip width. Then, when the starter says, "Take your mark," curl your fingers around the front edge of the starting block. Your hands can be placed either between your feet or outside them, whichever feels more comfortable. Bend your knees slightly, and move your center of gravity forward without losing your balance.

Concentrate on listening for the starting signal, usually a gun or horn. As soon as you hear the signal, snap your hands forward and push off the block with your feet. *Do not make a winding motion with your hands!*

The key to a successful start is to minimize the resistance you make when you enter the water. A big splash means a lot of resistance. So try to enter the water cleanly, with your body diving through the hole your hands made when they entered.

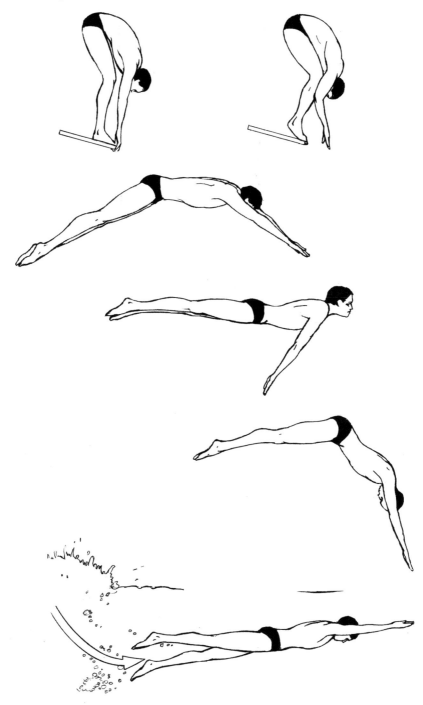

Figure 7.8. The Freestyle Start

Keep yourself in a streamlined position, head between your arms, as in the flip turn. Begin kicking vigorously, and angle yourself toward the surface of the water. After about three seconds you will surface, ready to take your first stroke.

TEN FREESTYLE TIPS

All the principles of efficient swimming outlined in Chapter 6 apply to the crawl stroke. Try to keep them in mind as you practice the stroke. In addition, the following ten tips will make learning the freestyle much easier.

1. Streamline your body.
2. Your arms provide most of the propulsion in the freestyle, so use an elongated **S**-shaped pull, the most efficient pattern there is.
3. Let your arm enter the water "quietly," fingertips first, elbow bent. Try to avoid slapping the water.
4. Keep your elbow high throughout the pull. This will enable you to exert the maximum amount of power.
5. *Accelerate* your arm throughout the pull.
6. Recover with a *bent* arm, elbow pointing straight up. Do not use a straight-arm recovery.
7. Roll your body at least forty-five degrees with every stroke you take. Doing so will increase your power and efficiency.
8. Avoid the mistake of breathing too early. Roll your head to inhale only after you see the opposite hand enter the water. Return your face to the water in time to see the recovering hand enter.
9. Learn to inhale on both sides. When practicing, try to breathe every third stroke.
10. Whether you use a two- or six-beat flutter kick, maintain a strong, steady rhythm.

8

THE BACKSTROKE

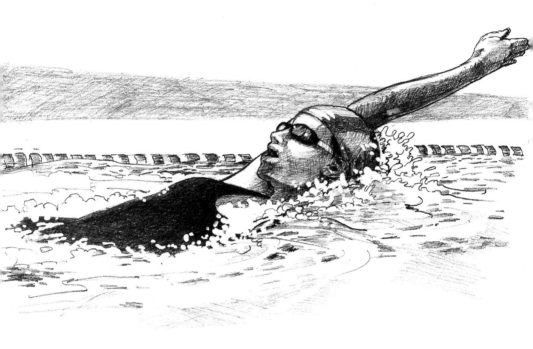
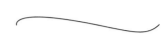

THE BACKSTROKE IS perhaps the most peculiar of the four major swimming strokes. It is, after all, the only stroke that is swum upside-down. In addition, unlike the other strokes, in backstroke you cannot see where you are going—only where you've been. It is no wonder that many a beginning swimmer, fearful of bumping his head on the pool wall, finds the stroke a bit disconcerting at first. But the back-stroke can also be reassuring. Since your face is always out of the water when you swim it, no special breathing technique is needed—you can breathe anytime you want to.

A BRIEF HISTORY

People have been swimming on their backs at least since the days of classical Greece and Rome. However, it was not until the twentieth century that the back *crawl* was invented. Before that the technique most likely used was what we now would call the *elementary backstroke*—essentially an inverted breaststroke. In 1794, for example, the Italian writer Oronzio de Bernardi described a form of elementary backstroke in his volume on the art of swimming. In London three quarters of a century later, the marquis Bibbero was reported to have used a similar method to swim a mile in thirty-nine and a half minutes.

The modern backstroke, or back crawl, was unveiled by an American swimmer, Harry Hebner, at the 1912 Olympic Games in Stockholm. Hebner used his revolutionary technique to carve more than three seconds off the Olympic record and defeat his favored German rivals. Olympic officials were aghast at Hebner's unconventional style and wanted to disqualify him. But U.S. officials intervened, correctly pointing out that the rules required only that a swimmer remain on his back throughout the race. The U.S. view prevailed, Hebner's victory was preserved, and the modern backstroke was born. The new technique was so much faster and more efficient than the older style that within a few years it had replaced it completely.

The backstroke changed very little over the next seventy years, although a number of improvements in technique were made. In the early 1980s, however, several American collegiate swimmers began experimenting with a radically new style—at least for the first twenty yards of their race. The technique, introduced by world champion Jesse Vassallo, was inspired by studies of the way dolphins swim and by the efficiency of the dolphin kick in the butterfly.

At the start of a race, a swimmer would streamline his body and swim underwater for as long as he could, using a reverse dolphin kick. He would not use his arms at all. After about twenty yards he would pop to the surface, take three or four strokes, make the turn, then swim the rest of the race using the back crawl. Invariably, even in top competition, these swimmers would jump out to a quick lead on the first lap. And just as invariably, they would tire in the later stages of the race, go into oxygen debt, and fall behind.

It was not until 1987 that a swimmer perfected the underwater dolphin technique. David Berkoff, a junior at Harvard University, used it to win the national collegiate title in the 100-yard backstroke, smashing the national record by almost a full second. The exciting innovation became known as the Berkoff blastoff.

In 1988 Berkoff broke the world record for 100 meters twice before the Olympics, swimming the first thirty-five or forty meters of his race underwater. At Seoul, he lowered the mark a third time in leading off the U.S. medley relay team. Ironically, however, Berkoff finished second in the 100-meter race itself. Getting off to a slow start, he was unable to overcome the early lead of Japan's Daichi Suzuki, who himself was using the Berkoff blastoff.

After the Olympics officials tried to outlaw the new technique. In 1991 a rule change limited the distance that could be swum underwater to the first fifteen meters of each lap.

Despite Berkoff's revolutionary innovation, which many competitive swimmers now use for the beginning of their race, the backstroke itself remains unchanged. People may wish to emulate the grace and efficiency of dolphins. But short of equipping ourselves with gill slits through bioengineering, we will never be able to match the ability of our aquatic cousins to swim for several minutes without needing to breathe. For us the backstroke will remain a surface stroke.

BODY POSITION

In swimming the backstroke, you should adopt as streamlined a body position as possible. Counsilman suggests you think of yourself as lying flat on your back in bed without a pillow. The key to the ideal backstroke body position is placement of the hips. Your hips should be just a few inches below the surface of the water. If you hold them too low (a common mistake), your legs will drop and you will create excess drag. If you hold them too high, your legs will ride too high and much of your kick will be out of the water.

The position of your hips is governed mainly by how you hold your head. In the proper head position, your ears are barely submerged, and the water line is about at the middle of your head and below your chin. Your head is in almost straight alignment with your body. To maintain this position while swimming, keep your eyes open and focus on an object about forty-five degrees above the surface of the water.

If you throw your head back too far, your hips will rise and your legs will follow. If you tuck your chin in close to your chest, your hips will drop and you will find yourself in a sitting position, creating a lot of unnecessary resistance.

There is some variation in the ideal backstroke body position, depending on a person's buoyancy. If you float easily and are unusually buoyant, tuck your chin slightly toward your chest. This will keep your hips from rising too high. If you are less buoyant than most people, try tilting your head back slightly. This will keep your hips from sinking too low.

ARM PULL

In the backstroke, as in freestyle, you propel yourself forward by using first one arm, then the other in a continuous, rhythmic, flowing motion. As in all the strokes, it is important to remember to push against water that is not moving. To do this most efficiently, your hands must describe an elongated S-pattern (see Figure 8.1).

As the stroke begins, your arm is extended straight backward and your hand enters the water directly above your shoulder. If you think of your body as a clock, with your head pointing to twelve o'clock, your hands should enter the water at about one and eleven o'clock.

The little finger enters the water first, the thumb last, and your palm faces outward. Many beginners tend to hold their palms upward as their hands enter the water. This causes unnecessary resistance, breaks the flow of the stroke, and prevents the hand from being positioned properly for the next phase of the stroke. So make sure your palm faces outward. As your arm enters the water, its momentum will carry it about eight to twelve inches below the surface before you begin to push backward.

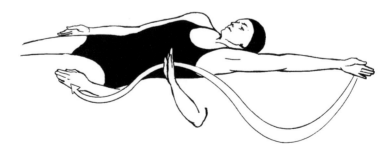

Figure 8.1. The Elongated S-Pattern of the Backstroke Arm Pull

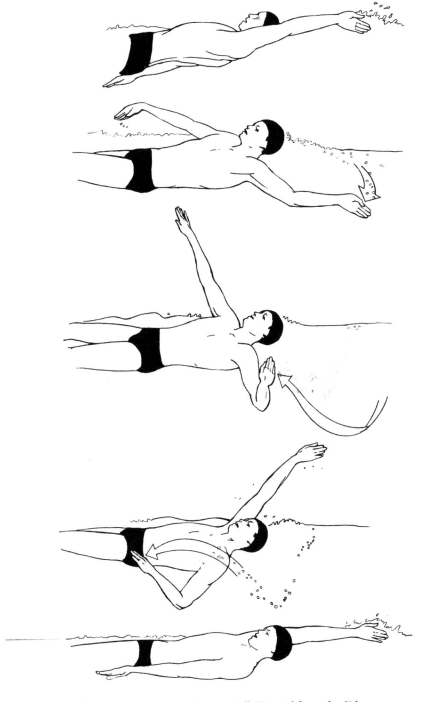

Figure 8.2. Phases of the Backstroke Arm Pull, Viewed from the Side

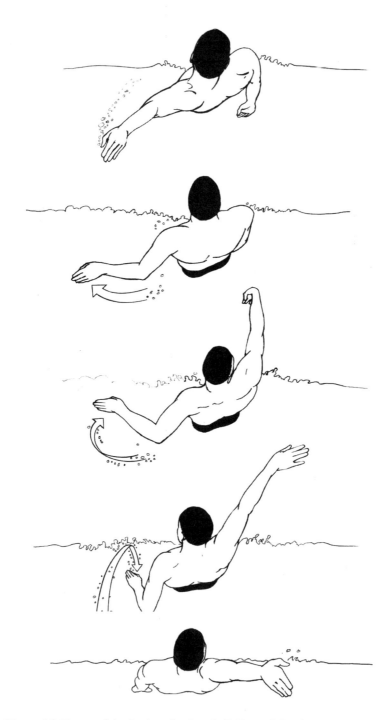

Figure 8.3. Phases of the Backstroke Arm Pull, Viewed Head-on

As in freestyle, a bent elbow and a natural body roll contribute greatly to the efficiency of the backstroke. Until the 1960s many swimmers used a straight-arm backstroke pull. However, simple mechanics, along with analyses of underwater films of world-class backstrokers, point unmistakably to the superiority of the bent-elbow technique. To demonstrate why this is so, Counsilman suggests you perform the following do-it-yourself test:

Put your feet in a tube, and float on your back with one arm at your side and the other overhead. Using the overhead arm, take several backstroke arm pulls holding your elbow straight. You will find you are pulling yourself around in a circle. Next, keeping the tube around your legs, swim a length of the pool, alternating arms but again keeping your elbows straight. You will find yourself moving in a wide zigzag pattern (much to the annoyance of the people trying to swim next to you). Now, repeat the two exercises using the bent-arm pull. You will find a tremendous reduction in your sideways motion. The bent-arm pull will propel you forward (rather than laterally) much more effectively.

To recap: your arm is extended back in a straight position directly above your shoulder; your right hand enters the water at eleven o'clock, little finger first and palm facing outward; as your arm follows your hand, it sinks a few inches before the pull begins.

Now, as you push your arm back, the bend in your elbow increases until it reaches ninety degrees at the midpoint of the stroke. From this point on, the bend gradually decreases until, at the end of the stroke, your arm is extended straight. At the very end of the S-shaped pull, your hand pushes downward. Figure 8.2 illustrates the phases of the arm pull as viewed from the side. Figure 8.3 depicts the same sequence, viewed head-on.

BODY ROLL

To do the bent-arm pull properly, your hips and shoulders must roll simultaneously about forty-five degrees to the side of the arm that is pulling, while your head remains in position. (A fun drill to help you achieve a stationary head position as your body rolls: place a quarter on your forehead, then swim backstroke, one length of the pool at a time. Try to complete each length without the quarter falling off your forehead.) The final downward thrust of the hand assists this rolling motion. Do not deliberately try to roll. If you do this stroke properly, your body will roll naturally.

The body roll is important because it permits the proper bend of the elbow, which in turn increases your arm's leverage for the pull. It also reduces drag by lifting your other shoulder out of the water during the recovery phase.

As you finish the arm stroke, your hand should turn so that your thumb leaves the water first, again to diminish resistance. During the recovery, keep your elbow absolutely straight, with your palm facing your body. Then, as you bring your arm directly over your shoulder, rotate your hand so the little finger can enter the water first. You are now ready to begin the next stroke.

The speed of your recovery arm should be equal to the speed of your pulling arm. As one arm is entering the water, the other should be exiting. By synchronizing your arms in this fashion, you will move forward in a continuous, flowing motion.

THE KICK

The backstroke kick is analogous to the flutter kick used in freestyle. But because you are swimming on your back, it is the *up*beat phase of the kick that provides most of your propulsive force. As in freestyle, the kick not only propels you forward but also stabilizes your body position.

The most efficient backstroke kick is the six-beat kick—six kicks of the legs for every complete cycle of the arms. During the upbeat

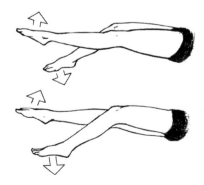

Figure 8.4. Phases of the Backstroke Kick

phase, your knee should be bent, with your toes turned slightly inward. During the downbeat, your knee should be kept straight. Figure 8.4 illustrates the phases of the backstroke kick.

The backstroke kick is quite natural and comes easily to most people. The most common mistake I have observed occurs when the knees are brought up toward the body and break the surface of the water. This results in a kind of bicycling motion—a very ineffective way to kick in the water, unless, of course, you are on a bicycle.

BREATHING

As mentioned earlier, breathing presents few problems in the backstroke, since your face is always out of the water. It is best, however, to establish a consistent breathing pattern: inhale and exhale once during each arm cycle. If you breathe haphazardly, you will tend to breathe too shallowly and start panting, especially as you become tired. This will only make matters worse.

I like to inhale as one arm reaches the highest point of its recovery and exhale as the other arm does the same. Other people inhale and exhale as each arm begins its recovery. It doesn't matter which pattern you adopt, so long as you are consistent.

PUTTING IT ALL TOGETHER

You have learned each part of the backstroke—the correct body position, the bent-arm S-shaped arm pull, the six-beat kick, and the proper way to breathe. Now you are ready to put it all together. The sequence of drawings in Figure 8.5 illustrates the proper way to do the backstroke.

THE FLIP TURN

Until recently, the backstroke flip turn was the most difficult turn to perform. But in 1991 changes were approved that made it both much easier and faster than before.

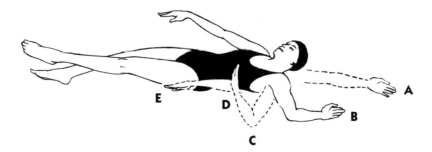

Figure 8.5. The Backstroke: Putting It All Together

A. The left arm has just entered the water at a point directly over the shoulder. The legs are kicked up and down in the flutter kick.

B. The left arm sinks downward as the pull begins and while the right arm starts its recovery directly upward.

C. The elbow of the pulling arm continues to bend as it is pulled backward. The recovering arm recovers directly upward.

D. The pulling arm pushes backward and downward, while the legs continue their flutter kick.

E. The pull ends with the palms pressing water toward the bottom of the pool, while the recovering arm enters the water in a line directly over the shoulder.

I must admit that, like many other Masters swimmers, I had trouble with the old backstroke flip turn. Because I didn't know precisely where I was, sometimes I would turn too close to and other times too far from the wall. I would always anticipate the turn with anxiety, usually slowing down as I approached it. In 200-yard races, I would often use the slower, open turn to avoid blowing the entire race on a poor turn.

All that is changed now. The new rules allow a swimmer to roll over onto his stomach and take one stroke just before the turn, which means he knows exactly how far from the wall he is; and they permit him to make the turn without touching the wall with his hand. Now I nail almost 100 percent of my turns, and I no longer hesitate as I approach the wall.

Sounds fine, you may be thinking. But how do I know when I'm approaching the wall if I'm not allowed to turn over and look until just before I make my turn? That's a fair question. The answer, as so many song lyrics tell us, lies up above.

Have you ever noticed the flags near the ends of most swimming pools? Called *backstroke flags,* they are placed at a precise distance from the end of the pool to signal backstroke swimmers that they are approaching the wall. In the standard twenty-five-yard pool, the flags are five yards from the end. In fifty-meter (and twenty-five-meter) pools, the flags are five *meters* from the end. (Five meters is about seventeen inches longer than five yards.)

Before learning the backstroke flip turn, swim a lap of backstroke and *count the strokes you take from the time the flags are directly overhead until you reach the wall*. Do it several times, just to be sure. I usually take three full strokes from the flags to the wall in a twenty-five-yard pool, three and a half in a fifty-meter pool. You may find that it takes you four, or perhaps five, strokes. Knowing how many strokes it takes from the flags to the wall is critical in performing the turn, as will be explained.

The backstroke flip turn is very similar to the freestyle flip turn described in Chapter 7. To do the turn, you must execute a complete somersault. But unlike in the freestyle turn, you do *not* twist your body, after the turn. The drawings in Figure 8.6 illustrate the phases of the backstroke flip turn.

As you pass under the flags, begin counting your strokes. Let's say you know it takes you four strokes to reach the wall. After completing your *third* stroke, roll over onto your stomach and, simultaneously, take another (freestyle) stroke. Keep both arms at your sides, palms facing downward, and do not kick while on your stomach.

As you roll over, you will be able to see where you are in relation to the wall. If you have timed your turn correctly, go immediately into your somersault. If you are still too far from the wall, let your momentum carry you closer before flipping. The somersault is the same as in the freestyle flip turn: duck your head and shoulders, add a little dolphin kick, and press down with your palms.

With your body in a tight tuck position and your arms still at your sides, complete the somersault by bringing your legs above the water.

You will now be on your back again. Plant your feet on the wall and push off with your legs. As you explode off the wall, bring your arms forward and streamline your body.

While you are gliding, begin kicking vigorously before coming to the surface. If you are very flexible, use a strong *reverse dolphin kick* while you are underwater, making sure you thrust from the hips. (The dolphin kick is described in detail in Chapter 10.) If you are only normally flexible, you may find it faster to use the backstroke flutter kick. Experiment to see which kick is more effective for *you*.

The rules permit you to swim up to fifteen meters underwater on your start and at each turn. But to do so requires a tremendously

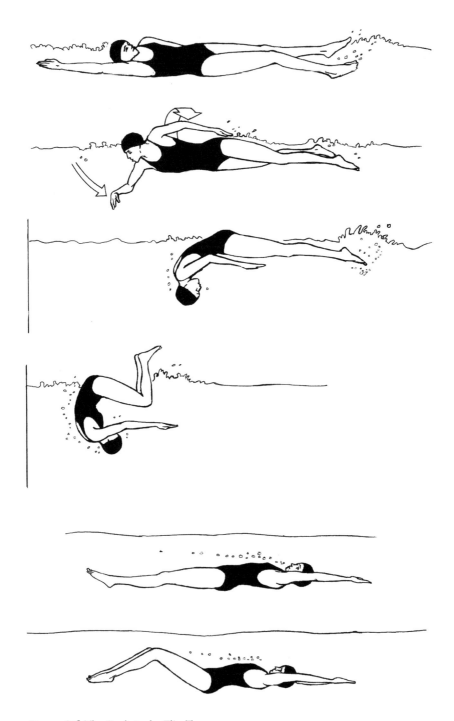

Figure 8.6. The Backstroke Flip Turn

large lung capacity. I recommend that you try three or four reverse dolphin kicks before your head pops to the surface and you begin stroking again. That should take you a good six or seven yards. If you find being underwater that long causes you to run out of air, try taking *fewer* kicks off the turns until you build up your lung capacity.

THE START

The backstroke is the only event that begins in the water rather than from a starting block (see Figure 8.7). Current rules require that your feet remain submerged during the start—you are not permitted to curl your toes over the edge of the pool.

Place your feet on the wall (or touch pad), with your toes just below the surface of the water. Then grip the bar of the starting block with your hands. When you hear the starter's command, "Take your mark," pull yourself up in a crouching position. Because it is tiring to hold this position, do not take this stance until you hear the command.

At the sound of the gun or horn, tilt your head back and swing your hands sideways in a circular motion. Push off the wall with your legs and arch your back slightly so you can clear the surface of the water.

As with the freestyle start, a clean entry is essential to maintain your momentum. Enter the water hands first, then upper torso, then legs, trying to have all your body parts go through the same hole. Holding a streamlined position, take several short, hard flutter kicks and come to the surface, ready to begin stroking.

You may want to try the faster Berkoff blastoff technique. If so, hold a streamlined position, with your arms extended behind your head. Then take several quick, shallow dolphin kicks before surfacing. Don't be discouraged if you have trouble learning this skill. It is tiring and requires a great deal of flexibility.

TEN BACKSTROKE TIPS

Try to keep the principles of efficient swimming outlined in Chapter 6 in mind as you practice the backstroke. In addition, the following ten tips will make learning the backstroke much easier.

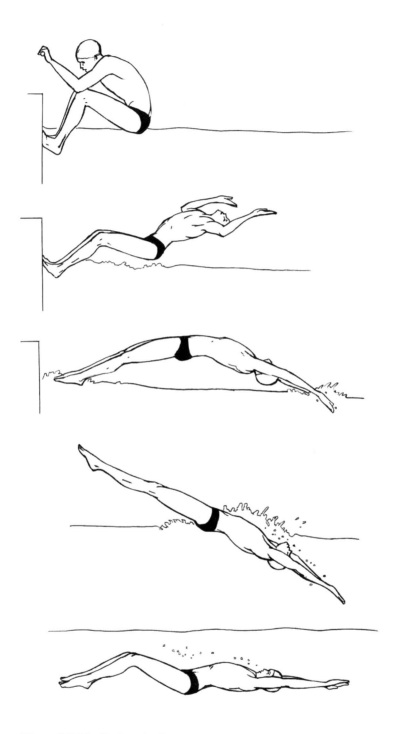

Figure 8.7. The Backstroke Start

The Backstroke

1. Adopt a streamlined position, with your hips just a few inches below the surface of the water.
2. Keep your head in almost straight alignment with your body, with the water line coming at the middle of your head just below your chin.
3. Remember that you propel yourself forward by pushing against still water. The best way to do this is by using an elongated **S**-shaped arm pull pattern (see Figure 8.1).
4. Your hands should enter the water, little finger first and palm outward, directly above your shoulders at one o'clock and eleven o'clock.
5. Although it may feel strange at first, keep your elbow bent throughout the pull to exert maximum power.
6. *Accelerate* your arm throughout the pull.
7. A natural body roll will increase the efficiency of your arm stroke.
8. Use a six-beat kick for every complete arm cycle. Bend your knee during the upbeat phase of the kick, and keep it straight during the downbeat.
9. Establish a consistent breathing pattern: inhale and exhale once during each complete arm cycle.
10. Before doing a backstroke flip turn, know how many strokes it takes you to swim from the backstroke flags to the wall.

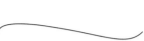

9

THE BREASTSTROKE

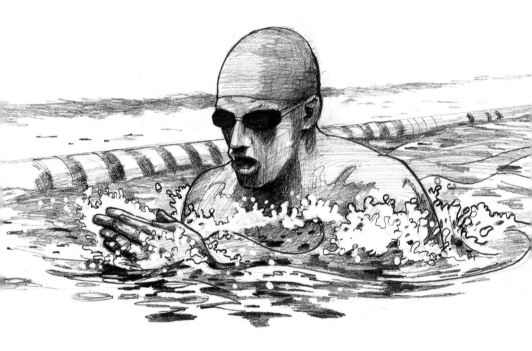

BREASTSTROKE IS THE enigmatic stroke. Regarded by novices as the easiest stroke, it is acknowledged by experts to be the most difficult. The breaststroke is used for relaxation by casual swimmers, but when swum competitively, it burns more calories than any other stroke, with the possible exception of the butterfly.

A BRIEF HISTORY

Breaststroke is both the oldest stroke and the newest one. Depictions of people swimming the breaststroke dating back thousands of years have been found on rock drawings, friezes, and pottery throughout the world.

This is the stroke sixteenth-century French author François Rabelais had his giants, Gargantua and Pantagruel, swim as part of their daily physical training program. And when he wasn't fomenting revolution, offering folksy advice, or flying his kite in the rain, it was the stroke utilized by Benjamin Franklin, one of the top swimmers of his day, in his frequent aquatic forays across the Thames.

Few people today realize that when Matthew Webb became the first person to conquer the English Channel in 1875, he used the breaststroke. The overarm stroke, which was just making its way into European consciousness, was deemed inelegant and certainly not suitable for proper gentlemen and ladies. In the past seventy years, however, only one swimmer, a German, has used the breaststroke to swim the channel. Of all the competitive strokes, it is both the *least* efficient and the slowest. When swum correctly, though, it can be surprisingly fast.

Since the breast and the butterfly became distinct strokes in the mid-1950s, the breaststroke has undergone more change by far than any other stroke. The past thirty years have seen coaches emphasize a wide variety of styles of arm pull, recovery, leg kick, head and body position, and timing.

Should the arm pull be wide, long, and narrow, or short and resemble a sculling motion? During the arm recovery, should the palms face outward, inward, or upward in a prayerlike position? Should the kick be wide or narrow? Should the body ride high or low in the water? Can the head dip below the surface of the water or not? Should the body remain flat throughout the stroke, or should it undulate in a dolphinlike movement? At what point should the swimmer breathe? When in the stroke cycle should she kick? In recent years, sophisticated biomechanical studies have answered many of these questions definitively. In other cases, technique still seems to be a matter of individual choice. This chapter will present the most up-to-date thinking on how to swim the breaststroke efficiently, indicating where variations appear to remain a matter of choice or comfort.

To complicate matters, top competitors have achieved success in the breaststroke using two basic styles—the conventional, American-style breaststroke and the undulating or dolphin breaststroke. In the late 1980s, still another style—the wave-action breaststroke—was developed by Hungarian coach Jozsef Nagy.

In addition, there have been a number of successful variations on the two basic styles. This is not the case with the other strokes. For example, the leg kick is more important in breast than in the other strokes, so some swimmers with especially strong legs emphasize the sweeping action of the breaststroke kick, known as the *whip kick*. Other swimmers rely more on a powerful arm stroke. To find the style with which you are most comfortable will require some experimentation.

All the successful variations, however, are based on a general style that was first used in the early 1960s. The man credited with creating the modern breaststroke is Indiana University's Chet Jastremski, coached by the legendary Doc Counsilman. In 1961 Jastremski introduced a radical new style, which featured a rapid, continuous turnover of the arms. He also changed the kick forever, doing away with the wide frog kick and substituting a narrower whip kick. This eliminated the glide that had previously characterized the breaststroke.

The results of these changes were electrifying. Jastremski became the first swimmer to crack the one-minute barrier for the 100-yard breaststroke. At the national championships that summer, he devastated the world records in the stroke, slicing four seconds from the 100-meter mark and carving over seven seconds off the 200-meter standard. By the 1964 Olympics, however, the rest of the world had caught up to Jastremski, and he was only able to win the bronze medal in the 200-meter event.

Although the breaststroke can be swum successfully using a variety of styles, this chapter will emphasize the basic principles that apply to effective swimming of the stroke no matter which variation you employ. As you learn the breaststroke, try to incorporate these principles into the style you adopt.

THE ENIGMATIC STROKE

Fitness experts claim that swimming the breaststroke burns fewer calories than the other strokes, but studies of competitive swimmers show that when done correctly it burns *more* calories than the rest—

with the possible exception of butterfly. Why? Because unlike in the other strokes, in the breast there is no easy over-the-water arm recovery to allow the swimmer a brief rest. Thus, he is constantly overcoming resistance.

In the United States, Canada, and Australia, youngsters are introduced first to the crawl stroke, or freestyle. In Europe, however, the breaststroke is the first stroke taught. Consequently, Europeans—primarily Russians, Hungarians, and Germans—have traditionally reigned supreme in breaststroke competition.

Natural Breaststrokers

Many swimmers and coaches believe that breaststroke is unlike the other strokes in that there are "born" breaststrokers. If you are not a natural breaststroker, you will have difficulty with the stroke. You may learn to swim it competently, but you will never achieve the grace and speed of a born breaststroker. Strangely, people who are natural breaststrokers often have difficulty with the other strokes. Likewise, many swimmers who are outstanding in the three other competitive strokes struggle with the breaststroke. For this reason, more often than not the breaststroke is the key to the individual medley race, in which a swimmer swims each of the four strokes.

How I Became a Breaststroke Swimmer

I am one of the lucky ones, a natural breaststroker. In 1957, as a thirteen-year-old freshman, I went out for my high school team, the Livermore (California) Cowboys. Swimming was the major spring sport at Livermore High, and the Cowboys were the perennial league champions. The stands were always packed for our home meets. All the best-looking girls were there. Ever since I could remember, I had been the best swimmer among my peers. This, I decided, was where I would make my mark: high school stud swimmer. It came as a shock when I was cut from the junior varsity squad after only a few days' practice.

Two years later I was bigger, stronger, and a cocky upperclassman. I decided to give it another go. This time I would not fail. On the first day of tryouts I slipped on my green Cowboy swimsuit and dove into the pool. "All right, you scrubs," barked Don Couch, the coach and my history teacher, "let's warm up with thirty-two laps freestyle." No problem, I thought to myself. I took off. After five laps, my arms were growing numb and my legs were begging for oxygen. I was exhausted, but I still had twenty-seven laps to go! And that was just the warm-up! I was doomed. In desperation, I switched to the only stroke I knew that would keep me afloat and moving, a sort of proto-breaststroke.

Having adopted this face-saving strategy, I tried to remain inconspicuous, but to no avail. I looked up, and there was Coach Couch hovering menacingly above me. "Whitten," he commanded, "get out of the pool." This is it, I told myself. I was busted, humiliated, cut before the end of the warm-up on the first day of tryouts.

I hauled myself out of the water and waited for the inevitable. "Whitten," he intoned from afar, "you're never going to be a freestyler, but you have a pretty good natural breaststroke kick. With some work, I think you have a chance to make the varsity in the breaststroke." I couldn't believe my ears. Expecting the coup de grace, I had been granted a reprieve.

So just like that I became a breaststroker. It wasn't easy that year. Mike Stocks was our top breaststroker. A senior, he was the league champion and record holder and had placed fifth at the state sectional meet the year before. Our number-two guy, Peter Becker, was no slouch either. A junior like me, he had finished third at the league championships as a sophomore. But I didn't care. I was on the team.

Coach Couch was right; I *was* a natural breaststroker. I worked hard and kept improving. Midway through our undefeated season, I had passed Peter and become the team's number-two breaststroker. At the league championships, I finished second behind Mike.

After the championships we had one dual meet left, against a team from another league. It was a sentimental occasion, Mike's last high school meet. He had decided he would work in his family's garage and not go on to college.

The final race of Mike's high school career was the 100-meter breaststroke. The gun went off, and we dove in. As we turned at the halfway mark I noticed, to my astonishment, that Mike and I were even. How could this be? We battled stroke for stroke until the final ten meters. Then I began to pull away. I reached for the wall. I won! My first breaststroke win ever! Not only that, but I had broken Mike's school and pool record. I couldn't believe it, the crowd couldn't believe it, the coach couldn't believe it, and Mike couldn't believe it. But he was gracious and congratulated me on my win and new record.

I kept on practicing. Spring turned to summer, then fall, then winter. Every day would find me in the pool. I continued to improve. By the next spring I was one of the top high school breaststroke swimmers in the nation. I went on to earn All-America honors, then set two national Junior Olympic records and several other national age-group records. I was sought after by several colleges and the next year was named to the U.S. national team. Although the breaststroke came naturally for me, I also learned to swim the other strokes fairly well—all, that is, except the backstroke. That achievement would be delayed until I was well into my Masters career.

For natural breaststrokers, the stroke is injury free. I have been swimming the stroke for thirty-five years, on average about five days a week, and I have never experienced problems. But because the stroke requires quite a bit of ankle and knee flexibility, some people may suffer knee strain. For this reason it is a good idea to begin swimming breaststroke gradually.

In breaststroke, timing is everything. Once you have mastered the rhythm of the arms, legs, and breathing, the stroke will flow almost effortlessly and you will feel as if you and the water are one. But first you need to learn the separate skills that compose the stroke. The following sections will discuss each phase of the breaststroke: body position, breathing technique, arm pull, and leg kick. Practice each phase separately until you have mastered it, always keeping in mind that it is part of a larger whole. Finally we will put it all together. With practice and some coaching, you will feel the rhythm of the stroke as you glide gracefully through the water.

BODY POSITION AND BREATHING

In the *conventional breaststroke,* your body lies flat on the surface of the water in a streamlined position. You begin and end each stroke cycle with your arms and legs extended, and the water at about your hairline. Your hips remain at or near the surface throughout the stroke, with your shoulders rising only slightly out of the water at the highest point of the stroke. As will be shown later, both hips and shoulders undulate slightly during the stroke cycle (see Figure 9.1).

In breaststroke, unlike the other strokes, breathing assists proper timing, so *remember to breathe on every stroke.* As your hands begin to separate, your head naturally starts up. When your arms are

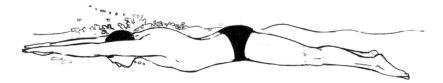

Figure 9.1. Body Position in the Conventional Breaststroke

sweeping inward and your head and shoulders are at their highest point, inhale with your chin just above the water surface (see Figure 9.2). Then, with your face in the water, exhale smoothly as your hands glide forward.

Until recently, breaststroke rules required a swimmer to keep his head above the water surface throughout the stroke. But current rules specify only that the head must break the surface of the water during some part of each cycle. This allows the swimmer to duck his head under the water, permitting a greater dolphinlike undulation and hence greater speed.

The *dolphin breaststroke* has been used by East European swimmers since the early 1970s. In the West, its use was pioneered by Britain's 1976 Olympic champion, David Wilkie, and by American Tracy Caulkins. Though more difficult than the conventional style, the dolphin breaststroke is probably more efficient. In this style, your body position changes during each phase of the stroke.

To swim the dolphin breaststroke, lower your hips and bring your shoulders upward, forward, and well out of the water as you sweep

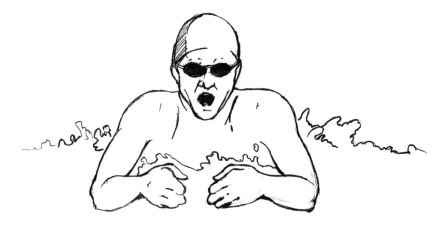

Figure 9.2. Breathing During the Breaststroke

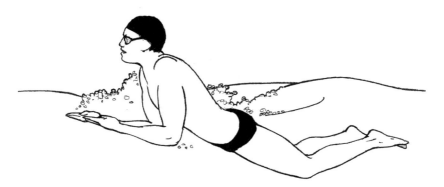

Figure 9.3. Body Position in the Dolphin Breaststroke

your arms inward. Breathe just as you complete the in sweep. Then return your head to the water as your arms extend forward in the recovery (see Figure 9.3).

ARM PULL

In the breaststroke, both arms pull simultaneously under the water in a heart-shaped pattern, *the elbows always remaining high* (see Figure 9.4).

The arm stroke consists of five phases:

1. a wide outward sweep
2. the catch
3. a downward sweep
4. an inward sweep, followed immediately by
5. the recovery

In the next few pages I will describe each of these phases. But remember that the arm pull and the recovery are one continuous motion, and that your hands should *accelerate* as they sweep outward until they come together under your chin, then slide gently forward.

What follows may seem complicated, but it really is not. Canadian coach Paul Bergen describes the breaststroke arm stroke as "like wiping the inside of two big bowls." Keep that overall description in mind as I detail each phase of the stroke.

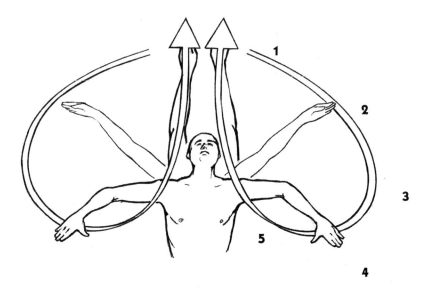

Figure 9.4. The Heart-shaped Pattern of the Breaststroke Arm Pull

The Out Sweep

Begin the stroke with your body in a streamlined position and your arms stretched forward about six inches below the surface of the water. Your elbows are extended. By flexing your wrists turn your palms out and back at about a forty-five-degree angle.

The Catch

As your hands sweep outward just past your shoulder width, you can feel them grab or "catch" the water. At this point, your hands, about two inches below the surface, gradually change pitch, from out and back to out, *down,* and back. Your thumbs are now pointing down. This change lifts your upper body high in the water and allows your head and body to surge over your arms.

The Down Sweep

After the catch is made, you begin the down sweep. Sweep your hands down and out in a circular path, remembering to accelerate throughout. Your elbows should remain high. Think of them as two shafts, with your hands rotating around them like propellers.

The In Sweep

The in sweep produces much of the lift and arm propulsion in the breaststroke. After your hands reach their deepest point, they continue their circular motion, sweeping inward as they rotate around your elbows. Still accelerating, your hands sweep first down and in, and then in, up, and back. During the down sweep and in sweep, the pitch of your hands gradually changes from out and down to in and up. Your elbows follow your hands down, in, and up until you finish the in sweep by squeezing them in under your chin.

The Recovery

When your hands are nearly together under your chin, begin the final stage of the stroke, the recovery. As you release the pressure your hands are exerting on the water, slide your hands smoothly forward together, remembering always to keep them streamlined. At this point your palms should be facing either upward or inward. I prefer to have them face upward. This position helps me bring my elbows within the plane of my shoulders. You might want to try both positions and choose the one that feels more natural to you.

When your arms move forward, the pitch of your hands will change quickly from upward (or inward) to downward. Finally, your arms are fully extended, about six inches below the surface of the water, and you are ready for the next stroke.

As mentioned earlier, it sounds complicated, but it's not. Practice each phase, then put them all together in a single rhythm:

out, down, in, recover
out, down, in, recover
out, down, in, recover

Figure 9.5 illustrates the complete sequence of the breaststroke arm pull, as seen from the front.

In teaching the breaststroke arm pull, I have found two common errors: (1) people pull their arms back too far during the down sweep; and (2) they hesitate as they lift their heads to breathe at the completion of the in sweep.

The arms should be pulled back only to a point at which they are parallel with the chin. If you pull them back too far, you will sink in

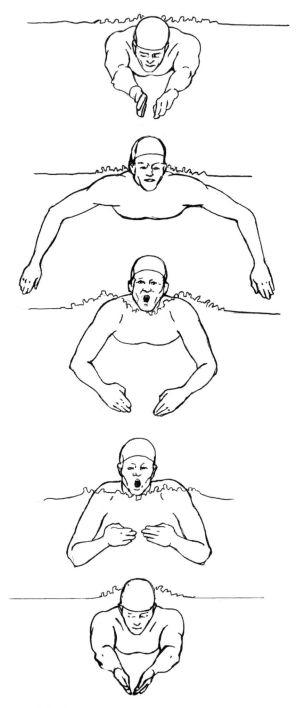

Figure 9.5. Phases of the Breaststroke Arm Pull, Viewed from the Front

the water and thus encounter increased resistance during the recovery. Similarly, there should be no hesitation in the arm pull. If you hesitate as you breathe, you will lose much of your forward momentum. (If you want to glide, you can do so as your arms shoot forward during the recovery.)

THE KICK

In the breaststroke kick, you first raise your heels toward your buttocks. Reach out with your feet as far as you can. Then, with your toes pointing out, kick back and together at the same time (see Figure 9.6).

Before Doc Counsilman revolutionized the breaststroke in 1960, most breaststrokers used the wedge, or frog kick. Here, the feet acted like paddles in a rowboat. The swimmer first swept his legs outward in an inverted **V**, then squeezed them together.

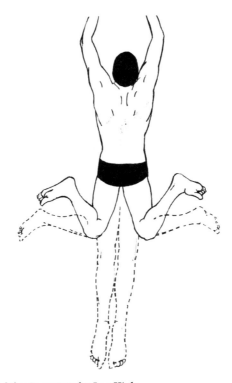

Figure 9.6. Pattern of the Breaststroke Leg Kick

Today all breaststrokers use the *whip kick*. With this technique you rotate your feet outward, downward, and then inward in a circular path. The whip kick is far more efficient and powerful than the frog kick because you use your feet more like the propeller blades of a motorboat than like paddles.

The whip kick consists of a recovery, an out sweep, down sweep, in sweep, and glide. There is no hesitation between these phases, and it is easiest to describe them as one continuous motion.

Begin your kick with your legs outstretched and your toes pointed. Then bend your knees and raise your feet toward your buttocks. Do

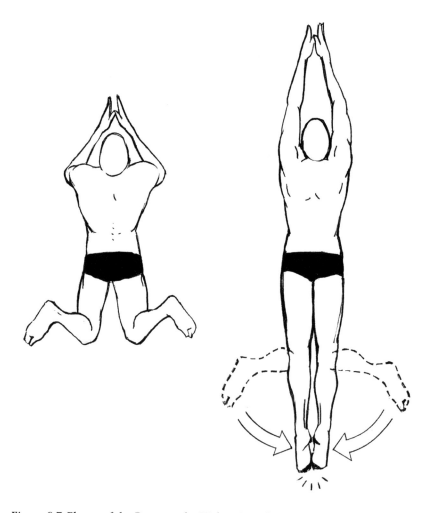

Figure 9.7. Phases of the Breaststroke Kick as Seen from Behind

not draw your knees up under your body. This is the most common error people make while learning the whip kick, and it creates a tremendous amount of resistance.

As your feet come up, your knees will separate until they are about shoulder width apart. When your heels are above your buttocks, point your toes outward. (This may feel awkward at first, but your muscles and tendons will eventually get used to the position.)

Immediately whip your legs down, back, and around in a circle until they are completely extended. This motion constitutes the propulsive phases of the kick. Figure 9.7 illustrates the phases of the breaststroke kick.

There are three important things to keep in mind as you are kicking: (1) Try to emphasize the *downward,* rather than the backward movement of your feet. This will increase your propulsive force and raise your hips in a dolphinlike motion. (2) Keep your toes pointed outward throughout the circle. (3) Just as you do with the arm stroke, remember to *accelerate* throughout the propulsive phases of the kick.

You have completed the kick when your feet come together. At this point, remember to streamline your body: straighten your knees, point your toes, and bring your feet up to the level of your hips.

PUTTING IT ALL TOGETHER

As mentioned earlier, even more than in the other strokes, the key to a fluid, efficient breaststroke is *rhythm*—the correct timing of the arms, legs, and breathing. When you've got the rhythm, each phase of the stroke will move in glorious synchronicity with every other phase. If you do not have the rhythm, the stroke will seem awkward and feel herky-jerky.

I believe the easiest way to learn the breaststroke is to take it in the following order:

1. Learn the whip kick.
2. Learn the arm stroke.
3. Learn the timing of the breathing.

When you are comfortable with each of these skills, you are ready to put it all together. The proper timing of the breaststroke is illustrated in the drawings in Figure 9.8.

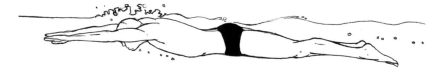

Figure 9.8. The Breaststroke: Putting It All Together
A. Begin with your arms and legs fully extended, your feet together, and your body fully streamlined.

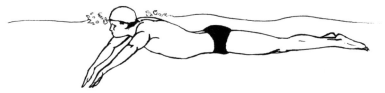

B. Begin the out sweep of the arms while your legs remain extended.

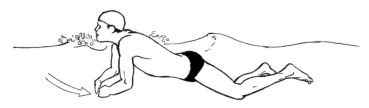

C. As your hands complete the in sweep, lift your chin upward and forward to breathe. At the same time, bring your feet up toward your buttocks.

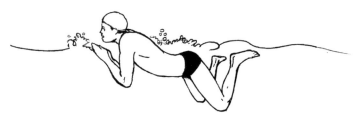

D. When your hands begin to glide forward in the recovery, whip your feet down, back, and around in a circle. Lower your chin into the water and exhale.

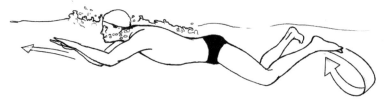

E. As your arms reach their full extension, your feet come together and your body is in a fully streamlined position.

THE TURN

Although flip turns are not permitted in breaststroke, the breaststroke turn is very important in competition. A good breaststroker can travel ten yards or more on each turn before taking her first stroke. In a twenty-five-yard pool, that amounts to almost half the distance of the race, so it is essential to learn to do the turn correctly. The sequence of drawings in Figure 9.9 illustrates the phases of the breaststroke turn.

Try to time your turn so that you approach the wall during the recovery phase of your stroke. Your body is stretched out in a streamlined position, your head is low in the water, and your eyes are fixed on the wall. Then, *while your body remains horizontal, touch the wall simultaneously with both hands.* This is very important in a race. If you dip your shoulder before touching the wall, or if you touch with one hand before the other, you will be disqualified.

As soon as you touch the wall, drop your lead arm. You will probably find you are more comfortable dropping the same arm for all your turns; I always drop my right. As you tilt your upper body away from the wall, your momentum carries your feet to the wall, preparing them for the push off.

Plant your feet *sideways* on the wall, and take a deep breath. Throughout the change in direction, keep your body low in the water, your head just above the surface. Many novices try to lift their bodies well out of the water, an entirely wasted motion.

With your body still tilted, release contact with your arm and submerge your head. Push hard off the wall, and immediately extend your body into a streamlined position. Your head should be slightly lower than your feet.

Breaststroke rules permit a swimmer to take one complete pull and kick underwater after the start of a race and after each turn. Because the breaststroke is faster under the water than on top, you should master the technique of the *pull out,* the last phase of the breaststroke turn.

After you have pushed off the wall, turn your palms outward and glide until you feel on the verge of slowing down. Then pull your arms down to your thighs, using a keyhole pattern, and you will surge forward.

Glide again until you feel yourself about to lose momentum. Then, as you simultaneously kick hard and bring your arms forward in a streamlined position, point your body toward the surface. As your head breaks the surface, you are ready to take your first stroke.

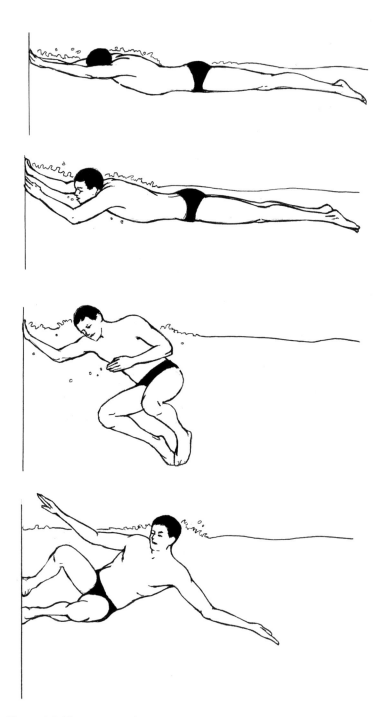

Figure 9.9. The Breaststroke Turn

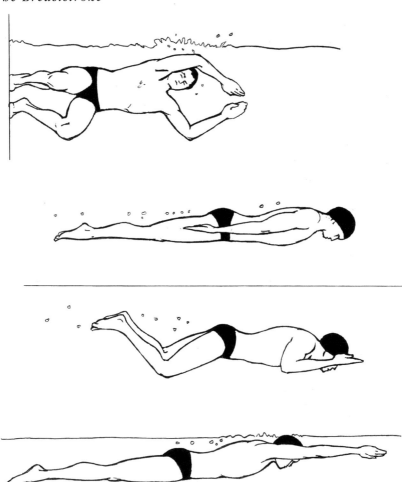

The timing of the pull-out phase of the breaststroke turn takes practice. Although I have been swimming the stroke for over thirty-five years, I still count to myself on every turn. It goes like this:

PUSH OFF "One, two, three . . ."
PULL DOWN "One, two, three . . ."
KICK. SURFACE.

If you do the turn properly, you should be underwater for about four to six seconds. Because you are swimming hard between turns, you will need to be able to hold your breath that long without going into oxygen debt, especially at the end of a 200-yard race. The best way to build your lung capacity is to practice the breaststroke turn properly every time you swim. During practice, you may find yourself tempted to cut the pull out short. Resist! In the long run, you will find that doing proper breaststroke turns will enhance your lung capacity well beyond what you thought possible.

THE START

The breaststroke start is performed almost exactly like the freestyle start (see Chapter 7). The only difference comes *after* you enter the water. Because in the breaststroke you are allowed to take a complete pull and kick under the water, let yourself dive a little deeper than you do in the freestyle.

The rest of the sequence is exactly like the breaststroke turn: glide, then pull down, using a keyhole pattern. Glide again. Then bring your arms forward as you kick, angling toward the surface. As your head breaks the surface, you are ready to take your first stroke. If you do this properly, you will travel more than half the length of the pool before taking your first stroke on the surface.

TEN BREASTSTROKE TIPS

The basic principles of efficient swimming that you learned in Chapter 6 apply equally to the breaststroke. However, the following ten tips will be helpful to keep in mind as you learn the breast.

1. Breathe on every stroke. In breaststroke, unlike the other strokes, breathing assists the timing.
2. Keep your elbows high throughout the arm stroke.
3. The arm stroke is basically a sculling motion. Many people pull back too far. Pull back only as far as your shoulders, so that your hands come together under your chin in the in sweep.
4. *Accelerate* your arms throughout the stroke cycle. Most beginners slow down or stop their hands as they come together in the in sweep.

5. There is no hesitation in the arm stroke at all. Glide only when your arms shoot forward during the recovery.
6. When beginning your kick, raise your heels toward your buttocks. Do *not* bring your knees under your chest.
7. *Accelerate* your feet with a strong whipping action throughout the kick, until your ankles come together and your legs are fully extended.
8. Breath at the proper time: just as your arms complete the in sweep.
9. Make sure to streamline your body between strokes.
10. Always practice the *complete* breaststroke turn during your workouts.

A FINAL NOTE: THE "WAVE-ACTION" BREASTSTROKE

When you watch the Olympics, the world championships, or the NCAA finals, you will notice that most of the swimmers are using a breaststroke technique slightly different from that just described. The new "wave-action" breaststroke was developed in the mid-1980s by Hungarian coach Jozsef Nagy and first used successfully by his student Jozsef Szabo to win the 200-meter breaststroke at both the 1987 world championships and the 1988 Olympics. Since 1989 American Mike Barrowman, another Nagy protégé, has used the technique to win world and Olympic titles and has repeatedly lowered the world record.

The wave-action technique builds on the body position in the dolphin breaststroke. In the dolphin breaststroke, the shoulders and

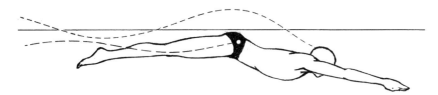

Figure 9.10. The Dynamics of the Wave-Action Breaststroke. The shoulders remain above the water through most of the stroke, leading to an above-water motion of the back. The buttocks make a much flatter wave than do the shoulders.

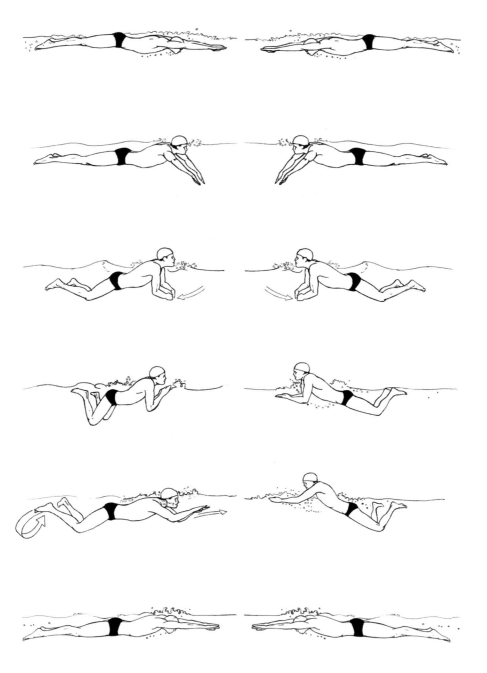

Figure 9.11. A Comparison of the Conventional (left) and Wave-Action (right) Breaststrokes.

upper body come well out of the water at the end of the in sweep. At this point, a wave-action breaststroker generally recovers by thrusting his arms *over the water*. His body follows in an exaggerated dolphin or wavelike motion. Figure 9.10 illustrates the wave-action technique.

The major differences between the conventional breaststroke and the wave-action breaststroke are these: in the conventional style, the swimmer remains horizontal during the leg recovery. His shoulders are underwater, and his hips stay near the surface. In contrast, the wave-action breaststroker brings his shoulders out of the water, keeping his hips down and his body inclined from shoulders to knees. In all other phases of the stroke, the body position is basically the same for both styles. Figure 9.11 compares the conventional breaststroke with the wave-action style.

The wave-action breaststroke requires both a tremendous amount of flexibility and upper-body strength. It is definitely not for beginners.

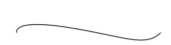

10

THE BUTTERFLY

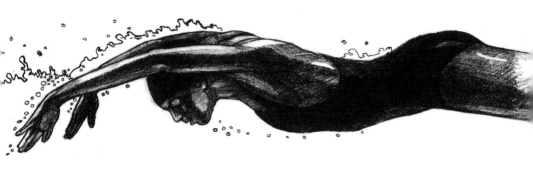

THE BUTTERFLY IS perhaps the most spectacular swimming stroke—powerful, dramatic, graceful, sinuous, and very fast. In fact, although the butterfly almost certainly will never surpass the freestyle in speed, the current world records for the stroke are about as fast as the freestyle records were only twenty-five years ago.

The fly, as it is popularly known, is swum with an undulating body movement. Both arms are brought forward together over the water, then brought back simultaneously and symmetrically. For every arm stroke, there are two kicks, with the legs moving up and down simultaneously in the dolphin kick.

A BRIEF HISTORY

Unlike the other strokes, whose origins go back hundreds and even thousands of years, the butterfly is a creation of the twentieth century. There is some controversy over who deserves the title of father of the butterfly—several American, German, and British swimmers of half a century ago appear to have valid claims.

The butterfly was conceived about 1930, when breaststroke swimmers Erich Rademacher of Germany and Henry Myers of the United States realized there was nothing in the rules to prevent them from recovering their arms over instead of under the water. They combined this over-the-water arm recovery with the breaststroke kick and soon discovered that, though it was tiring, they could go faster with it than they could with the conventional breaststroke—at least for short distances. The new technique caught on quickly and by the 1940s threatened the breaststroke with extinction.

Shortly after Myers popularized the new arm stroke, Coach Dave Armbruster of the University of Iowa began having his swimmers experiment with a novel leg action—the fishtail, or dolphin kick. One kick per stroke. Although it was illegal in competition, Armbruster found it was even faster than the new butterfly-breaststroke. Coincidentally, Jack Hale—whose remarkable international swimming career spanned the 1930s, '40s, and '50s and who now is one of England's top Masters swimmers—was experimenting with the same kick at the time.

By the early fifties many breaststroke swimmers were trying to find ways to incorporate the faster dolphin motion into the end of their kick. But how to do so legally? Under the rules, a swimmer was not allowed to break the horizontal plane with his feet. Adding a dolphin motion at the end of the breaststroke kick clearly broke the horizontal plane.

The issue finally came to a head at the 1952 Olympics in Helsinki. As the competitors filed past the spectators for the 200-meter breaststroke final, all eyes were on the world-record holder, Germany's Herbert Klein. The sentimental favorite, Klein was a German Jew who had somehow survived the horrors of a Nazi concentration camp and was now reaching for Olympic glory.

A tall, muscular man in his late twenties, Klein stood on the starting block, all concentration, the blue number tattooed on his arm a poignant symbol of the painful obstacles he had had to overcome. The gun went off. As the race progressed, it was obvious that most of the competitors were using some version of the dolphin kick. But Klein was doing so most conspicuously. "Clunk, clunk, clunk, clunk." With each stroke Klein's feet made a heavy "clunk" sound as they broke the surface of the water.

Klein finished third. Despite his illegal kick, the judges refused to disqualify him or any of the other competitors.

After the Olympics, the pressure to legitimize the dolphin technique became so great that the butterfly and breaststroke were officially designated as distinct strokes. The breaststroke was redefined to permit only an underwater arm recovery (although this was modified in 1989). The new butterfly technique called for an over-the-water arm recovery combined with an up-and-down leg action. The only similarities remaining between the two strokes were that both prohibited swimming under the water and both called for simultaneous movements of the arms and legs. The separation was now complete; the modern butterfly had been born.

At about the time Klein was making waves in Helsinki, the final stage in the development of the butterfly was unfolding 3,000 miles away. One warm autumn day in 1952, a muscular sixteen-year-old freshman decided to try out for the Springfield (Massachusetts) College swim team. It was a decision that would eventually land him in swimming's International Hall of Fame. William Yorzyk had been a nonswimmer throughout high school, but Coach "Red" Silvia quickly sized the boy up as a potential champion. Under Silvia's tutelage, Yorzyk began experimenting with a "double-dolphin" kick—*two* kicks for each arm cycle. It worked.

At the U.S. national championships in 1956, Yorzyk burst upon the international swimming scene with his double-dolphin, setting four world records. He went on to win a gold medal at the Melbourne Olympics that summer, outstroking the field in the 200-meter butterfly by an incredible four seconds. Dr. Bill Yorzyk is now in his early sixties. A teammate of mine in the New England Masters Swim Club, he can still swim the butterfly in times many collegians would envy. Among his peers, he remains far and away the fastest flyer in the world.

BODY POSITION

Performed correctly, the butterfly is a thing of beauty, a marvel of human skill, strength, and coordination. However, for many people it is also the most difficult stroke to learn, as well as the most fatiguing. For this reason, even more than with the other strokes it is essential that you remain streamlined as you master each of the techniques that make up the butterfly.

In swimming the fly, your body should lie as flat on the surface of the water as possible. You must remember to hold your hips high, no deeper than a few inches below the surface. Your hips will sink if your kick is too deep, if you raise your head too high to breathe, or if you push the water down during the arm pull. As soon as your hips begin to sink, your legs will follow. As your body moves toward a vertical position, the amount of drag increases, and the butterfly quickly becomes almost impossible to perform.

You should not try deliberately to achieve the undulating body movement so characteristic of the butterfly. This rhythmic motion is a result of the dolphin kick and the recovery and stroking action of the arms. If your stroke and kick are done correctly, the undulation will follow naturally.

ARM PULL

The butterfly arm pull is similar to that of the freestyle. The major difference, of course, is that in the fly both arms pull simultaneously. This means that compared with your freestyle pull, your butterfly pull will be shallower simply because you cannot roll your shoulders when both arms are pulling at the same time. (This lack of body roll is the chief reason the fly is unlikely ever to be faster than the crawl stroke.)

One of the most common mistakes people make in swimming the fly is trying to push the water straight back. It is tempting to do this, because it seems it would be the most effective way to propel yourself forward. Not so; as in all the strokes, you must always strive to push against *still* water. The most efficient way to do this in the butterfly is to have your hands describe an imaginary keyhole or hourglass pattern (see Figure 10.1).

Begin the stroke as your arms enter the water just wide of your shoulders, with your hands facing outward at about a forty-five-degree angle. Your arms are almost totally extended, with your elbows slightly higher than your hands so you can "catch" the water after the entry.

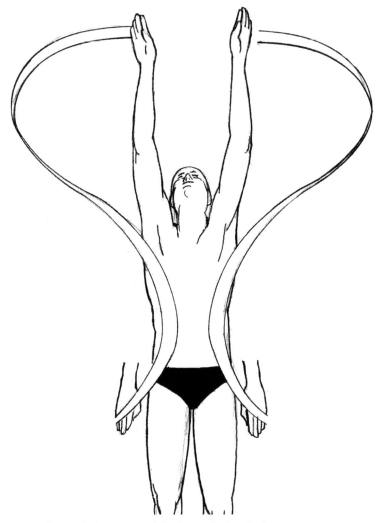

Figure 10.1. The Keyhole Pattern of the Butterfly Arm Pull

Once you have caught the water, begin the pull—first outward, then down and back—and start to bend your elbows. As your hands sweep around the top of the "keyhole" and then toward each other, the elbow bend increases. It reaches a maximum of about ninety degrees when your hands come to within six inches of each other. During this time your palms gradually change position until they are facing slightly inward.

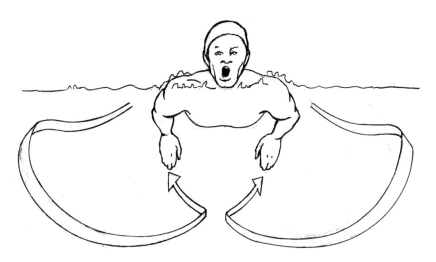

Figure 10.2. Phases of the Butterfly Arm Stroke, Viewed from the Front

In the final phase of the stroke, your hands thrust almost straight backward past the hips. As you complete the arm stroke, the bend in your elbows decreases gradually and your palms face backward. Figure 10.2 illustrates the complete sequence of the butterfly arm stroke as seen from the front.

The final arm thrust (along with the second dolphin kick) should help drive your shoulders and upper arms out of the water, leaving only your wrists and hands under the surface. You are now ready for the overwater arm recovery.

The butterfly arm recovery is a rounding-out motion. Unlike the freestyle recovery, in which the elbows are held high, the fly recovery is executed with the elbows barely clearing the surface. This helps maintain a flat body position while minimizing the energy needed to lift both arms at the same time.

In performing the butterfly recovery, your arms should remain loose and relaxed. Allow the momentum generated by the underwater pull to carry your arms out of the water and forward, in a low, semicircular sweep. As you complete the recovery, your elbows become almost fully extended and your palms face down.

You've done it, by Jove, you've done it. Your first full butterfly stroke! And just like Pablo Morales (well, almost). Now you're ready for the next stroke, and the next, and the next.

THE KICK

The *dolphin kick* consists of an up-and-down kicking motion by both legs simultaneously. The leg action is basically similar to that of the flutter kick. But because both legs move together, the hips are able to play a much more prominent role in propulsion. This characteristic makes the dolphin kick the fastest and most efficient of all kicks.

In performing the dolphin kick, spread your feet slightly and keep your ankles extended but relaxed. Foot and ankle flexibility is important in maintaining the fluid action of the kick.

The kick itself consists basically of a downbeat and an upbeat. In the downbeat, you bend your knees slightly, and your hips rise just as your knees reach their full extension. In the upbeat, you straighten your knees out. Figure 10.3 illustrates the phases of the dolphin kick.

Perhaps the most common mistake novice swimmers make in learning the dolphin kick is bending the knees excessively during the upbeat. This usually happens because of holding the feet and ankles too stiff. The result is a static action, which slows the stroke down and makes the arm stroke difficult. The solution is simple: allow your feet and ankles to relax, and go with the flow of your body.

Learning the Dolphin Kick

According to experts like Cecil Colwin, a top Canadian swim coach, the easiest way to learn the dolphin kick is to practice it using a kick

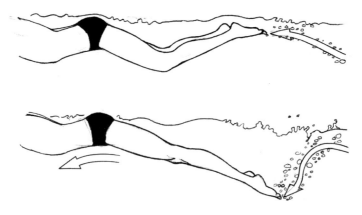

Figure 10.3. Phases of the Dolphin Kick

board. Hold the board out in front of you, with your hands about one third of the way along its length. Keep your hands together, relaxed, with your palms facing down.

As you begin to kick, remember *not* to push down on the board. Keep your shoulders low and your hips high. This position will permit your body to undulate naturally with the kick. Try to avoid excessive up-and-down movements of your shoulders and back. If you find yourself bobbing, hold your back straight and concentrate on kicking from the hips.

Once you have the kick down pat, you are ready to learn to coordinate it with the arm stroke.

Timing

In the modern butterfly, there are two dolphin kicks for each arm cycle. The timing of the kicks is critical to maintaining a streamlined body position, countering resistance, and supplying continuous propulsion—in short, to swimming an efficient fly.

The downbeat of the first kick occurs just as your arms enter the water. This causes your upper body to drop lower in the water than

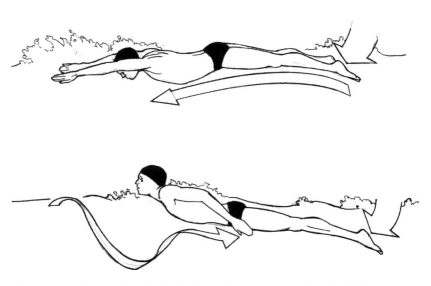

Figure 10.4. Timing of the Dolphin Kick. The downbeat of the first kick occurs as the arms enter the water. The downbeat of the second is during the final thrust of the arm stroke. It is during the second downbeat that you must inhale.

your hips, resulting in the characteristic undulating motion of the butterfly.

The downbeat of the second kick takes place during the final phase of the arm stroke, just as your hands are pushing back and up. Timed properly, it helps drive your shoulders out of the water for the recovery. At the same time, it allows you to raise your head to breathe (see Figure 10.4).

It seems that one of the two kicks is always larger than the other, depending on how fast you are swimming. When you sprint the butterfly, the second kick is larger than the first. But when you cruise the fly at a more leisurely pace, the first kick is the stronger.

BREATHING

In butterfly more than in any other stroke, the timing of breathing is important. Swum correctly, the butterfly is a rare combination of power and grace—literally poetry in motion. But like its namesake, it can be a fragile creature. Each of its parts—the arm stroke, the leg kick, the body motion, and the breathing—fit together to form a rhythmic, flowing, almost organic whole. When even one part is out of sync, the entire stroke is affected. If you breathe at the wrong time, your streamlined body position will immediately be altered, resistance will increase, and your stroke will deteriorate rapidly. So you must breathe at precisely the right moment.

But when is the right moment? The correct time to inhale is at the highest point of your stroke—*near the very end of the arm pull and during the downbeat of the second kick* (see Fig. 10.4). As you inhale, extend your neck and push your chin slightly forward, but do not lift it from the water. Try to curl your lips outward so water does not enter your mouth.

As soon as you have inhaled, return your face to the water an instant before your hands enter to begin the next stroke. As the arm pull progresses through its keyhole pattern, exhale slowly through your mouth and nose. Just before you are ready to breathe again, give a forceful puff of air. Now, as you complete the final thrust of the arm stroke, your face will lift out of the water and you can inhale again.

In butterfly, unlike in breaststroke, you do not need to breathe every stroke. How often you breathe is partly a matter of personal preference and partly a function of your conditioning, your lung capacity, and how far you are swimming. The farther you swim, the more often you need to breathe. However, the less often you need to breathe, the easier it is to maintain the proper body position. Assume, for instance, that you decide to breathe every second stroke. Simply hold your breath throughout the first arm cycle. Then inhale and exhale during the second arm cycle.

I generally breathe every third or fourth stroke when swimming a sprint of 50 yards or meters. In a 100-yard race, I breathe every other stroke. On those rare instances when my usually well-buried masochistic streak rears its ugly head and I convince myself to swim a 200-yard fly, I find I need to breathe every stroke except for the first and last laps.

No matter what the distance, strive to maintain a consistent breathing pattern. Mark Spitz, for example, always breathes every second stroke in the 100-meter butterfly. When he swam the 200-meter fly, he adopted a 2-1-2-1 pattern: two strokes then a breath, one stroke then a breath, and so on. In any event, what is important is to establish a consistent pattern. Do not try to swim as far as you can on the first breath, then come up gasping for air. It doesn't work.

While almost all butterflyers breathe to the front, occasionally you will see a swimmer who breathes to the side, as in the freestyle. No swimmer using this unorthodox style has been more successful than America's Melvin Stewart. In 1991 Stewart established a global mark for the 200-meter fly at the world championships. A year later he reasserted his dominance of the event by garnering Olympic gold, outstroking his nearest pursuer by almost two seconds.

Does this mean that it is best to breathe to the side when swimming the fly? Probably not. Pablo Morales, who won the 100-meter fly at the Barcelona games, breathes to the front. So do Qian Hong of China and America's Summer Sanders, winners of the women's 100- and 200-meter events at the '92 Olympics. So too did all the other 1992 finalists in all four Olympic butterfly events. Why? Because breathing to the front is a more fluid, natural motion when swimming the butterfly. It takes less effort and is more efficient.

Not only that, but the rules require that when you swim the fly you maintain a level position in the water at all times. When you breathe to the side, there is a tendency to roll. Stewart is able to maintain a flat body position while breathing to the side because he is endowed with unusual strength and flexibility. There is no harm in trying side breathing if you want to, but the chances are you'll find front breathing far easier.

To sum up:

1. Inhale at the very end of the arm stroke.
2. Breathe only as often as you need to.
3. Establish a consistent breathing pattern.

PUTTING IT ALL TOGETHER

By now you have learned all the aspects of the butterfly: the stream-lined body position, the "keyhole" arm pull, the double-dolphin kick, the undulating body movement, and the proper breathing technique. As has been emphasized repeatedly, however, swimming a fluent butterfly depends on the ability to coordinate each of these skills with the others. This stroke is one of those phenomena about which it can truly be said that the whole is much more than the sum of its parts.

Cecil Colwin suggests learning the stroke in the following order:

1. Learn the dolphin kick.
2. Learn the arm stroke.
3. Coordinate the kick and the arm movement without the head action.
4. Coordinate the arm movement and the head action without the kick.

Once you have mastered steps 3 and 4, you are ready to put it all together. Figure 10.5 illustrates the proper way to swim the fly, as seen from the side and head-on.

One of the problems people encounter in learning to swim the fly is that it requires both coordination and strength. After taking just a few strokes, most people simply lack the strength necessary to do the stroke properly. The result is that they lapse into what my good friend Emmett Hines, coach of the H_2Ouston Swims Masters Club, calls the ButterStruggle. Hines, the 1993 U.S. Masters Coach of the Year, wryly defines the ButterStruggle as a less than graceful series of jerks and spasms that occur after fatigue has robbed a swimmer of his ability to do the butterfly correctly. "Watching it," he notes with a Texas drawl, "is kinda like watching a cat cough up a fur ball—it's painful to see, but there ain't a whole lot you can do for it at the moment."

Fortunately, there *is* a training technique that can help you over-

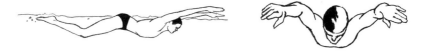

Figure 10.5. The Butterfly: Putting It All Together
A. The arms enter the water at shoulder width with the elbows straight. The feet kick downward in the first kick.

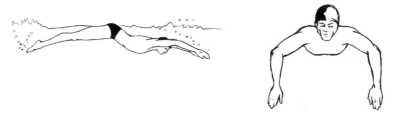

B. The hands press in an outward and downward direction, with the elbows held high and kept bent.

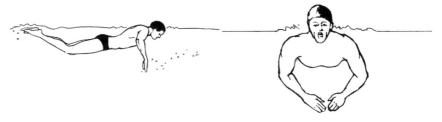

C. The hands almost come together under the chest, and the elbows are bent at right angles.

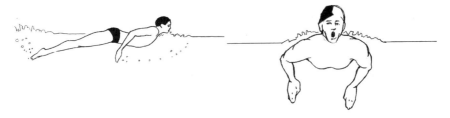

D. As the arms finish the pull, the second kick is made and a breath is taken.

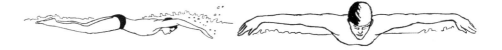

E. The arms are recovered over the water, and the head is lowered so the face is down.

come it. Hines calls it half fly. To do the half fly, all you need is the ability to swim at least one proper stroke of butterfly and the rest of a lap freestyle.

Here's how it works. Let's say you are swimming 200 yards. After the push off, take one stroke of butterfly, then finish the lap using freestyle. After the turn, do the same thing for the next lap, and so on.

As this gets easier, take *two* strokes of butterfly at the start of each lap. Once you are comfortable swimming the entire distance with two strokes of fly per lap, move up to *three* strokes—always being sure to drop back at the first hint of ButterStruggle. In this way, you can gradually improve your ability to swim the butterfly properly over longer and longer distances.

THE TURN

The butterfly turn is very much like the breaststroke turn (see Chapter 9). Where it differs comes *after* the push off.

Approach the wall with your head low and your body stretched out in a streamlined position. Then touch the wall with both hands simultaneously. As soon as you touch the wall, drop one arm. Tilt your upper body away from the wall, allowing your momentum to carry your feet to the wall, preparing them for the push off. Plant your feet *sideways* on the wall, and take a breath.

With your body still tilted sideways, release contact with your arm and submerge your head. Push hard off the wall, and immediately extend your body into a streamlined position. Take two dolphin kicks, then bring your arms through the underwater pull (Figure 10.6). Surface and start stroking.

THE START

The butterfly start is performed almost exactly like the freestyle start (see Chapter 7). The only difference comes after you enter the water. At this point take two or three short, hard dolphin kicks, then come to the surface ready to begin flying.

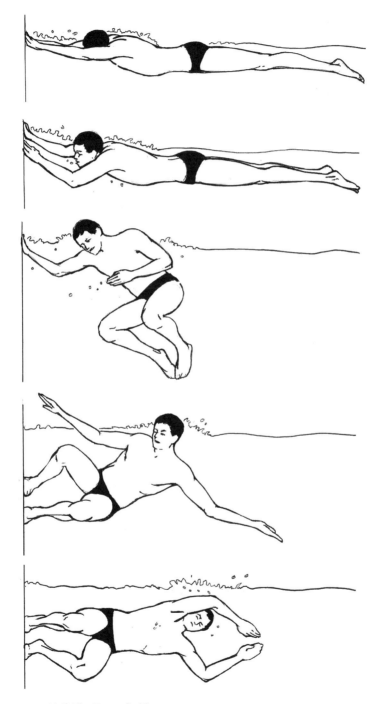

Figure 10.6. The Butterfly Turn

TEN BUTTERFLY TIPS

All the principles of efficient swimming outlined in Chapter 6 apply to the butterfly. Try to keep them in mind as you practice the stroke. In addition, the following ten tips will make learning the butterfly much easier.

1. Lie as flat on the surface of the water as possible, holding your hips high.
2. Do not try deliberately to achieve the characteristic undulating body movement of the fly. It will come naturally if your stroke and kick mechanics are correct.
3. Remember that you propel yourself forward by pushing against still water. The best way to do this is by using the "keyhole" arm stroke pattern. Do not pull straight back.
4. Do not slap the water with your hands but enter sharply, with your hands facing outward at about a forty-five-degree angle. Your hands should enter the water just outside shoulder width, arms almost totally extended and elbows slightly higher than your hands.
5. Your recovery should be made with a *low,* semicircular sweep over the surface of the water.
6. Keep your arms loose and relaxed as you recover. If you tense them, your muscles will tire quickly.
7. Use two dolphin kicks for each stroke.
8. The downbeat of the first kick occurs just as your arms enter the water, the second as your hands push back in the final thrust of the stroke. The timing of the kicks is crucial.
9. Breathe at the highest point of your stroke, near the end of the arm pull and during the downbeat of the second kick.
10. Establish a consistent breathing pattern.

A FINAL NOTE: THE BUTTERFLY-BREASTSTROKE

Before we move on, I should say a word about the butterfly-breaststroke. In competition (with the exception of Masters), the butterfly can only be swum using the dolphin kick. However, many Masters swimmers, as well as most noncompetitive swimmers, prefer to swim the fly with a breaststroke kick.

The Butterfly

The butterfly-breaststroke is not nearly as fast or efficient as the modern butterfly, but for many people, especially those with a powerful breaststroke kick, it can be much easier to learn. Also, because it allows you to rest during the glide after each kick, it is not as tiring as the fly.

In the butterfly-breaststroke, the arm stroke is exactly the same as in the butterfly, and the kick is the whip kick used in the breaststroke (see Chapter 9). The kick should occur just before the arms enter the water—precisely when the first downbeat is made in the conventional butterfly. You also breathe just as you do in the fly, inhaling during the final phase of the arm stroke.

I find the butterfly-breaststroke useful during the early part of the season, when I'm trying to round myself into shape. If I am swimming the fly and find I'm tiring badly, I throw in a lap of butterfly-breaststroke rather than stopping and resting. That way I can pick up the fly at the next turn and keep going.

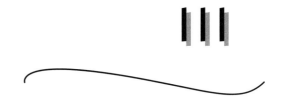

BECOMING FIT

11

SWIMMING AND SEXUALITY: HOW TO ENHANCE YOUR LOVE LIFE

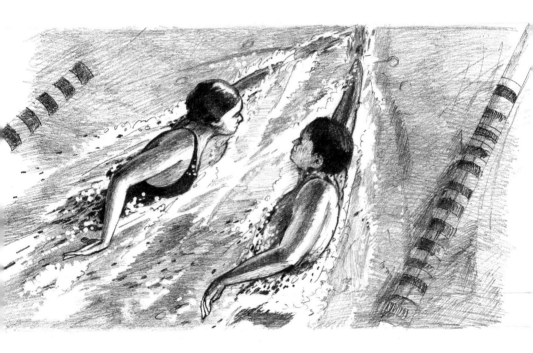

IT DOESN'T MATTER if you are twenty, forty, sixty, or even older: if you want an active and rewarding sex life, start swimming.

The first section of this book provided a lot of good news about the benefits of exercise in general and swimming in particular. No matter your age, regular workouts can improve your health, increase your resistance to disease, help you lose weight, increase your energy level, reduce stress, make you more confident, and even increase your creativity. But that's not all. There is even better news.

A pioneering study I conducted beginning in 1986 demonstrates conclusively that swimming can profoundly improve your love life. Since I presented the study results at a scientific meeting in Atlanta in 1988, several other researchers have confirmed these findings.

We found that middle-aged and older men and women who exercise regularly have sex lives much more like those of people a great deal younger.

Lisa Browning,* of Santa Monica, California, is typical of the people we studied who reported their sex lives reinvigorated after they began swimming. A vivacious, forty-six-year-old middle manager, Lisa began swimming at the local Y five years ago. "I was disgusted with the way I looked and felt," she told me. "I was fast sinking into a middle-age morass—flabby, no muscle tone, tired all the time. I felt *old*.

"Love life? It was ancient history." She laughed. "In twenty years of marriage, our love life had gone from exciting to routine to almost nonexistent. It was lifeless, tedious, dull."

One morning she decided it was now or never. "I'm just too young to feel like this," she told herself. That same afternoon she took the plunge.

"It was hard in the beginning, let me tell you," she recalled. "Those first few days were tough. I was ready to give up. Swimming just two laps was exhausting." But she stayed with it and gradually improved.

Today Lisa swims almost two miles four days a week, and last year her husband, Bob, joined her. She feels ten years younger and reports that her energy level has increased dramatically. "I'm not tired anymore. I feel good about myself. I even wear the same size clothes I wore in college. I have more energy—for work, the kids, my husband. The best part is that our love life is exciting again. It's fantastic!"

AGING AND SEXUALITY

In American society, sex is regarded as an activity for the young and attractive. The idea of older, or even middle-aged, couples engaging in sexual activity often evokes uneasiness. Young people in particular are embarrassed by the thought of their grandparents, or even par-

*Not her real name.

ents, engaged in sexual passion. They acknowledge grudgingly that their parents must have made love once, if only to produce them. Or even several times—to produce their siblings. But that was long ago. Surely they hop into bed nowadays only to get a good night's sleep.

Studies of aging and sexuality generally have shown that with advancing years comes a decline in frequency of both intercourse and other forms of sexual activity. More than forty-five years ago, Alfred Kinsey and his colleagues were the first researchers to examine systematically the effects of aging on sexual behavior. They learned that, contrary to popular opinion, interest in sex continues well into late adulthood. But they also discovered that as men and women grow older, their sexual activity decreases. More recent studies have confirmed these trends. However, other researchers, including me, believe that decreased sexual activity may be a result of poor health and cultural attitudes and expectations rather than a direct consequence of aging.

SWIMMING AND SEXUALITY

Ever since the advent of the fitness boom, advocates of swimming, running, and aerobics have claimed that vigorous physical exercise can rejuvenate the declining sex lives of older people. When I searched the professional literature, however, I was unable to find a single study that addressed this issue. Apparently the fitness gurus were relying on anecdotal evidence—and perhaps more than a bit of wishful thinking.

My study was the first to look at the relationships among aging, sexuality, and vigorous physical exercise.

How the Study Was Done

I surveyed 160 Masters swimmers, men and women between the ages of forty and eighty from throughout the United States. I wanted to discover if there was a relationship between vigorous exercise (swimming) and sexual interest and activity—specifically if individuals who exercise regularly have more active and fulfilling sex lives than others their age.

All the people I studied were healthy and in fine physical condition, unlike those in other studies on aging and sexuality. All had been swimming regularly for at least one year. Some had been competing continuously for ten to sixteen years. Their athletic backgrounds were varied: more than half had been competitive swimmers in their youth. A few were former Olympians, but many had never competed athletically before they joined the Masters program. In terms of present achievement, they ranged from average Masters swimmers to national champions for their age-groups.

Their training levels varied as well. At the low end were those who swam only forty-five minutes a day for three days a week. At the high end were a few individuals, mostly men, who were swimming two to three hours daily six days a week. Some supplemented their swimming with weight training, biking, running, or aerobics. On average, these swimmers trained about an hour a day, four to five days per week.

I divided the subjects into two age groups: forty to forty-nine and sixty and over (most of these were sixty to sixty-nine). A four-page survey was sent to 254 randomly selected Masters swimmers. One hundred and sixty responses were received, an extremely high response rate of 63 percent. The subjects remained anonymous unless they said yes to a request for a follow-up, in-depth personal interview. Twenty swimmers agreed to be interviewed, and twelve brought along their spouse or partner.

What I Wanted to Learn

My study attempted to answer the following basic question: *Is there a positive relationship between vigorous physical exercise (swimming) and sexual interest and activity?*

If I found such a relationship, I also wanted to know:

- *Is the relationship linear?* That is, does more training result in an ever-improving sex life?
- *Does the level of sexual interest and activity continue over more than two decades—from the forties through the sixties?*
- *How much do these older athletes* enjoy *their more prolific sex lives?*
- And, finally, *What accounts for these more active sex lives?*

Sexual Interest
In terms of sexual interest, my findings were consistent with those of other studies over the past forty years. Contrary to popular stereo-

types, people retain a high level of sexual interest throughout their life span; for most of us, the spirit remains willing no matter how weak the flesh becomes. My subjects reported a level of sexual interest slightly higher than the levels found in other studies. Probably their good health accounts for this difference.

Sexual Activity

It is in the area of sexual activity—particularly frequency of intercourse—that I found some of the most dramatic results. In my study 97 percent of those in their forties and 92 percent of those sixty and older reported being sexually active with a partner (see Table 11.1). These figures are higher than those found in other studies, and of those who were not active, all but one had suffered the loss of a partner through death, disablement, or divorce.

TABLE 11.1.
Percentage of Swimmers Reporting Being Sexually Active
(with a Partner)

	Forties	Sixties and Older
Men	98%	94%
Women	94	89
Average	96	92

Among the subjects who were sexually active, 100 percent in all four categories, men and women in their forties, and men and women sixty and older, reported having sexual intercourse *at least* once a week. How unusual is that? Edward M. Brecher's 1984 study of sexually active people over fifty found only about two thirds reporting intercourse at least once a week (see Table 11.2). Father Andrew Greeley, professor of sociology at the University of Chicago, reported in 1992 that 37 percent of married men and women over sixty made love once a week or more. Carin Rubinstein found in 1985 that 47 percent of the women over forty she studied reported having intercourse once a week or more.

My swimmers made love an average of 7.1 times per month—about the same as twenty-six- to thirty-three-year-olds in the general population. This is several times higher than the figure for people their own age who do not exercise.

Apparently age has had little effect on the sexual appetites of the athletes I studied. When I compared swimmers in their sixties with

TABLE 11.2.

Percentage of Sexually Active Adults Reporting Intercourse at Least Once per Week

Brecher's Study of General Population

	Fifties	*Sixties*	*Seventies*
Men	90%	73%	58%
Women	73	63	50

Whitten's Study of Swimmers

	Forties	*Sixties*
Men	100%	100%
Women	100	100

TABLE 11.3.

Frequency of Intercourse Among Swimmers Studied (times/month)

	Forties	*Sixties*
Men	7.6	7.1
Women	7.0	6.6

TABLE 11.4.

Percentage of Sexually Active Adults Reporting a High Level of Sexual Enjoyment

Brecher's Study of General Population

	Fifties	*Sixties*
Men	90%	86%
Women	71	65

Whitten's Study of Swimmers

	Forties	*Sixties*
Men	100%	98%
Women	94	88

those in their forties, I found very little decline in how often they had intercourse (see Table 11.3).

Sexual Enjoyment

Not only are my physically active subjects making love more often but they seem to be enjoying it more. Ninety-four percent of the swimmers I studied report a high level of enjoyment. This is quite a bit higher than in Brecher's study (see Table 11.4). The differences between the women in the two studies are particularly striking. For example, 88 percent of women over sixty who swim reported a high level of enjoyment. Contrast that with only 65 percent of the women in the general population.

Is More Better?

Having established a strong link between regular swimming and increased sexual activity and enjoyment, I turned my attention to another question: Is the relationship linear? Does more and more exercise lead to an ever more bountiful sex life?

Sorry, workout fanatics. My data provide no support for any such relationship. There seems to be a threshold level of exercise that produces an enhanced love life. This level corresponds to the lower end of training intensity in the swimmers I studied—three days a week, forty-five minutes a day. Beyond this level, increasing your training apparently does not result in ever-increasing sexual interest or activity.

In fact, whereas moderate exercise apparently revs up the libido, it may be that too much exercise virtually shuts down the sex-hormone factory in both men and women. A study of triathletes by researchers at California Polytechnic University in San Luis Obispo found that doubling men's workout time from 90 to 180 minutes per day significantly lowered testosterone levels and sperm counts. Many of these men completely lost interest in the one activity they used to like even more than swimming, cycling, or running.

Why? When you exercise too much, your brain is unable to produce as much of the hormone FSH. This causes a man to make less testosterone. As a result, he loses interest in (and often cannot make) love.

The same thing happens to women who exercise too much. When a woman overexercises, it upsets both her hormonal balance and her ability to become sexually aroused, according to Barry J. Klyde, an endocrinologist with New York Hospital–Cornell Medical Center. Too much exercise reduces the amount of estrogen a woman produces, which can cause her to stop menstruating. This condition is frequently seen in female distance runners. An inadequate supply of estrogen can also produce the symptoms of menopause in younger women. Sexual desire may diminish as the vagina shrinks. The vaginal lining thins, and lubrication ceases. All these effects contribute to common female sexual dysfunction—painful or uncomfortable intercourse.

My study supported these conclusions. I found that when men and women engage in extremely heavy training—eighteen hours a week or more—sexual desire decreases. This is not surprising. If you have ever engaged in very heavy training, you know that the last thing on your mind when you get home from working out is making love. Instead, you can't wait to get some food inside you and then plunk your tired body down on the nearest sofa or bed.

Scientific research leaves no doubt that regular exercise in the form of swimming can enhance your love life. But beyond a certain level of training, if you want to improve your sex life, spend more time with your partner, not in the pool.

Other Studies

Since my study on exercise, aging, and sexuality was first presented, several studies have endorsed my conclusions. Researchers at the University of California at San Diego compared two groups of sedentary, middle-aged men. One group was placed on a nine-month program of moderate aerobic exercise; the other group maintained their lethargic habits. The exercisers reported a dramatic increase in the frequency of their lovemaking that the couch potatoes did not report. The researchers noted that as the men became more fit, their sex lives improved accordingly. How's that for an incentive to swim?

Another study, conducted by Linda De Villers, a Santa Monica, California, psychologist and sex therapist, polled some 8,000 women. Almost half reported an increase in sexual arousal, activity, and enjoyment after beginning regular exercise programs. In her practice, De Villers reports, "It is unusual to have somebody in therapy for low sexual desire who is a regular exerciser."

What Accounts for These Results?

In a very real sense, swimming is a sort of sexual Fountain of Youth, allowing people to indulge in sex just as often at age sixty as they did at age thirty. But what accounts for this astonishing fact? Are there important hormonal factors that account for it? Can it be explained mainly by psychological factors? Or is it a combination?

The Testosterone Hypothesis

Many studies have shown that moderate physical exercise produces increased levels of the male sex hormone, testosterone. This occurs in both men and women. It may be that this hormone accounts, at least in part, for our results. But I am skeptical: testosterone levels remain elevated for only a short while after exercising. Furthermore, the relationship between testosterone level and sexual activity in humans (as opposed to other species) is not direct. Increases in testosterone are associated with increases in aggressive behavior, but such an influence on sexual behavior has not been established. Men with testosterone levels below a certain threshold are unable to perform sexually. After the threshold is achieved, however, there seems to be no increase in sexual activity. Although the testosterone hypothesis seems an unlikely explanation for the increased sexual activity, future studies will continue to look for a connection between the two.

The Growth Hormone Hypothesis

Another possibility, not yet explored, has to do with the production of human growth hormone (hGH). Chapter 5 pointed out that human growth hormone leads directly to physiological changes associated with youth: an increase in muscle, a decrease in body fat, an increase in the elasticity of skin, and so on. This is true whether the hGH is produced naturally by the body or injected. Human growth hormone is secreted in bursts by the pituitary gland during and immediately after vigorous exercise, and also during deep sleep.

An increase in hGH production makes the middle-aged and even older person younger in a number of critical respects. One of the characteristics of younger people is that they engage in sex more often than older people. So it is possible that increased sexual interest and activity are by-products of the increased production of hGH. This intriguing hypothesis, too, awaits further study.

Psychological Factors

What about psychological factors? One of the sorry realities of modern life is stress, which, as mentioned in Chapter 3, is a major factor implicated in heart disease. Stress also often leads to depression. According to Dr. Helen Singer Kaplan, director of the Human Sexuality Program at the New York Hospital–Cornell Medical Center, chronic stress can be devastating to sexual functioning, turning lovemaking from a pleasurable sharing of intimacy into an impossible act. Even mild stress dulls the zest for life.

Body image also plays an enormous role in sexual feelings, according to Dr. Shirley Zussman, director of the Association for Male Sexual Dysfunction in New York. The improved self-esteem that comes from a healthier, more attractive body carries over into sexual situations, she says. "The way you view yourself and the way you appear in your mate's eyes is very important. If you feel your partner sees you as desirable, you're more able to free yourself and enjoy the sexual experience."

Dr. De Villers agrees. Sexual confidence and satisfaction are highly correlated with a fit body, she says. For example, she points out, many women are reluctant to assume the female-superior position during lovemaking, even though it is often the most satisfying position. The reason is a brittle self-image. "They complain, 'He can see my fat stomach.' "

Swimming helps you lose excess body fat and sculpt an attractive, vital body that you will be happy to have your partner see. This changed perception of yourself will increase your self-esteem. If you are confident about yourself, you will have a better time in bed.

In my study the Masters swimmers reported that they often receive indications that they are forestalling, or at least slowing, the "normal" aging process. They have more endurance and are stronger than before they began exercising, confirmed by the fact that many of them are actually swimming faster as they get older. They socialize with attractive younger people, who respect them and their accomplishments. At the pool they see many people with appealing, fit bodies, people who give them positive feedback about their own attractiveness. Indeed, they say they look better and feel better about their bodies. It's no wonder they feel sexier too.

Social psychologists Ellen Berscheid and Elaine Walster studied physical attraction in men and women. Not surprisingly, they found that people are sexually and romantically attracted to those they find physically attractive. This is true both before and after marriage.

William Griffith found that arousal of sexual desire leads to an increased sexual attraction to people seen as physically attractive and an increased aversion to those perceived as physically unattractive. Applied to the effects of aging on physical attractiveness, he argues that, in both men and women, normal aging is associated with declining physical attractiveness as defined in our society. Robert Redford and Linda Evans notwithstanding, our standards of beauty are closely linked with youthfulness.

In my study, I asked the subjects to rate themselves for physical attractiveness compared with others their age. I asked them to use a five-point scale, ranging from very attractive to very unattractive, with 3 being "about average." The results were astonishing: eighty percent rated themselves in the top two categories; 20 percent rated themselves as average. None rated themselves below average. Clearly these are people with strong self-images, people who feel good about themselves.

Is there any basis in reality for these extremely positive self-assessments? Perhaps there is something in pool water that bloats egos. Apparently not. In the interviews as well as written surveys, I asked the swimmers' partners to rate their physical attractiveness. These "significant others"—husbands and wives, boyfriends and girlfriends—rated the swimmers as even more physically attractive than the swimmers had rated themselves.

It is evident that the swimmers I studied view themselves as younger than their chronological age and more attractive than others their age. Equally significant, the most important people in their lives agree.

Psychological and Physiological Interactions

Stress and depression are physiological as well as psychological factors in decreasing sexual interest and activity, for, as Dr. Klyde points out, these psychological states force the body to secrete more of the hormone cortisol, which suppresses the production of sex hormones. In turn, the increased cortisol upsets the neurotransmitters in the brain responsible for stable emotions, leading to greater stress and depression. Stress also causes constriction of peripheral arteries, preventing blood from flowing to the genitals and inhibiting arousal.

Numerous studies have shown that aerobic exercise is a powerful antidepressant and is great for relieving stress. Like other forms of exercise, swimming promotes the release of endorphins, the hormones that make you feel good. Feeling good, in turn, decreases the amount of cortisol you secrete, restoring to normal your production of sex hormones as well as the neurochemical balance that affects your emotions.

Being overweight also contributes to impotence through physiological as well as psychological mechanisms. Says endocrinologist

Klyde, "Excess fat converts the male sex hormone testosterone into the female sex hormone estrogen. As a result, desire wanes, frequency and firmness of erections decrease, and the breasts [in males] may enlarge." Swimming reverses this condition. "Fat is reduced, the breasts shrink to normal, and more testosterone is produced. This resuscitates the libido, which revives the erections."

THE BOTTOM LINE

A recent Gallup poll showed that active Americans are driven by a common goal. They are swimming, running, walking, biking, and dancing because they believe that exercise transforms their lives. It helps them to become the best human beings they can be. Recent studies, mine among them, show that the benefits of exercise extend far beyond the enhancement of one's physical and emotional well-being. Whatever your age, swimming can revitalize your love life.

I think the final word should go to a Florida woman who called in to a radio program on which I was being interviewed recently. Responding to a description of the results of my study on aging, swimming, and sexuality, and to my comment that in our society sex among older people is often regarded as not quite dignified, savory, or even "proper," she said, "Honey, I'm ninety years old. I swim every day. I love to make love. And, sugar, I don't care what anyone says: I'm going to heaven!"

12

WOMEN AND SWIMMING

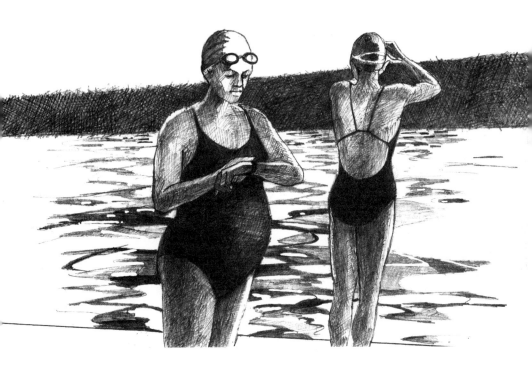

As DISCUSSED IN previous chapters, swimming provides bountiful and life-enhancing benefits. It makes you stronger, healthier, more energetic, and more productive; it reduces stress, keeps your body fit and youthful, and improves your mental functioning; it can help you quit smoking; it provides protection against heart disease, diabetes, possibly some forms of cancer, arthritis, asthma, and a host of other debilitating diseases; it makes you more confident, attractive and sexy; in sum, it can extend your life and improve its quality.

All these benefits accrue equally to men and women, to young and old. But swimming offers some additional benefits for women only.

SWIMMING AND PREGNANCY

The time: August 1991. The place: Elizabethtown, Kentucky. As thirty-two-year-old Bonnie Glasgow Rhodes stroked smoothly up and down the fifty-meter pool at the U.S. National Masters Swimming Championships, it quickly became clear that she was right on target for a new world record in the 400-meter individual medley.

The 400 IM is swimming's most demanding race: 100 grueling meters each of butterfly, backstroke, breaststroke, and freestyle. Stirred on by the roar of the crowd, Rhodes never faltered. When the Austin, Texas, accountant and mother of two finally slammed into the touch pads, she had carved a whopping six seconds off the old record. Not a bad day's work—especially for a woman who was four months pregnant.

Another record of sorts was set in 1992 by another thirty-two-year-old, Leslie Craven. Leslie, who swims for both fitness and competition, competed in the 200-yard freestyle only two days before giving birth to a healthy eight-pound baby boy (of course, the tuck in her flip turns wasn't as tight as usual). Three days after giving birth, Leslie was back in the pool again. "I tried to swim every day of my pregnancy," she recalls. "It felt wonderful—relaxing and soothing."

Not every pregnant woman, of course, can set a world Masters swimming record, and not every woman will want to swim up to the moment of delivery. But the near-weightless environment of swimming can provide important benefits for virtually every pregnant woman—keeping her muscles toned, relieving the physical and emotional stress of carrying a heavy burden around for several months, eliminating backaches, increasing the flow of oxygen to her baby, and (because her muscles are strong) helping make the delivery easier.

Kimberly Fagan of Tulsa, Oklahoma, had suffered from chronic back pain since her early teens. When she found out she was expecting for the first time, her doctor, fearing that pregnancy would exacerbate her back problems, recommended that she get in the water and swim several days a week. "It was amazing," she recalls. "Within a week the backaches just disappeared. I felt better when I was pregnant than I did before. It's been several years now, and as long as I swim on a regular basis, I no longer have any problems with my back."

No one had to convince swim coach and instructor Judy Bonning, of Coral Springs, Florida, about the benefits swimming provides pregnant women. She had seen them firsthand many times during her coaching career. So when the thirty-seven-year-old became pregnant for the first time, she not only continued her daily swims but started a class for pregnant women. Within weeks she had over thirty women in the program. As word of its success spread, more and more women signed up. "Within a month it was one of the most successful programs we had going," Bonning recalls. "We had more women signing up than we could accommodate."

According to Dr. Desider Rothe, clinical professor of obstetrics and gynecology at the New York Hospital–Cornell Medical Center, "Not only is swimming the best all-around exercise there is but it is especially well-suited to the needs of pregnant women." Dr. Jane Katz, author of *Swimming Through Your Pregnancy,* explains why this is so: "Swimming helps you enjoy your pregnancy and prepare for labor and delivery by gently toning and strengthening your body. Not only will your labor and delivery be easier, and your pregnancy more enjoyable, but after you give birth your recovery and return to fitness and figure will be quicker."

Of course you should consult your doctor before swimming through your pregnancy. But only a tiny minority of women should find themselves barred from swimming for medical reasons. In fact, nowadays most obstetricians are aware of swimming's benefits and encourage a mother-to-be to get in the swim, both for her sake and for the sake of her unborn child.

A recent study conducted by the Melpomene Institute in Minneapolis demonstrated just how dramatic these benefits can be. The study compared three groups of young expectant mothers: those who swam for exercise while pregnant, those who ran, and those who did no exercise at all. The two groups of women who exercised experienced important advantages over the sedentary women: they had easier deliveries, suffered less from postpartum depression, and regained their normal weight and figures much more quickly.

There was, however, one major difference between the swimmers on the one hand and the runners and nonexercisers on the other. This was in the area euphemistically termed by the study negative outcomes. *Negative outcomes* means spontaneous abortions and stillbirths. The swimmers had only one fourth as many of these heart-breaking experiences as the women in the other two groups.

SWIMMING AND BREAST CANCER

Every three minutes a woman in the United States learns she has breast cancer. Affecting the lives of nearly 500 women each day, this relentlessly expanding wave engulfs almost 200,000 American women each year. In 1993, some 46,000 women died of the disease, and the number keeps growing.

Experts estimate that an American woman today stands a frightening 1 in 9 chance of developing breast cancer. This represents a big increase over the 1 in 20 odds of only two decades ago. It is no exaggeration to say that breast cancer has become an epidemic.

The Causes of Breast Cancer

Many medical researchers now believe that the skyrocketing increase in the rate of breast cancer is largely a result of our sedentary, high-stress life-style and our high-fat diets. That is the bad news. The good news is that these factors are within our control. You can lessen your likelihood of contracting breast cancer through regular exercise, such as swimming, and through eating a balanced diet, both of which reduce body fat. Of course no one can guarantee that if you eat right and swim every day, you won't get breast cancer, but these two factors alone will significantly tilt the odds in your favor. What's more, recent evidence seems to suggest that if you do contract breast cancer, your likelihood of surviving will be greatly improved if you exercise regularly and eat a healthy, balanced diet.

There are three major identifiable causes of breast cancer: (1) family history, (2) dietary fat, and (3) percent body fat. There are also minor causes: age (the older you are, the more likely you are to contract the disease); early onset of puberty; late menopause; delayed childbearing; and a previous history of cancer. In addition, many people believe that pollution and other changes in the environment have contributed to the rise in the incidence of breast cancer over the past few decades.

Let's look at each of the major causes.

Family History

The odds of getting breast cancer are two to three times higher for a woman whose mother or sister had the disease. The risk is even higher if that relative developed cancer before menopause or had cancer in both breasts. You cannot determine who your relatives are, of course, but if you know that your genetic background places you at unusual risk, you can improve your odds of avoiding the condition by swimming on a regular basis and by the decisions you make about your diet, birth-control methods, and postmenopause hormone therapy. Likewise, you can improve your chances of detecting the condition at an early stage by performing regular, careful breast self-examinations and by following your physician's recommendations regarding how often you have a mammogram done.

Diet

Several major epidemiological studies have singled out dietary fat as a possible culprit in breast cancer, particularly for postmenopausal women. Other studies suggest that the large number of calories typically consumed in a high-fat diet may represent the real underlying risk. In an attempt to settle the controversy, three National Cancer Institute researchers, led by biostatistician Laurence S. Freedman, reanalyzed one hundred animal experiments, in many cases pooling data from various studies before hunting for statistical trends. In an article published in *Cancer Research* in 1990, they concluded that fat and calories pose independent breast-cancer risks.

A study of Finnish women, described in the November 1990 issue of the *American Journal of Clinical Nutrition,* analyzed dietary questionnaires filled out at least twenty years before by 3,988 healthy women aged twenty to sixty-nine and found that the 54 participants who later developed breast cancer showed a "consistently higher" average percentage of fat-derived calories. Dividing the entire sample into thirds based on the proportion of fat in the women's diets, the authors calculated that the subgroup eating the most fat had a breast-cancer risk about 70 percent higher than the subgroup eating the least. Unfortunately the study lacked any data about the exercise habits of the women.

Chapter 4 discussed how a low-fat diet with a balance between carbohydrate and protein produces hormonal effects that protect against heart disease and other deadly illnesses. It also pointed out that certain vitamins—particularly vitamin A, especially in the form of beta carotene, vitamin C, and vitamin E—may protect against cancer, including breast cancer. Recent research seems to indicate that these vitamins provide this protection by preventing cellular and genetic damage. Taken together, these data strongly suggest that a low-fat, high-fiber diet, balanced between carbohydrates and proteins and rich in fruits and vegetables, may help prevent breast cancer.

Body Fat

Some years ago researchers discovered that when Japanese women emigrated to the United States, their incidence of breast cancer increased severalfold, mirroring the rate among native-born Americans. Obviously genetic factors could not explain this alarming rise, so the researchers concluded that it was caused by the fact that the immigrants abandoned the low-fat diet they ate in Japan in favor of an American high-fat diet.

It is, however, not only the high dietary fat you eat but what becomes of it after you eat it that is responsible for increased breast-cancer risk. According to Dr. Barry Sears, obesity, or high body fat, leads to high insulin levels in the blood. In turn, this results in a decrease in the sex hormone binding factor. Therefore, the amount of free estrogen in the bloodstream is increased. It is this free estrogen that is directly associated with breast cancer.

What happens is the free estrogen searches for estrogen receptors. These receptors can be found in large numbers in the breast tissue, and they cause these cells to grow. Among the cells the free estrogen finds are potentially malignant cells. The normal cells produce prostaglandins, which counterbalance this growth; the malignant cells do not produce the prostaglandins, so they begin to reproduce unchecked. The result is breast cancer.

According to Sears, the level of body fat that is associated with a significantly increased risk of breast cancer is 35 percent. That is well above the 22 percent threshold that defines a physically fit woman and the 17 to 21 percent for female Masters swimmers of all ages. Unfortunately, 35 percent is the average figure for American women.

The idea that maintaining lifelong physical fitness can help protect against breast cancer was supported by a long-term study of former college female athletes published by Harvard epidemiologist, Rose Frisch and her colleagues in 1992. Compared with women who were nonathletes in college, the former athletes remained more active throughout their lives, had lower body-fat percentages, and were less likely to develop breast cancer.

Another study, published in 1992, in *The New England Journal of*

Medicine, also singled out the role of body fat in the development of breast cancer. A team of researchers led by Dr. Thomas Sellers of the University of Minnesota School of Public Health reported that high levels of body fat increased the likelihood that women whose genetic background placed them at risk would develop breast cancer.

Not only does obesity increase the risk of a woman developing breast cancer but it also increases the risk of the cancer's recurrence. In a study of women with breast cancer headed by Dr. Ruby Senie of the Centers for Disease Control, 32 percent of obese women developed cancer recurrences, compared with 19 percent of normal-weight women.

The drug Tamoxifen is most often used to treat breast cancer. It is a powerful agent that blocks the uptake of estrogen from the breast tissues. But Tamoxifen has significant noxious side effects, and the same result can be achieved *before* cancer has developed by keeping insulin levels down. The easiest way to do this is through regular exercise and eating a balanced diet.

All it takes is a little discipline. Given the stakes, that's not too much to ask.

OTHER FEMALE CANCERS

Breast cancer is not the only form of this deadly scourge that can be prevented by swimming. Research at the Harvard School of Public Health showed that women who remained physically active throughout their lives were two and a half times less susceptible to cervical and other cancers of the reproductive system.

Again body fat seems to be a triggering factor. "These women were leaner in every age-group than sedentary women," notes Dr. Frisch, who also directed this study. "Because body fat makes estrogen, leaner women make less estrogen, and of a less potent kind." As with malignant breast cells, estrogen triggers cell division in the cervix, creating a greater opportunity for abnormal change. According to Dr. Frisch, aerobic activities such as swimming will burn off body fat, keep you lean and trim, and help protect you against these cancers. She recommends swimming at least thirty minutes three days a week.

One of the major health problems women face is osteoporosis: bone loss after menopause, when their bodies reduce production of estrogen, the female sex hormone. This reduction of bone mass, which affects more than half of American women over fifty, makes the bones break easily, leading to hip fractures, crushed vertebrae, and other painful problems.

Over the years, many studies have demonstrated that moderate exercise can slow or prevent the rate of bone loss, but until recently conventional wisdom had it that only weight-bearing exercises, such as running or aerobics, could produce this desirable effect. A 1994 study conducted by Esther Goldstein at Hebrew University–Hadassah School of Public Health and Community Medicine in Jerusalem suggests otherwise.

The study involved two groups of volunteer postmenopausal women over the age of fifty. Goldstein demonstrated that swimming and water aerobics add to bone mass in middle-aged women *better* than conventional, land-based exercise—thus providing an effective activity to mitigate the effects of osteoporosis.

A 1987 study by a Portland, Oregon, endocrinologist, Eric S. Orwoll, showed that swimming provides the same bone-saving protection in men. When their bone-mineral content was compared with that of seventy-eight nonexercising subjects the same age who were getting either mineral supplements or a placebo for another study, the swimmers clearly had a large edge. Diet could not account for the differences, since calcium and protein intake was the same for both groups. His findings, says Orwoll, "can be a boon for people who have difficulty with weight-bearing exercise—and for the large number of people who just enjoy swimming."

Another study, conducted by Dr. Richard L. Prince and others from Sir Charles Gairdner Hospital in Nedlands, Australia, and published in *The New England Journal of Medicine* in 1992, found that combining exercise with low doses of estrogen was the most effective way of preventing bone loss among older, postmenopausal women. Women who took estrogen while engaging in light exercise increased their bone density by about 3 percent per year. In addition to strengthening bone, the supplements prevent heart disease and relieve hot flashes and other unpleasant symptoms of menopause. A combination of exercise and doses of calcium also slowed bone loss but was not as effective as the exercise-estrogen combination. The most effective combination of all is exercise plus calcium and estrogen supplements.

The good news about exercise and osteoporosis is not confined to older women. A 1992 study published in *The Journal of the American Medical Association* showed that even though they have stopped growing, women can build stronger bones throughout their twenties by engaging in exercise such as swimming and by taking in adequate amounts of calcium. This is the first time scientists have shown that bones can continue to gain mass and strength after they have stopped growing longer in late adolescence. The scientists at Creighton University School of Medicine in Omaha found that exercise and calcium increased the young women's bone mass by 5 to 6 percent. These figures provide hope that a combination of exercise and a diet rich in calcium can actually *prevent* osteoporosis later in life.

SELF-ESTEEM: A TALE OF TWO WOMEN

One of the lamentable realities of modern American society is that its structure seems to foster low self-esteem among many women. Although this deplorable situation clearly is changing, it is still a fact of life for countless American women and girls. Even the most talented and accomplished of women are not immune from this modern social malady. Research by psychologist Matina Horner demonstrated that low self-esteem can produce an actual fear of success. Even Gloria Steinem, whose accomplishments as a writer, editor, and feminist leader have been equaled by few, admitted in her book *Revolution from Within: A Book of Self-Esteem,* that she suffered from low self-esteem and saw herself as both unaccomplished and physically plain. Swimming is one way many women have found to deal with low self-esteem. The feelings of strength, competence, accomplishment, self-reliance, and physical attractiveness the sport engenders have helped thousands of women overcome the debilitating effects of low self-esteem. Here are the stories of two such women.

Katherine Casey

Katherine Casey is an attractive forty-five-year-old teacher at Lakes High School near Tacoma, Washington. She is an avid Masters swimmer who also manages to find time to coach swimming, diving, track and field, and gymnastics. Now happily remarried, not many years ago she was a battered wife.

"I was married to my first husband fourteen years," she told me. "One of the reasons I was attracted to him was the fact that he was so athletic. I felt that his participation in athletics would enhance our relationship, since I was also very involved in swimming and coaching. I even coached at the high school he had graduated from. I thought he understood my participation in athletics. That was the way it seemed while we were dating."

Once they were married, Katherine was shocked to discover that her athletic activities were no longer okay, that her husband had taken a proprietary view of her and the way she spent her time. "It began very subtly," she recalls. "First with the sense of dissatisfaction with me, refusing to kiss me hello when he came home from work, refusing to participate or go with me to my sporting events, trying to keep me from my friends, refusing to talk to me, yelling at me." Her husband's behavior eventually escalated into his hitting things, breaking furniture, denting her car, physically threatening and abusing the children, and finally physically assaulting her.

"I spent years wondering what was wrong with me," she confided. Only two things kept her going through this rough time: "my teaching assignments and my swimming." When the battering began, Katherine finally got out of the relationship.

"You know where I went the next weekend? I packed up the kids and went to a swim meet. I was sick and injured, but I had to swim! It was the last thing I was hanging on to." She remembers that day well; instead of laughing and talking with her swimmer friends, she hid in the corners so no one would see her bruises until she could get makeup back on her face. But Katherine soon came to understand that she had no cause to feel shame because of her husband's actions. And swimming played a part in her recovery, confirming for her that she was really okay, still the person she had been, that she was worthwhile. "My last shreds of self-esteem needed that support and confirmation," she recalls.

Katherine is still swimming today. One of her workout partners is Walt Reid, her husband of four years, whom she met at a swim meet. "To this day," she remarks, "swimming is a source of physical and inner strength for me. I so much depended on it for my self-esteem and sense of power and strength during those bad times that it's become as necessary a part of my life as eating and sleeping. Putting my head down in the water, stretching out and feeling power return to my muscles strengthens my belief in myself. It clears my brain and empowers me to do whatever I have to. Nobody can take away the good feelings I get each day from swimming."

Susan Livingston

Looking at her, it is hard to imagine that this tall, athletic, graceful, confident woman once suffered from low self-esteem. At age fifty-five, Susan Livingston could easily pass for an attractive forty-year-old. As one talks with her, this feeling is reinforced. She is gracious, knowledgeable, and assertive. She knows what she wants in life and how to go after it, but always with style and class.

Susan, who has three grown children, operates a successful bed-and-breakfast in scenic Marblehead, Massachusetts. She supplements her income as a seamstress specializing in wedding gowns. But her real passion is swimming. Although you would never know it from talking with her, Susan is one of the top women swimmers her age in America.

In keeping with the dominant values of her time, Susan married right after graduating from Smith College and immediately settled down to being a housewife and raising a family. "I never had to do anything that brought me in touch with the grown-up world," she recalls, "not even balance the checkbook. My husband took care of everything. My only job was to be the perfect wife and raise our three children."

When her Ozzie-and-Harriet marriage began breaking up in 1983, Susan was devastated, and totally unequipped to function in a changing world. It was then, quite by happenstance, that she started swimming. A natural, she has been at it ever since. Today, she says, "I couldn't live without it."

When Susan was in college, there were no competitive athletic programs for women, but she did join Smith's synchronized swimming team. Years later she describes herself as "swimming laps with my limp, delicate hands and my head out of the water, as synchro swimmers do, just exercising. I happened to go to a pool when a Masters swimming practice was going on. I just fell into it. Coach Jack Hayden kind of tucked me under his wing, and a month later I was competing."

Susan has been swimming ever since, and in ten years has racked up over forty New England records in the forty-five to forty-nine, fifty to fifty-four, and fifty-five to fifty-nine age-groups. In 1985 she won a national title in the 200-meter backstroke and in 1991, at the age of fifty-three, recorded lifetime best times in several events. But she doesn't worry about her times. "I swim for fun, fitness, and friendship, and I love every minute of it: the practice, local meets, traveling all over the country to the nationals each year, making interesting new friends. It's been a great time."

With her divorce had come a kind of identity crisis, Susan says. "If you weren't somebody's wife, then who were you? Swimming helped me with that. In becoming a swimmer I developed my own identity and a new set of friends who respect me for who I am."

Susan comes by her talent naturally; she is a fine all-around athlete, and her father was a national collegiate swimming champion at Yale. But she had had no previous experience in competition. Perhaps feelings associated with her divorce had something to do with her drive during the first few years she swam in Masters competition. "Now I have nothing to prove. I'd love to go faster, but I do well enough for me."

Along with her new sense of who she was came self-esteem. She says, "Through swimming, I learned I could do anything I set my mind to: swim faster, balance a checkbook, manage my own portfolio, repair the roof, haul the garbage to the dump, or start a successful business. Through swimming I've finally found myself."

13

THE SPORT OF A LIFETIME:
SWIMMING FROM 8 TO 108

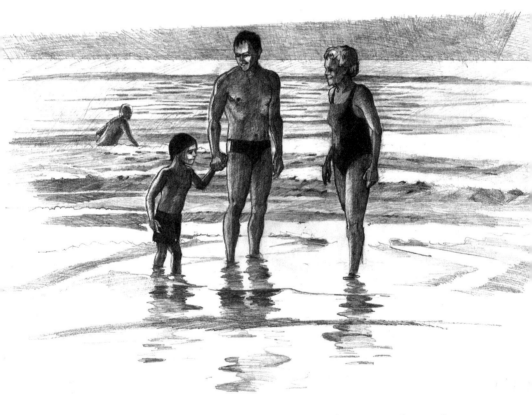

ELSEWHERE IN THIS book I have talked about the fitness revolution that has swept America and many other nations since the early 1970s. Despite the fact that this revolution has affected only a minority of men and women, it has had a major impact on our nation's health statistics: death rates from heart disease have declined significantly, and many Americans are now living longer, healthier lives.

Sadly, one large and important group of people has been left almost untouched by the fitness revolution: America's children. Put simply, American kids are grossly out of shape. As a result of inactivity, too much television, poor nutrition, and lack of parental guidance, they have become little butterballs. And they are becoming fatter and less active every year.

THE CHUBBING OF AMERICA

A 1992 survey of children between the ages of three and seventeen conducted by Louis Harris for *Prevention* magazine found that 34 percent of kids were significantly overweight, compared with 24 percent only seven years earlier. Thirty-nine percent of boys are overweight, while 30 percent of girls are too heavy.

Not only that, but the older kids are chubbier than the younger ones: 22 percent of children under twelve were overweight, while a depressing 57 percent of thirteen- to seventeen-year-olds were too fat. Because the study looked only at weight and not body-fat percentage, these figures may even underestimate the extent of the problem. Many children, particularly girls, have what appears to be a healthy weight but because of inactivity carry too much body fat. A "huge number of kids" have developed weight problems by their teen years, says Thomas Dybdahl, director of research for *Prevention*. "By the time they are eighteen or twenty, weight control may already be a losing battle for millions of people."

Other studies bear out these alarming conclusions. According to the National Association for Sport and Physical Education, 40 percent of children aged five to eight are obese, are inactive, or have elevated blood pressure or cholesterol levels—all major coronary-risk factors. As many as half the nation's schoolchildren are not getting enough exercise to develop healthy hearts and lungs. One study shows that more than half of all female grade-school students and about a quarter of their male counterparts cannot perform a single pull-up. Another found that some 33 percent of school-age boys and 50 percent of girls could not run a mile in under ten minutes.

Still another study, directed by Wynn F. Updike of Indiana University, concluded that student fitness declined precipitously between 1980 and 1990. This study, involving an estimated 9.7 million schoolchildren, compared performance on four tests of strength, endurance, and flexibility. It found that in every test, students in 1990 performed significantly worse than their peers only a decade earlier—for example, it took them a full minute longer to run a mile.

THE TERRIBLE PRICE OF INACTIVITY

The consequences of this corpulence and inactivity are devastating and will be long-term. According to a study spanning sixty years and published in 1992 in *The New England Journal of Medicine,* being overweight during the teenage years can lead to life-threatening chronic disease in adulthood, even if the individual later sheds the excess weight. In fact, the study indicated that adolescent obesity was even more strongly linked to health risks than being overweight in adult life.

The lasting effects of the chubbing of America's teens are most pronounced among boys. Those in the heaviest quarter of the population in weight relative to height were found to be more likely to suffer fatal heart attacks, strokes, colon cancer, and other health problems before their seventieth birthdays. Men who were overweight as teenagers had death rates nearly double those of men who had been slender during adolescence.

Women who were overweight as teens were found to be at greater risk of developing arthritis, atherosclerosis, and diminished physical abilities. By the time they reached their seventies, these women had trouble coping with the tasks of daily living—climbing stairs, lifting objects, or walking a quarter of a mile.

The study's director, Dr. Aviva Must, an epidemiologist at the Human Nutrition Research Center on Aging at Tufts University in Boston, concluded that it is essential that we prevent overweight in our youth by reducing dietary fat to no more than 30 percent of the calories consumed and by increasing the amount of exercise undertaken. Fortunately these goals can be easily achieved.

STARTING YOUNG

One of the intriguing things about human beings is that we are born knowing how to swim. Place a young child in a bathtub or pool and he or she will paddle around with gusto. You won't see an Olympic-level butterfly or backstroke, but the baby will be swimming. After about six months, the swimming reflex disappears unless it is nurtured.

In recent years programs have been established in different parts of the world to do just that nurturing. In San Diego, for instance, the late multisport coach Murray Callan taught children to swim for almost fifty years. Most of his students came to him before their third birthday.

Callan, a member of the National Swim School Association, demonstrated repeatedly that six-month-olds can easily be taught to swim. Over the years he taught thousands of children to do so. He believed that the benefits of early swimming include better motor skills and improved respiratory function. "A baby who swims early," said Callan, "usually crawls sooner. Babies who are early swimmers also tend to be healthier babies."

Another advantage is that the youngsters become "pool safe," reducing the possibility of an accident. A child is considered pool safe when he or she can fall or jump in and then swim unassisted to the side of the pool. Parents should always remain vigilant, however. Never assume that your young child is completely pool safe.

Callan began by gently placing the infant in ninety-five-degree water in a face-up position. The warm water is soothing and relaxing, and the position ensures that the baby is in no danger of drinking or inhaling the water. As soon as she feels the water on her body, she responds naturally with fluid swimming motions, the back of her head and bottom bobbing on the surface.

Callan did not teach strokes to children under the age of two. Before then they squirm through the water, using one arm or two, one leg or two, eventually arriving at their destinations. "Don't ask very young children to do anything that interferes with their fluid movements" was his advice. After the age of two he began teaching stroke technique.

Generally it takes a six-month-old baby about a year to learn to swim. One-year-old children learn in about six months. Two-year-olds take about four months, three-year-olds about three months, four-year-olds about two months, and children between five and eight only about one month. If you would like information about early childhood swimming programs in your area, contact the National Swim School Association (see Appendix F).

The Ideal Sport for Kids

Children and adolescents must get regular exercise, not only to build lean, trim, attractive bodies but also to develop strength, endurance, agility, and flexibility. As well, good exercise habits established young and nurtured through childhood last for a lifetime, providing health benefits for as long as we live. Perhaps no sport is better for accomplishing all this than swimming.

One key to reaping swimming's benefits for children is to make it fun. There is no reason for young children to engage in heavy training. If the sport becomes drudgery, a child eventually will tire of it and want to quit, losing the pleasant associations with the sport that can provide lifelong benefits. By contrast, if swimming remains fun, children will look forward to practice, and they will be more likely to continue swimming throughout their lives. When my son was in school, I had to drag him out of the pool to get him to come home for dinner. Alexa Schuler, an eleven-year-old girl I know, can't wait to get to her daily practice session. In fact, when she doesn't do her chores at home or finish her homework, her parents threaten that she won't be able to go to practice until her responsibilities are met. This always does the trick.

Health and Fitness Benefits

While an alarming and growing number of America's youth are living a life of indolence and sloth, with calamitous consequences for their futures, many others—hundreds of thousands of youngsters across the nation—are enrolled in organized swimming programs. Their future—and their present—looks very different indeed. A study published in 1991 showed, not surprisingly, that these swimmers are likely to be quite a bit leaner, stronger, and healthier than nonswimmers. They are also less likely to become sick and when they do get sick to recover faster.

Academic Success

There is more: despite devoting an average of five to ten hours per week to working out, youthful swimmers tend to do much better than their peers in their schoolwork.

These results come as no surprise to those of us who have been around the sport for many years. Each issue of *Swimming World* magazine contains short feature articles on four or five youngsters who have achieved outstanding success in swimming for their ages. Almost without exception, these boys and girls between ten and sixteen are also honor students and active in both other sports and other extracurricular activities. In fact, it is almost *expected* that young swimmers will also be outstanding students. This admirable behavior pattern continues through college. In almost every college in the country, members of the swim team have higher graduation rates and higher grade-point averages than other athletes and nonathletes, despite the extra hours they spend in training.

My son, Russell, is a good example of this phenomenon. He began swimming at age seven and continued through college. During that time he also excelled in a variety of other sports, especially gymnastics (in which he also competed in college) but also judo, track and field, volleyball, and basketball. He began taking guitar lessons at the same time he started swimming, and now he composes and performs his own music. Throughout his school career he was an outstanding student, especially in his final three years in college. During that time, he also managed to earn his pilot's license.

One of the happy side effects of swimming is that it teaches self-discipline. Nowadays few other activities do. Few children will grow up to become Olympic champions, but they all can grow up to be winners in the much more important game of life. Besides its many health benefits, swimming teaches its young practitioners important lessons in managing a busy schedule. It also inculcates a sense of responsibility, commitment, and organization that lasts a lifetime.

Few Injuries

Some other sports may confer some of these advantages on young athletes, but swimming has that additional major advantage that will appeal to parents: it is almost injury free. Although an increasing number of American youth are remaining sedentary, the minority that do exercise are becoming more prone to injury. According to orthopedists and pediatricians across the nation, sports-related injuries are cropping up with alarming frequency in children. These injuries usually are caused by overuse, improper technique, poor equipment, and the inability of immature bones, tendons, and joints to handle the stress being placed on them by heavy athletic training and competition.

Such injuries usually respond well to rest, but if ignored they can result in major and at times permanent problems. According to Dr. Barry Goldberg, director of sports medicine at Yale University Health Services, "If kids are caught up in a situation where there is pressure to play through the pain or tough it out, these injuries tend to progress to chronic injury and sometimes lifelong disability, which is really a crime."

Because it takes place in water, a much less stressful environment, swimming results in relatively few children's injuries.

TYPICAL CHILDREN'S SPORTS INJURIES

Baseball: Little League elbow (inflammation where tendon and bone meet at inner elbow); tendinitis and bursitis of shoulder.

Basketball: Schlatter's disease (knee pain resulting from inflammation).

Football: Head injuries, spinal injuries.

Gymnastics: Stress fractures of lower spine and forearms.

Running: Stress fracture of the shinbone, Sever's disease (inflammation where the Achilles tendon attaches to the foot, showing up as heel pain).

Soccer: Sever's disease (see above).

Tennis: Tendinitis (inflammation of tendons) of shoulder and elbow ("tennis elbow").

Age-Group Swimming

Perhaps the most successful sports program for kids is the U.S. national age-group swimming program. There is nothing quite like it in any other sport. Presently more than 220,000 youngsters between the ages of eight and eighteen are enrolled in the United States Swimming (USS) program. Several hundred thousand other kids are involved in similar, less competitive programs in YMCAs, boys' and girls' clubs, Jewish community centers, and country clubs. It is very much because of these programs that the United States has dominated swimming at the international level since the late 1950s, although many other countries are now establishing similar programs.

How the Program Works

There are USS age-group programs in every state of the Union, plus Puerto Rico and Guam. Canada has a similar program. In age-group swimming, boys and girls train together but compete separately. Children are divided into five age-groups: ten and under, eleven and twelve, thirteen and fourteen, fifteen and sixteen, and seventeen and eighteen. Most areas have an eight and under age-group as well, but USS has wisely decided not to make this age-group an official category. Swimmers are rated by their ability in each event, according to national time standards. These standards are C, B, A, AA, AAA, and AAAA. Swimmers even at the B level are impressive athletes. Kids who are A swimmers or better are simply awesome.

U.S. Swimming compiles a list each year of the top sixteen swimmers nationally in each event and age-group. Perusing past lists of top-sixteen swimmers is like reading a who's who of later world and Olympic champions: Janet Evans, Summer Sanders, Tracy Caulkins, Jenny Thompson, Pablo Morales, Mark Spitz, and so on. The program also publishes the national records for every event and age-group. The records as of 1994 appear in Appendix E.

At the local level, meets group swimmers according to ability: B swimmers swim in B meets, A swimmers in A meets, and so on. Once a swimmer has achieved a new time standard, she can no longer compete against lower-rated children (until she moves up to the next age-group). Thus, kids are always competing against their peers in terms of sex, age, and ability.

The top swimmers in each region compete twice yearly in regional championships. Those meeting even tougher national standards can go on to the junior national championships. The cream of the older swimmers, those who meet still tougher standards, can then compete at the senior national championships. (If you would like information about age-group swimming programs in your area, you can contact United States Swimming, Inc. The address and phone number are listed in Appendix F.)

The Birth of Age-Group Swimming

The national age-group program, arguably the most valuable legacy in the history of youth sports, formally began in 1951, but its roots extend back several decades. In 1913 Carl Bauer arrived in the United States from Germany with credentials to spare. As a young man he had distinguished himself in swimming, water polo, soccer, gymnastics, and rowing. All these talents he carried on a six-foot, 190-pound frame, which he kept fit by swimming every day.

After beginning his work in Chicago, he moved to St. Louis in 1917 to become swim coach of the Missouri Athletic Club (MAC), remaining there until his retirement fifty years later. It was at the MAC that Bauer devised an age-group training regimen for the boys' team in 1918. He was convinced that there was a correlation between age and ability; unfortunately, in the 1920s the top officials of the Amateur Athletic Union weren't buying the idea. By the late 1940s, Bauer had become one of the most successful coaches in the land, guiding his team to several national championships, and soon many in swimming started to listen to his ideas more closely.

Beth Kaufman, a swimming mom and Marin County (California) Red Cross water safety chairman, was one of them. In 1950 she convinced AAU officials that a test of Bauer's age-group idea was in order. The following January the first age-group meet was held. The entry fee was twenty-five cents. The meet proved such a success that the program went national the following year. Kaufman, who came to be known as the mother of age-group swimming, became its first chairman, remaining in the position for the next ten years. As an age-grouper myself in California, I remember her well as a thoughtful, enthusiastic, maternal presence at many of the major meets.

Under Kaufman's guidance, the program proved a phenomenal success. She demonstrated conclusively what she had always suspected—that with training and competition geared to age, kids would progress at a more reasonable pace and perform longer in the sport.

It did not take long for results to pour in. In the 1955 Pan-American Games, Mary Lou Elsenius became the first age-group swimmer to win an international gold medal. In 1960 age-group alumna Chris von Saltza was the top medal winner of the Rome Olympics, winning three gold medals and one silver. By 1964 every single member of the U.S. Olympic team was an age-group alumnus, and the United States had thrown down an aquatic gauntlet for the rest of the world.

MASTERS SWIMMING

The crowd's chattering turned to a hush of anticipation as the starter called the swimmers to their marks. Eight muscled bodies leaned from the starting blocks. At the sound of the gun they were off, stroking furiously down the fifty-meter length of the pool. A quick touch, push off the wall, pull underwater, and then back again. As the winner strained for the electronic touch pad, a roar went up from the crowd: just over one minute and fifteen seconds. A new record!

The picture is a familiar one. You have seen it a hundred times before on *Wide World of Sports* and similar programs. Only this time it was different. This time the beaming, ecstatic face of the winner belonged not to a twenty-year-old college student but to forty-five-year-old Manuel Sanguily. The scene was the Brown University pool, site of a special national swimming competition, the U.S. National Masters Swimming Championships. Sanguily, a physician living in Tarrytown, New York, had just smashed the world record for the 100-meter breaststroke for men in his age-group.

Throughout this book I have talked about Masters swimming, a phenomenally successful national swimming program devoted to fitness and competition. Its enthusiasts come in both sexes, in all ages, from nineteen to one hundred plus—in all colors and sizes, from every part of the country, from all walks of life. They include bankers, truck drivers, secretaries, psychologists, doctors, housewives, firemen, blacksmiths, judges, writers, artists, nuns, lawyers, clowns, herpetologists, priests, policemen, presidential candidates, cabinet members, rabbis, teachers, accountants—you name it. There are former Olympic greats, like Tracy Caulkins, and there are tens upon tens of thousands of people who never swam competitively before—some who were unable to swim even one lap a year ago. They swim for many reasons: for health, to lose weight, to reduce stress, for the challenge of training and competing, to renew old rivalries and friendships, to make new friends, to look better and feel better, and they all swim for the sheer fun of it.

The Origin

This is not your typical fast exercise fad, in one year and out the next. The brainchild of Dr. Ransom Arthur, former dean of the University of Oregon Medical School, Masters swimming lets swimmers pursue all the motives just listed and puts the emphasis on lifelong physical fitness. It began in the 1960s, when Dr. Arthur and his colleagues at the Naval Medical Neuropsychiatric Research Unit in San Diego developed prototype swimming programs for adults in the area. Unfortunately, like Carl Bauer before him, Arthur met with little success when he attempted to sell the idea nationally to the AAU and the President's Council on Physical Fitness. Finally, in 1969 he interested John Spannuth, then head of the American Swim Coaches Association, in sponsoring a meet.

Growth

The first Masters meet, held in Amarillo, Texas, in May 1970, drew some sixty-five competitors. Today there are programs in every state and in more than seventy other countries, including all the traditional swimming powers, such as Germany, Japan, Australia, and Russia, and even such unlikely aquatic redoubts as Bangladesh, Pakistan, Fiji, New Guinea, and the United Arab Emirates.

Since 1970 Masters programs have been initiated in other sports, but swimming remains far and away the most popular. The first World Masters Games, held in Toronto in 1985, featured competition in over twenty sports, but more than half of the 5,000 participants were swimmers.

Every year two national championships are held, a short-course (twenty-five-yard pool) meet in May, and a long-course (fifty-meter pool) meet in late summer. Each usually draws upward of 1,500 competitors. National and world top ten rankings are compiled for every event and every age-group, and world records are certified by FINA, swimming's international governing body. Since 1984 there has been a world-championship meet every two years, typically with 4,000 to 5,000 participants. These meets have been held in New Zealand, Japan, Australia, Brazil, the United States, and Canada. Future meets are scheduled for England and Germany. (For information about Masters swimming programs in your area, contact United States Masters Swimming, Inc. The address and phone number are listed in Appendix F.)

How It Works

All the standard events—freestyle, backstroke, breaststroke, butterfly, individual medley, and relays—are included in a Masters meet. There are even several events unique to Masters swimming: 50-yard and 50-meter sprints for backstroke, breaststroke, and butterfly; the 100-yard individual medley; and coed relays, in which teams are composed of two men and two women. Competition is held in five-year age-groups: for example, men thirty-five to thirty-nine and women fifty to fifty-four. In the United States, the youngest age-group is nineteen to twenty-four. Elsewhere, Masters begins with the twenty-five to twenty-nine age bracket.

In many other sports athletes are not defined as "Masters" until they are thirty-five or forty years old. But since the Masters swimming program places primary emphasis on the promotion of lifelong physical fitness for all, it draws people soon after they leave school and begin their careers. Of course, many top athletes continue to perform at the highest level throughout their twenties and thirties, and sometimes even into their early forties. But few of us are elite athletes, and it makes eminently good sense to have a program geared toward ordinary folks.

In the United States alone, more than half a million men and women have participated since the program began. Even more impressive is the far greater number of people who do not compete at all but simply swim to maintain their physical fitness. As has been noted, every survey conducted on physical fitness over the past three decades has concluded that swimming far outstrips in popularity and participation running, aerobics, tennis, and every other sport. These participants in swimming experience the many benefits the sport has to offer: enhanced health and fitness, resistance to disease, stress reduction, greater peace of mind, a more active love life, and an extended life span.

Mani Sanguily, the balding, charismatic physician who smashed the 100-meter breaststroke record for his age-group, is one of the nation's most popular Masters swimmers. In 1956 Sanguily was a flag bearer for his native Cuba at the opening ceremonies of the Melbourne Olympics. While studying for his M.D. at the Ohio State University School of Medicine, he won a gold medal at the Pan American Games and several U.S. national titles. In 1959 he set an American record for the 100-meter breaststroke with a time of 1 minute 14.7 seconds. Then, after almost two decades away from competitive swimming, Sanguily clocked 1:15 for the same event. Several years later, at the age of fifty-one, he duplicated this feat. Today, at the grand age of sixty-one, he has added only three more seconds to his time and is the fastest breaststroke swimmer in the world in his age-group.

Yet the thrill of this kind of victory is not what brought Sanguily back to swimming. "I'd always had this crazy desire to swim across the Hudson River," he told me. (In Tarrytown, New York, the spot where Sanguily wanted to cross, the river is two and a half miles wide.) "I didn't smoke, and I'd been playing tennis regularly, so I thought I was in pretty good shape. Wrong! The first day in the pool, I swam four laps and could barely climb out." After this painful experience, however, things got better. "I was surprised how easy it was to get my stroke back; soon I was going about three thousand yards a day."

The following summer Sanguily swam across the Hudson. Now his river crossing is an annual Labor Day event, a media occasion that draws hundreds of participants, as well as celebrities such as television commentator and former Olympic star Donna DeVarona.

Dr. Sanguily is an energetic man. In addition to his medical practice, he is a leading television spokesman for improving the nation's health care, particularly among Hispanic Americans, doing shows on topics such as diet, hypertension, and smoking. An asthmatic, he is also active in promoting awareness of asthma as a major health problem and of swimming as the best activity for controlling the disease. Despite having a schedule that would exhaust most people, Mani Sanguily gets in his 3,000 yards of swimming, four or five days a week.

GETTING OLDER, GETTING BETTER

The last several decades have become a new age for aging. On the one hand, scientists have begun seriously to probe the mysteries of the aging process. On the other, Masters athletes—particularly swimmers—have challenged socially accepted notions of aging by first testing, then stretching, and then exceeding virtually all the limitations associated with aging. The result is that a new consensus about aging is in the making.

We now know that it is indeed possible to remain physically, mentally, and sexually vigorous throughout middle age and well into the seventies, eighties, and even beyond. We know it because so many people do it. In fact, not only is it possible but I believe it should be considered normal. The key to having a healthy, vital, productive, and long second half century of life is a sound exercise program, such as swimming so consistently provides. This is true in youth, in early adulthood, in middle age, and especially in the later years.

SOME EXTRAORDINARY OLDER FOLKS

During my two decades plus of Masters swimming, I have come across many remarkable, vibrant, and robust older people, men and women who are living examples of what successful aging is all about. Some are top competitors, others swim solely for fitness. Whatever their background, profession, or life-style, they share an openness to new experiences and an extraordinary zest for life. Truly the young at heart, they are the wave of the future, pioneers and role models for the rest of us.

One of these people who comes immediately to mind is Gus Langner, who at ninety-one looks at least twenty-five years younger and has the strength and endurance of a man half his age. Gus holds many Masters world records, including every freestyle record for men ninety to ninety-four, and is able to swim a mile in about thirty-six minutes. He wakes up in the morning eager to squeeze every drop of living from the day. My friend Jack Geoghegan, fifty-two, a successful lawyer and top Masters swimmer in his own right, says in admiration, "When I grow up I want to be Gus Langner."

Then there is seventy-eight-year-old Mardie Brown, whom I told you about in Chapter 1, a great-grandma six times over, who lives on a farm in Palermo, Maine, with her husband, Don. Mardie, whose ready smile is her hallmark, has a figure most women in their thirties and forties can only dream about. Several years ago, while traveling to the World Masters Swimming Championships in Brisbane, Australia, the Browns made two stops. In Honolulu, Mardie took a few days to learn how to surf at Waikiki. Then it was on to Australia's Great Barrier Reef, where they spent several days of spectacular scuba diving.

My good friend Abe Olanoff, eighty-eight, was a wrestler in high school and college. "Never lost a match," he will tell you, "even when I wrestled in a higher weight category." Abe spends much of his time teaching swimming and leather working to the blind and helping older people undergoing physical rehabilitation. A lifeguard for many years, he has been involved in swimming for as long as he can remember, but it wasn't until after he retired in 1972 that he began swimming competitively. He has been at it ever since, recently setting three world records in the eighty-five to eighty-nine age-group.

Abe just "doesn't know from limitations." I recall a sight from 1991, which Abe himself might not remember because it was nothing unusual to him. After winning the 400-meter individual medley at the U.S. national championships, he gripped the edge of the pool and hoisted his body out of the water. No fuss, no bother, no strain. He was eighty-five years old, and he had just finished swimming's most grueling event, one hundred meters each of butterfly, backstroke, breaststroke, and freestyle. Instead of swimming slowly to the side of the pool and climbing out on the ladder, he just boosted himself out of the water. The young soldier from a nearby military base who was serving as a backup timer in Abe's lane was astonished; "Man," he said, "*I* have trouble doing that even when I haven't swum a race."

I could go on and on. I know many people in their sixties and early seventies whose current activities and accomplishments would astonish most folks, but I no longer consider them old. They have been around a good many years, but they are younger, in body, mind, and spirit, than most people many decades their juniors. I would like to tell you about two extraordinary people in their nineties who credit swimming with their incredible vitality.

Martha Munzer

Silver-haired Martha Munzer is a modern Renaissance woman. At age ninety-three, she is more involved in today's burning social issues and has more energy than most people half her age. Regarded as a pioneer and visionary by her peers and an inspiration by all who know her, Munzer is an author, dedicated educator, social crusader, liberated spirit, and plain old truth talker. She is also a lifelong swimmer who attributes her longevity and good health to her practice of swimming every day.

In 1992 she finished work on her tenth book, *Friends of the Everglades: A Living History*. It lays out the environmental crisis the Everglades faces today and recounts the story of Marjory Stoneham Douglas, who heads the organization that is trying to save this unique national treasure. One of her other books, *Pockets of Hope,* is about poor towns throughout the United States that have picked themselves up by their collective bootstraps and transformed themselves into vital, successful communities, often being forced to overcome deep racial prejudice to do so. Six of her other books are about environmental issues and are aimed at young readers.

I met Munzer when she was attending the seventieth reunion of her class at the Massachusetts Institute of Technology. The first woman to earn a degree in electrochemical engineering, she was one of only 20 women in a class of over 2,000. She created quite a stir at the reunion when she insisted on taking her daily swim—this one in Henry David Thoreau's Walden Pond. "I don't know what all the fuss was about," she says with wide-eyed innocence. "The meetings and the parties were great, but I couldn't miss my daily swim. I love to swim, and all I wanted was for someone to drive me out to Walden Pond."

Munzer's love of swimming started when she was a little girl in Far Rockaway, New York, on Long Island. She says, "In the summer I swam in the ocean almost every day. That's when I developed my deep love of the sea." She recalls that bathing suits were a lot different back then: "You had to be completely covered, your legs couldn't show, you even had to wear a hat when you swam. It's a lot better now." She still swims religiously every day, either in the ocean or at a pool near her home in Lauderdale-by-the-Sea, in Florida. "I'm no Janet Evans," she admits, "but I do about twenty laps a day."

Walden Pond is by no means the most unusual place Munzer has swum over the years. She enjoys recounting some of her more exotic aquatic encounters. "About ten years ago I was in Edinburgh, Scotland, and I went swimming in the Firth of Forth. The water was very cold, much colder than Walden Pond, and I was the only one in."

But that wasn't the coldest water she has swum in. "No"—she smiles—"that was in Ketchikan, Alaska, back in the sixties. I was working on a book then, and I was taking a boat around the southwestern part of Alaska. The boat would stop at all the little towns, and the first stop was Ketchikan. I had about an hour, so I jumped off, found a cab, and told the driver to take me to a spot where I could go for a swim. He said, 'Lady, we don't swim in Alaska,' and I said, 'I do,' so he took me to a place on the ocean where the little Indian kids swim. The children were amazed to see me dive in, and the taxi driver thought I was out of my mind, but I had a great time."

There is no doubt in Munzer's mind that regular swimming has contributed to her good health and longevity. "Most people my age have trouble getting around by themselves. I'm not saying I'm as strong as I used to be, but I feel like a woman of sixty." Her prescription: "All I can say is, keep learning, keep marveling, keep laughing—and never stop swimming."

Tom Lane

I met Tom Lane, now one of the nation's oldest Masters swimmers, back in 1978, when he was a lad of eighty-four. I remember how impressed I was by his positive outlook. "Every day I look in the mirror," he told me then. "I say, 'My goodness, that's young Tom Lane in there.'" Fourteen years later I showed up at his doorstep in San Diego, tape recorder in hand, to conduct an interview. The tall, square-shouldered, white-maned gentleman was apologetic when he arrived five minutes late. "Sorry," he said, "I was out shooting nine holes of golf."

Lane exercises every day, and he looks it. Aside from golf ("I always walk the course, never take a cart"), he lifts weights, does calisthenics, bowls, puts the shot, tosses the javelin, and slings the discus, but his favorite form of exercise is swimming. He also continues to manage his own stock portfolio with great success and listens to music and tapes of favorite books. The fact that a bout with glaucoma in 1986 left him blind has not deterred him a bit. "It just presented a new challenge," he says with a smile.

Today, at the age of one hundred, Lane could easily pass for a healthy man in his early seventies. The retired patent lawyer has set Masters records in the backstroke, breaststroke, and freestyle in three age-groups. One of his goals was to become the first person over a century old to compete in Masters competition, but in 1993 he was preempted by two older swimmers. "I've always liked competition, and always liked swimming," he told me. "My mother taught me how to do the breaststroke when I was four. I compete mostly with younger men now; there aren't that many men in my age-group."

But as Masters swimming has continued to grow in popularity, Lane's earlier records have gone by the wayside. "The number of older participants increases each year," he says, "so these young bucks are coming up and breaking my old records. But that's fine. Records are made to be broken. Now that I've moved up to the one hundred and over age-group, though," he says with a gleam in his eye, "my records may last for a spell. Not too many fellas that age are up for a good swimming race. My philosophy has always been, 'If you can't beat 'em, outlive 'em."

Lane is an inspiration for younger people who feel that old age is synonymous with a sedentary life-style. He says that for many people retirement is when an active life can begin, when you can throw yourself into what you really like to do. His coach, Barbara Dunbar, says that Lane is an inspiration for younger people: "It's inspiring for them to see that at a hundred and blind, Tom Lane is strong, extremely bright, and very lucid. It's good for them to see older people in great shape having a good time."

14

GETTING IN SHAPE:
THE INS AND OUTS
OF TRAINING

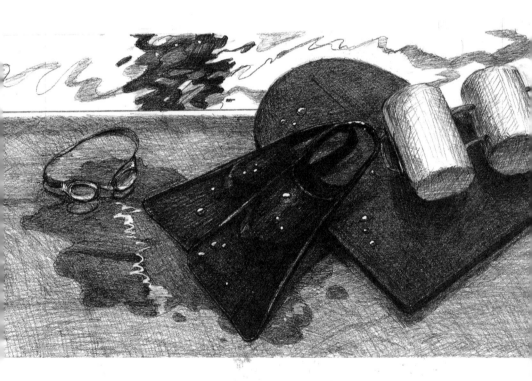

THE MOMENT OF truth has arrived. You have mastered the fundamentals of one or more of the four competitive strokes and even learned how to do a flip turn. Your doctor has given you a green light, and it is time to begin reaping all the benefits swimming can offer you. It is time to start your training. But before you get into the pool and begin churning up the laps, let's get acquainted with the equipment you will be using and with some key training terms and concepts.

TOOLS OF THE TRADE

Pace Clock

To get the most out of your training, you will want to learn how to read a pace clock. It's very easy, especially for those of us who grew up before digital watches. Nowadays most pools are graced with a big pace clock, with large, black second and minute hands (see Figure 14.1); some pools have two of them, one at each end. Since much of your training will consist of timed swims, including interval sets, you will need to know how to use the clock, so take a few minutes to acquaint yourself with it.

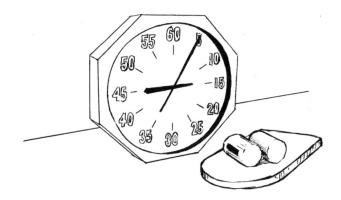

Figure 14.1. The Pace Clock

Later in this chapter we'll discuss interval training in detail. For now, let's say you are doing a set consisting of five 200-yard swims in which you begin each swim every three and a half minutes (5 × 200 on 3:30). You start the set when the second hand is "on the 60" or "on top"—that is, when it is pointing straight up. Your first 200 takes 2:50. You will start the next 200 "on the 30," giving you forty seconds of rest.

Kick Board

One of the most important pieces of training equipment you will use is the kick board. Rectangular in shape, with rounded edges, kick boards usually are made of a light, buoyant material. They vary in size, but most often are about twenty by ten inches, large enough to maintain your body position while you are kicking but small enough to handle easily.

A kick board is used when you want to concentrate solely on your kick. Grip the board about two thirds of the way up, one hand on each side (see Figure 14.2). If you grip the board too near the bottom, your legs will tend to sink. If you grip the top, your body will lie on the board, and your buttocks and feet will come out of the water, an unnatural position for swimming.

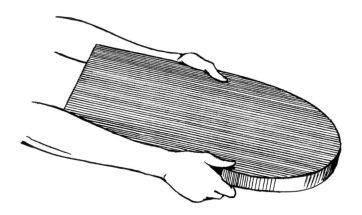

Figure 14.2. The Kick Board

Kicking is an important part of swimming technique, and swimmers find using a kick board, which supports you in the water as you practice kicking technique, an excellent way to tone leg muscles fast. Isolating the leg muscles while maintaining proper body position, a kick board allows you to build leg strength and improve your technique. In addition, because the leg muscles have such bulk and are so far from the heart, the heart must pump a large volume of blood to supply them with oxygen, and this raises your heart rate, an essential element of any aerobic workout.

Do not be discouraged if when you first use a kick board you seem to be making little headway through the water for the energy you are expending. Progress will come quickly if you keep at it. A good friend of mine wanted to incorporate kicking into her exercise program to firm up her thighs and buttocks. The first day it seemed to take her forever to kick one lap of the pool (twenty-five yards). Indeed, if I hadn't been there to encourage her, she might have given up. The next day she kicked two laps, with a short rest between them, and each lap was considerably faster than the one that had been so agonizing the day before. On the third day she made two laps without resting. By the end of two weeks, she was kicking sixteen laps without resting.

Pull Buoy

Pull buoys are used for arms-only swimming, or "pulling." Although they come in a variety of shapes and sizes, most pull buoys are made of a light, buoyant, foamy material and consist of two small cylinders (usually five to seven inches in length and about thirteen inches in circumference) connected by an adjustable cord (see Figure 14.3).

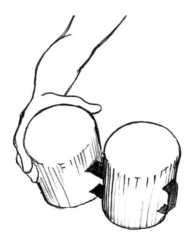

Figure 14.3. The Pull Buoy

You will use a pull buoy when you want to concentrate solely on your arms, either to improve your stroke technique or to increase the stress on your arms and shoulders to strengthen them. Pull buoys are often used in conjunction with other pieces of equipment, such as hand paddles and drag suits.

Place the buoy between your thighs and grip it tightly. Then, simply stroke with your arms without kicking your feet. Because the buoy is buoyant, it will keep your legs elevated, maintaining a proper body position. Try not to let the buoy slip down your legs, because this will adversely affect your body position. Although it may take a little practice, you will even be able to do flip turns while using a pull buoy.

Once you become adept at pulling, you will find that you can go remarkably fast. In fact, many people can pull long distances using just their arms—faster than they can swim. This is because the buoy elevates their legs so that no energy is spent maintaining the heavy leg muscles in a proper streamlined position.

Like many swimmers, I often incorporate pulling in my workout. Sometimes I pull during my warm-up, concentrating on stroke technique and hand position and focusing on breathing bilaterally. At other times, I do a "pull set" (for example, 5 × 100 on 1:20—five 100-yard swims leaving every minute and twenty seconds) as one of the interval sets in my workout.

Hand Paddles

Using hand paddles is a form of aquatic resistance training, an excellent way to strengthen the muscles of the arms, shoulders, chest, and upper back. Usually made of a hard, plastic material, hand paddles come in a variety of shapes but are basically rectangular. On top they have two arcs of rubber tubing (see Figure 14.4). Simply slide your fingers through the first arc, place your middle finger through the second, and you are ready to go.

Because the paddles make your hand larger, you encounter greater resistance as you move them through the water. This not only works the specific muscles you need for swimming but also causes your heart to work harder. One of the key values of hand paddles is that they force you to move your hands correctly, elbows high, in the S-pattern described in Chapters 6 through 10. If you drop your elbows, you will immediately find that your paddles "slip" and you get no propulsion at all.

A constant temptation with paddles is to grip the edges with your thumb and little finger, thus guiding them through the water and preventing slipping. But this defeats one of their major purposes: to force you to stroke properly even when your muscles begin to tire—and when you first start using paddles you will tire very quickly.

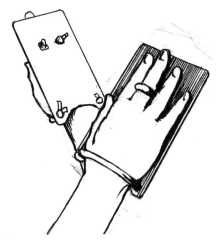

Figure 14.4. Hand Paddles

Paddles are often used along with a pull buoy. This results in even greater stress on your upper-body muscles. But a word of caution: build up the distance you swim using hand paddles gradually. At the first sign of pain or soreness, stop. Don't push it! For many people, particularly adults, the additional shoulder stress can result in injurv.

Fins

You probably thought that fins were used only by snorkelers and scuba divers. Or perhaps you have seen them simply as toys for children playing in the water. But in recent years fins have become an important piece of equipment used both in training and in teaching certain techniques.

Swim fins work by increasing the surface area of your feet, letting you exert more pressure on the water. This in turn helps you move faster. There are several benefits to using fins, among them that they help you develop leg strength, allow you to practice swimming at race speed, and increase your ankle flexibility (see Figure 14.5).

Fins are also an excellent way to accelerate the healing of a sprained or strained ankle. According to a recent study in *The Physician and Sportsmedicine* by Dr. James Larson, kicking with fins helps you recover strength and range of motion. The water dampens sudden stress while the fins provide additional resistance to rebuild ankle strength.

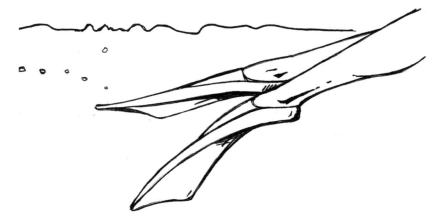

Figure 14.5. Swim Fins

Occasionally I incorporate kicking with fins into my warm-up or as a set in my workout. For example, my warm-up may include a 500-yard backstroke kick with fins, in which I make sure I go at least ten yards underwater using a reverse dolphin kick on every turn (eight to twelve kicks). This improves my ankle flexibility, helps me think about my turns, and increases my lung capacity. Sometimes I will try to make each one hundred yards faster than the one before, or I may do a set of freestyle, backstroke, or butterfly kicks with fins. A typical set would be five or ten 100s, leaving every 1:20.

A problem with using fins in workouts is that they tend to become addictive. They are so much fun that you may find yourself coming up with excuses for using them more and more. Resist! I limit my fin use to two or three times a week, and a maximum of 1,000 yards each time.

Swim fins are also useful in learning to swim the butterfly, back-stroke, and breaststroke correctly. In the butterfly they provide extra power and help develop the undulating motion that characterizes the stroke.

In the backstroke, they are doubly useful. As you are learning the stroke, fins will keep you from dragging your feet and assist you in maintaining the proper body position. They will also help you learn the "Berkoff blastoff," the underwater reverse dolphin kick many backstroke swimmers now use on their starts and turns.

Many coaches have their swimmers use fins when they are learn-ing the dolphin breaststroke or the new wave-action breaststroke (see Chapter 9). The fins are useful both in learning the rhythm of the stroke and in maintaining a high body position.

Training Fins

But plain old swim fins may be obsolescent. Since 1990 increasing numbers of swimmers at all levels have been using a new generation of training fins. The most popular are called Zoomers, a sort of superfin created for the serious swimmer. Zoomers are performance fins shorter than regular fins. They were invented by Marty Hull, a former California dentist who is now a full-time inventor and designer of exercise equipment (see Figure 14.6). He is also one of the top Masters swimmers in the world.

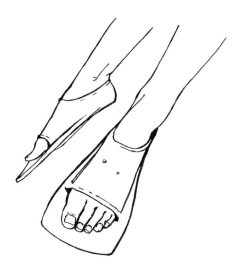

Figure 14.6. Zoomers, a New Superfin

Zoomers provide an effective, specific weight workout in the water. The idea behind them is simple: they allow you to employ the full range of motion you use when racing, at the same or slightly higher speeds, and with significantly greater force. The result is muscles built in the precise proportions needed for a particular swimming movement.

The highly successful Stanford University men's and women's teams use Zoomers during 40 percent or more of their workouts. Basically the fins are used two ways: during regular interval training and for high-speed sprinting. When worn during normal sets, Zoomers provide high-level cardiovascular conditioning, but because you go faster when wearing them, the rest intervals are a little longer than usual to allow for sufficient recovery.

Kicking sprints, called *shooters,* are done underwater without breathing. Swimmers use either a freestyle kick or a reverse dolphin kick (underwater). A set of shooters consists of ten to twenty one-lap (twenty-five yards or fifty meters) sprints swum all-out. Between sprints swimmers either rest or swim an easy lap or two.

Swimming sprints consist of a set of 25-, 50-, or 100-yard high-speed swims with sufficient rest between each sprint to recover.

By 1993 other manufacturers, including Barracuda, Force Fin, Hyperfin, and Speedo, had introduced their own training fins to compete with Zoomers.

Other Equipment

As mentioned in Chapter 6, many swimmers wear two, three, or even more suits while working out. This time-honored practice has a dual purpose: it allows you to extend the life of worn-out, threadbare swimsuits which, if worn alone, might well expose you to obscenity statutes; and it increases resistance while you are training. When the time finally comes to squeeze into only one Lycra suit for your big race, your body will seem lighter, and you will feel as though you are slipping through the water.

From time to time you may find yourself using additional paraphernalia as you work out. Many swimmers train with a drag suit, especially during the early part of the season. Developed by Doc Counsilman, it is worn over your swimsuit and features strategically located pockets that catch the water as you swim forward, greatly increasing the resistance you encounter. The harder you swim, the greater the resistance. Swimming even a few hundred yards while wearing a drag suit can be exhausting, especially at first. But it is a great way to build conditioning.

A new piece of equipment based on the same principle is the Swim Chute, a parachute manufactured by KYTEC. Here an adjustable parachute, attached by straps to your waist, is dragged behind you. Again: the harder you swim, the greater the resistance.

Some swimmers wear small weights around their wrists or biceps while training. Again, the theory is a familiar one: overload the muscles during training to build strength.

Another way to increase resistance and build strength is to place a small inner tube around your ankles. This prevents you from using your legs at all. Some swimmers like to use a tube in conjunction with a pull buoy, paddles, and a drag suit.

Bill Mulliken, an Olympic breaststroke champion and now a successful corporate lawyer in Chicago, often wears sneakers and tights when he practices his breaststroke kick. Other swimmers use webbed gloves to improve their feel for the water. Some of the gear you will need may be supplied by the pool where you train. The rest may be purchased in sporting-goods shops, through catalogs, or directly from the manufacturer. Appendix B provides a list of places from which you can order any of the paraphernalia just discussed.

The inventory of innovative swimming techniques and equipment is almost endless. One technique, which uses half-inch surgical tubing, is called "tethered swimming." After making loops at each end of the tubing, wrap the middle of it around a stationary object at the end of the pool. A ladder or starting block will do just fine. Next, slip the loops around your waist. Then start swimming. As you swim away from the edge, the tubing begins to stretch. When it is stretched as far as it will go, you must swim powerfully to prevent being pulled back.

A high-tech version utilizing the same principle involves the use of a flume. This is the aquatic equivalent of a treadmill. A swimmer swims against an adjustable current of water, trying to maintain position. A flume allows a swimmer to get a good workout even in a very small pool, and it helps a coach who wants to critique a swimmer's stroke technique.

One of the world's most sophisticated flumes, used to analyze the strokes of America's elite swimmers, is located at the U.S. Olympic Training Center in Colorado Springs. But many small pools around the country now feature flumes. Even small home pools can use them. In 1993 manufacturers introduced several low-priced flumes for use in backyard pools.

THE LANGUAGE OF SWIMMING

An important part of becoming a swimmer involves learning the "language" of swimming—the basic terms and concepts that are as much a part of the sport as "line drive," "pop up," "home run," "fungo," "spring training," and "sacrifice fly" are a part of baseball lingo. You have already been introduced to many of the basic terms in Chapters

6 through 10. Some terms and concepts are the same as in other sports—"interval training" and "split times," for example. Others are unique to swimming. In any event, learning this special language is both fun and easy, and you will find that in a very short time it will be almost second nature to you.

Interval Training

One of the techniques you will be using to enhance the quality of your workouts is called interval training. Swimmers have used this tool for over thirty years, and recently it has been adopted by runners. Although coaches and trainers have long been convinced of the value of interval training, and of its superiority over long swims or runs, it was not until 1992 that it became clear exactly why the technique is so effective. After all, both interval training and long swims (and runs) elevate the heart rate to within the training range. This means that both techniques provide similar, if not identical, cardiovascular benefits.

The reason interval training is so valuable can be explained with three letters: hGH. Human growth hormone is the key hormone discussed in Chapter 5 that is responsible for building muscle mass and reducing body fat. The hormone is secreted by the body during exercise, and it turns out, according to a study by William J. Kraemer of the Center for Sports Medicine at Pennsylvania State University, that the best way to maximize the secretion of hGH during exercise is to perform a series of relatively intense repetitions with limited rest between. In other words, interval training.

Interval training features the set. A *set* consists of a series of swims, each a certain distance, done at a specific time interval. Each individual swim is called a *repeat*. Here are some of the major types of interval sets.

Holding your repeats
In one kind of set, you will want to hold your repeats steady. For example, let's say that your fastest 200-yard freestyle is 2:30. You might want to do a set of six 200-yard swims, starting every three minutes and thirty seconds. If you swim at 80 percent of your current ability, a reasonable expectation, you will do each repeat in 3 minutes. That will give you 30 seconds' rest between each 200-yard swim. As you might imagine, the first 200-yard swim will be relatively

easy; in fact, you might be tempted to go faster than 3:00. Don't! Until you are in excellent shape, you'll find it progressively harder to hold each repeat at 3:00.

Naturally, when you start training your conditioning and endurance will leave a great deal to be desired. But as you get into better shape, you'll find sets like the one just described easy to do. At this point you will want to reduce the resting time between repeats.

Two months have passed. Your fastest 200-yard freestyle is down to 2:25 and you're in much better shape. Now, instead of doing a set of six 200-yard repeats on 3:30, you drop the interval to 3:15 and try to hold each repeat at 2:50. And so on.

LOFO

"Last one, fast one" is another way to enhance the training benefits of an interval set. These sets were a favorite of my coach, Peter Farragher. In a LOFO set you hold the first five repeats at your designated time (2:50 in the preceding example). Then you swim the final repeat all-out, as fast as you can.

A more advanced technique is the *descending set*. Here the objective is to swim each repeat a little faster than the previous one—not so easy, since you become increasingly fatigued. Descending sets are also useful in developing an internal sense of pace. When I swim an event, whether in practice or in a meet, I almost always know my time to within a few tenths of a second.

An alternate kind of descending set is the *descending rest interval*. Here you hold your time steady for each repeat, but you decrease resting time between repeats. For example, let's say that you want to swim 10 × 100 yards holding 1:20. After the first swim you rest for 50 seconds; you drop your rest to 45 seconds after the second swim, to 40 seconds after the third, and so on. Finally, you have only 10 seconds' rest before your last 100-yard swim.

In another kind of set, your aim is a *negative split* of each repeat. Negative splitting, which involves swimming the second half of any distance faster than the first half, is a valuable training and racing skill. Let's say your set consisted of 5 × 200 on 3:00. Your goal is not just to hold each 200-yard swim at 2:45 but to swim the second 100 yards of each repeat 5 seconds faster than the first; your first 100 yards might be 1:25 and your second 1:20. Now you must be aware not only of your overall pace but also of your pace for each segment of each repeat.

A further variation on the same theme is a *descending set, negative splitting each repeat*. Again, let's say your set consists of 5 × 200 on 3:00. Now you swim the first repeat in 2:45, with splits of 1:24 and 1:21. On the second repeat you finish in 2:42, with splits of 1:22 and 1:20, and so on.

Still another type of interval set is the *pyramid*. Here you hold your rest interval steady but gradually increase, then decrease, the distance of each repeat. Usually you also try to hold a steady pace. A typical pyramid set consists of a 100, 200, 300, 400, 300, 200, and 100-yard swim. Let's say your rest interval is 30 seconds between repeats, and you try to hold a 1:30 pace. You swim the first 100 yards in 1:30, then rest for 30 seconds. The next repeat is a 200-yard swim, which you do in 3:00. Rest another 30 seconds. Then swim 300 yards in 4:30, and so on. As you can imagine, it becomes progressively harder to hold your 1:30 pace. There are also many variations on the pyramid.

Distance per Stroke (dps)

Why does Matt Biondi swim faster than you—or me, or just about anyone? Part of the answer lies in his natural ability, his years of training, and his positive mental attitude. His height (six feet, six inches) is also an asset. But the key to Matt's success may well lie in the efficiency of his stroke.

I remember watching Matt compete in the 1987 NCAA championships. I was amazed when I counted his strokes in the 100- and 200-yard freestyle—sprint events—and found that he took only twelve long, smooth strokes per (twenty-five-yard) lap. Jeff Rouse, America's fastest backstroker in the early 1990s, uses only eleven or twelve strokes per lap. The top breaststroke and butterfly swimmers typically need merely six or seven strokes for each lap they swim. Clearly these athletes are on to something.

In contrast, fitness swimmers generally take twenty to twenty-five strokes to swim a lap of freestyle or backstroke. Breast and fly may take more than a dozen strokes. Novice swimmers take even more. Top-flight Masters swimmers usually use fifteen to eighteen strokes for a lap of free and back, and eight or nine for breast and fly.

A computer-aided study published in 1992 suggests that length of stroke is indeed a major key to success. Dr. Richard C. Nelson, a professor of biomechanics at Penn State University, looked at 500 swimmers who competed in the Seoul Olympics. He found that the faster a swimmer performed, the longer his or her strokes were. "It seems to indicate," he concluded, "that training should focus on establishing a maximum stroke length."

Actually, many coaches have been doing just that, at least since the 1970s. They call it *distance per stroke,* or *dps* for short. These coaches emphasize the importance of maintaining a long stroke even—or rather *especially*—as you feel yourself tiring. I count strokes almost every lap of every workout and in every lap of every race.

You might want to try it too. Swim a hundred yards freestyle at a moderately fast clip, remembering to count the strokes you take for each lap. Let's say you take nineteen, twenty, twenty-one, and twenty-one strokes and swim 1:30. Next, set yourself the goal of swimming the same time taking nineteen strokes for each lap. Feel yourself stretch each stroke as your arm enters the water and as you pull through the stroke cycle. Once you have accomplished that, try reducing the strokes to eighteen per lap. Then try to lower your time to 1:28 or 1:25, maintaining eighteen strokes per lap. And so on. This exercise will focus your mind on making your stroke as long and efficient as you can. The result will be that you swim more efficiently, faster and with less effort.

The Taper

Tapering is a key element in preparing for your most important meets. Most experts agree that it is not possible to "peak"—that is, swim the fastest you are capable of—more than twice a year, and having a successful taper, or "hitting your taper," as swimmers say, is a major factor in determining whether you will peak or not.

When you taper, you gradually decrease the amount of yardage you swim during each training session. At the same time, you rest longer both during and between your sets, and you increase the quality and intensity of your sprints. The idea is that after months of building strength and cardiovascular conditioning, you can peak by giving your body additional rest and by swimming in practice at close to race speed.

The taper begins several weeks before your big meet. Exactly how long it should last varies from person to person; you will have to learn what is best for you from experience. But among the important considerations are the yardage "base" you have put in over the previous several months, your age, and your body's ability to recover.

If I have been able to train consistently, a typical taper for me takes about three weeks. During that time I gradually decrease the distance I swim daily from about 4,000 to only 1,500 yards. Finally, the day before the big meet I may not swim at all.

Broken swims are often used during the taper to give you a sense of how fast you are likely to go in your big meet. In a typical broken swim, you take a brief rest at the halfway point, then an even shorter rest at the three-quarters mark. Your time is the total elapsed time minus the resting time.

When I do a "broken" 200-yard swim, I usually rest for fifteen seconds after the first 100 yards and another ten seconds after 150. In a "broken" 100, I rest for ten seconds at the fifty-yard mark and five seconds more at the seventy-five.

A typical broken 200-yard breaststroke for me is as follows:

100 yards—1:14 (rest 15 seconds to 1:29)
150 yards—2:06 (rest 10 seconds to 2:16)
200 yards—2:54

My time for the 200 yards is the total elapsed time (2:54) minus the 25 seconds I rested, or *2:29*. This is often a remarkably accurate predictor of how fast I will swim under race conditions.

One of the most distinctive rituals of swimming is *shaving down* before a big meet. Swimmers shave their legs, arms, and chest to decrease water resistance. Some high school and college swimmers also shave their heads, but wearing a cap provides the same benefit. I'm worried that if I shave my head the hair may never grow back, and I'm not ready yet for the Yul Brynner look.

Shaving was introduced on the international swimming scene at the 1956 Olympics by Australian sprinter Jon Henricks. He was so embarrassed at having denuded himself of body hair that he wore a robe literally until he mounted the starting blocks. "I looked like a plucked chicken," he said later. But the saucy Aussie blasted to victory in the 100-meter freestyle, swimming's glamour event, in record time. His teammates took notice and quickly followed suit. The result was that Australia dominated the competition as never before or since, winning every freestyle event for both men and women. But the secret was out; by the early 1960s, shaving down before the big meet had become a swimming ritual around the world.

And *ritual* is the right word. Many teams conduct "shaving parties" a day or so before their major competition. On the day of the meet, many swimmers can be found in the showers trimming the shave they did the day before to remove any hair that has grown in the interim.

Nonswimmers often ask if shaving really helps you go faster, or whether it is all in the mind. The unequivocal answer is *it really helps. And* it helps psychologically. Careful scientific studies have demonstrated repeatedly that shaving can reduce a swimmer's time by about 2 to 3 percent, depending on just how hirsute he or she was before shaving. Two or 3 percent can easily be the difference between winning and finishing last in the Olympics or the Masters world championships.

It also feels great! Although the total amount of hair removed probably weighs only a few ounces at most, you feel much "lighter" after shaving. You seem to glide effortlessly through the water like a dolphin. And, contrary to what I have been told hundreds of times, the hair is not coarser or darker when it grows back. It comes back just as it was before.

POOL ETIQUETTE

You are just about ready to begin training. But before you do, a brief word about pool etiquette is in order. Every day more people are getting in the swim. Indeed, in many parts of the country, pools are filled to capacity. These people range in ability from rank beginner to accomplished athlete; from individuals who are focused completely on their own movement up and down the pool to those who are continuously aware of the position of every person in their lane. To avoid conflict, and make everyone's experience more enjoyable, a number of conventions have grown up over the years. Here they are in brief:

Conventions

1. **Lane designations.** In most pools, lanes are designated as slow, medium, or fast. These are relative terms. Choose a lane compatible with your speed, then notify the others in the lane that you are joining them.
2. **Swimming pattern.** If there are two of you in a lane, you may opt to keep to one side of the lane; the other swimmer will stay on the opposite side. Three or more swimmers in a lane must *circle*

swim: In the United States, Canada, and most of the rest of the world, the custom is to stay to the right, that is to swim counter-clockwise. (As you might expect, in Great Britain, Australia, and a few other Commonwealth outposts, swimmers circle clockwise. When *will* these people get it right?)

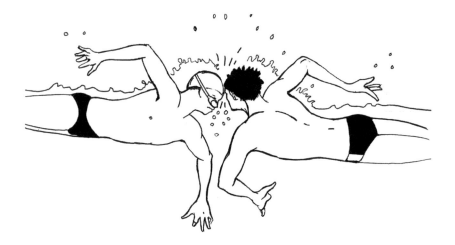

3. **Joining a workout.** If there is a workout set in progress, you may join only as a part of the set.
4. **Speed.** Slower swimmers must yield to faster swimmers.
5. **Passing.** Pass on the left (on the right in the United Kingdom and Down Under). Tap the foot of the person in front of you before passing. If you are being overtaken at the turn, stop, and wait until the other swimmer has pushed off.

In addition, observing several rules of common courtesy will be helpful.

Courtesy

1. Do not stand in front of the pace clock.
2. **Entering.** When you enter the water, never dive, jump, or push off into oncoming swimmers. Wait until they have made the turn and pushed off.
3. **Stopping.** If you need to stop, squeeze into the corner to the right of oncoming swimmers, so they will have sufficient room to turn.

4. Push off underwater. This will reduce the waves encountered by oncoming swimmers.
5. At all times be aware of what is going on within your lane. Also, try not to kick or swing your arms into another lane.
6. Keep your toenails and fingernails trimmed.

COME ON BABY, WORK OUT

If you observe these commonsense conventions and courtesies, every swim session should be an enjoyable, invigorating experience.

Now it's down to the real nitty-gritty: the workout. Here is where everything you have learned finally comes together. As mentioned before, one of the things that make swimming so interesting is the almost infinite variety of ways it allows you to work your body and cardiovascular system. As you read earlier in this chapter, in addition to practicing the four competitive strokes, you can use a kick board to work your legs, a pull buoy with or without hand paddles to concentrate on your arms and upper body, flippers to work on speed and ankle flexibility, or Zoomers to increase your yardage at race pace.

Training Specificity

I have always believed in the importance of *quality training* and *training specificity.* If you want to swim fast in competition, you have to swim fast in practice. Swimming endless laps at an easy pace, the aquatic equivalent of jogging, will make you stronger and improve your cardiovascular fitness, and these are important benefits of fitness swimming. But easy lap swimming will do precious little to help you swim faster. To swim fast, your body needs to adjust to the demands that fast-pace swimming will place on it. The only way this will occur is for you and your body to experience those demands during training.

The Workout

Ideally, you should train with a coach and a group of fellow swimmers. But if you are working out on your own, certain elements should be included in all your workouts. Appendix A provides a series of sample workouts at three levels: the fitness or lap swimmer, the intermediate swimmer, and the advanced or competitive Masters swimmer. Each workout lasts no more than one hour. But these samples are meant to be just that. After a while you will be able to write your own workouts, providing yourself almost infinite variety and enabling you to work on your strengths and weaknesses, or simply those aspects of swimming you enjoy most.

Most of the workouts I do follow a basic structure:

1. **Stretching.** Especially for the adult swimmer, and especially in the morning, it is important to do a few stretching exercises to limber up your muscles before you begin training. Take about five minutes to stretch your legs, shoulders, and back before entering the water.

2. **Warm-up.** This is an easy swim designed to get your muscles warm and your body in motion before beginning the major parts of your workout. Warm-up swims range from about 200 to 1,000 yards. Swimmers usually mix strokes and sometimes include some kicking or pulling.

3. **Kick, pull, or drill set (followed by an easy swim).** These sets are done to allow you to focus on and strengthen particular aspects of your swimming skills. To concentrate on your arm stroke, you may want to do a pull set using a pull buoy—say, 5 × 100 yards with 30 seconds' rest between each repeat. In addition, you might want to focus on your breathing pattern and try to increase lung capacity. If so, you can, try to swim the set alternating your breathing pattern: on laps 1 and 3 you may breathe every third stroke, whereas on laps 2 and 4 you will breathe every fifth stroke. I usually swim a pull set one day and a kick set the next. *Drills,* which are described briefly in Appendix A, are particularly useful in helping you improve your stroke technique, and even the greatest swimmers in the world incorporate drill sets into their workouts almost every day. After this set, swim an easy one hundred yards or so to warm down.

4. **Major set (followed by an easy swim).** This is the key focus of each workout. The major set will vary, depending on which stroke or strokes you want to concentrate on, how far along you are in your training, and, if you are a competitive swimmer, whether it is the beginning, middle, or end of the season. Accordingly, you may have only very short rests (5 to 10 seconds) between repeats (at the beginning or middle of the season) or long rests (at the end). The most important thing is to make sure that you put all your effort into each repeat. A favorite midseason set of mine is to swim 5 × 100 yards

breaststroke on 1:30, trying to descend each swim. When I am in good shape, I will start out at about 1:22 for the first one, then gradually bring my time down about half a second for numbers 2, 3, and 4, then try to blast the final swim at about 1:15. Following the major set, do an easy swim of about one hundred yards.

5. **Timed swim (followed by an easy swim).** Although not all coaches feature this element in their workouts, I like to include an all-out effort almost every time. This is usually a kicking or pulling swim (say 500 yards kicking or pulling) or an event that is *not* swum at meets (for instance, 500 yards backstroke). I keep a record of how I do each time, and my goal is to swim the event faster than I did the previous time.

6. **Sprints.** *If you want to swim fast, you have to practice swimming fast.* This is the rule of specificity of training. Although sprints are hard to do, especially near the end of a training session, it is important to include a sprint set in your workout at least twice a week. As mentioned earlier, many top swimmers now do their sprint sets with Zoomers. Two typical sprint sets are 5 × 50 yards freestyle with 30 seconds' rest and 8 × 25 yards free with 30 seconds' rest, trying to hold your breath for each sprint. (As you get in shape, you will find your lung capacity increasing significantly. During a taper, you may replace a sprint set with a broken swim.)

7. **Warm-down.** This is an important, often neglected, part of every training session. Swim a slow, easy 100 to 200 yards to allow your muscles to rid themselves of the lactic acid that has built up during the workout. An easy warm-down is essential to eliminate muscle soreness. A study published in 1994 indicates that it is also the key to avoiding a heart attack following intense training.

Planning Your Training Season

To keep track of your progress—and you will find that you improve very quickly, especially in your first few months of training—you should create a plan for yourself, one that is as specific as possible. This plan should include an overview of your season (if you intend to compete), your interim and ultimate goals (see the last section in this chapter), a regular training time, and a realistic training schedule.

One of the hardest things for adult athletes is finding time to train. After all, we are busy with our families and jobs. The only way to handle this situation is to make your training a high-priority item, a *given*. Set aside a specific forty-five minutes or hour—whatever is reasonable considering all the demands on your time—*and stick to it*. Yes, there will be times when something comes up that will keep you from the pool—a sick child or a business meeting that can only take place at a certain time—but barring these exceptions, stick to your plan.

Ideally you should try to work out with a group. Swimming with others is easier and more enjoyable than working out by yourself. Many community centers and Y's have Masters swimming groups that work out early in the morning, at noon, or after work. These groups are usually very supportive, with swimmers helping one another on stroke technique, pacing, and so on. But if you cannot find a group with a compatible schedule, train on your own.

TIPS FOR TRAINING

At last you are ready to begin training. Whether you are training simply to improve your cardiovascular fitness, because you aspire to conquer the English Channel, or because you want to compete in the Iron Man Triathlon, chances are you will use the freestyle most of the time. But try to incorporate the other strokes into your workouts as well.

Variety is the spice of life, and, as emphasized earlier, one of the most appealing things about swimming is the great variety of ways you can use it to work your body and cardiovascular system. I also suggest that you use flip turns during practice sessions. (Of course, if you are in an ocean or a lake, there won't be a whole lot of opportunities to do flip turns.) But doing them in practice will keep you from grabbing an extra second or two of rest on the turns, and it will help increase your lung capacity. For years I avoided doing flip turns on swims over a hundred yards. Then, six years ago, I simply made up my mind I would do them on every turn when I was swimming freestyle. Within a few weeks I had achieved my goal. Now it is simply a matter of course that I flip all my turns.

SETTING GOALS

In swimming, as in all athletic endeavors, it is important to give your-self something to strive for. You should set both interim and ultimate goals, and they should be both difficult and realistic. If your best time for the mile swim is twenty-six minutes, an ultimate goal might be twenty-two minutes. But you must face that you are not going to get there all at once. Set an interim goal of, say, twenty-five minutes, and make sure to savor that feeling of accomplishment when you achieve it. Then set out to reach your next interim goal—say twenty-four and a half minutes.

Your goal can be much more modest. If you haven't exercised for years, and were never much of a swimmer to begin with, your ulti-mate goal the first season might simply be to swim a mile without stopping. If you can only make two laps (50 yards) before becoming winded the first time out, don't be discouraged. Set an interim goal of twenty laps, or 500 yards. Each time you work out, say three times a week, decide to do a nonstop swim in which you try to go one lap farther than you did the previous time. It will be difficult at first, but eventually adding that lap will not be difficult at all. In just a few weeks you will have reached your first interim goal. Then set your next interim goal, 1,000 yards, without stopping.

Whatever your level of swimming, keep your eye on the prize—your ultimate goal—but enjoy that delicious feeling of success at each small step along the way.

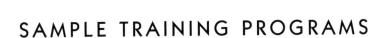

SAMPLE TRAINING PROGRAMS

COACHED MASTERS WORKOUTS are held in all fifty states in the United States and in every province in Canada. You can find out if there is an organized workout program in your area by calling the U.S. Masters Swimming national office (508-886-6631). If there are no programs near you or if the workout schedules do not match your schedule, you will have to work out on your own, or, preferably, with a partner.

This appendix provides a sampling of workouts and stroke drills to help you get the most out of the limited time you have available for getting—and staying—in shape. Most of the workouts have been adapted from those prepared by the coaching staff of the Southern California Aquatics Masters (SCAQ) swim team in Los Angeles. The goal is to optimize your time and efforts in the pool. Each workout is given at three levels:

- Fitness/Lap swimmer
- Intermediate swimmer
- Advanced Masters swimmer

The drills are for *everyone*. Swimming is unlike running in that technique can be as important as conditioning. This means that if you work diligently on perfecting your stroke technique, you can continue improving your times in your forties, fifties, and even sixties and seventies. Even

Olympic champions spend a few minutes every day working on their technique. The drills here will help you improve your skills no matter what your ability level.

WORKOUTS

Workouts for Beginners

Before you start doing the workouts described here, you should be able to swim at least 500 yards (twenty lengths of a standard, twenty-five-yard pool) without stopping. Once you've learned how to swim freestyle, or one of the other strokes described in Chapters 7 through 10, it will be fairly easy to build up to 500 continuous yards. Don't be intimidated. The trick is to increase your yardage gradually. If you can swim 50 continuous yards now, in a few weeks 500 yards will be a piece of cake.

The following is a program you can follow to build up to the 500-yard level. If you find them too easy, you may want to skip the first few workouts: *begin at your current level of ability and fitness.*

I recommend that you swim only three times a week at first. As always, if you are over thirty, be sure to have a medical exam before starting your program and once a year thereafter.

Here is a three-week program to get you ready for the fitness/lap swimmer level of training. The first workout will take you only ten to fifteen minutes. That's enough for the first time. By the time you finish the ninth workout, you'll be swimming almost a mile, and it should take you between forty and fifty minutes. Now, let's get started.

Workout 1
Swim 50 yards. Rest 1 to 3 minutes.
Kick 2 × 25 yards with a kick board, resting between laps.
Swim 50 yards.
Total: 150 yards

Workout 2
Swim 75 yards. Rest 1 to 3 minutes.
Swim 50 yards. Rest 1 to 3 minutes.
Kick 3 × 25 yards, resting between laps.
Swim 50 yards.
Total: 250 yards

Workout 3
Swim 100 yards. Rest 1 to 3 minutes.

Pull 50 yards with a pull buoy. Rest 1 minute.
Kick 2 × 50 yards. Rest 2 minutes between fifties.
Swim 100 yards.
Total: 350 yards

Workout 4

Swim 150 yards. Rest 1 to 2 1/2 minutes.
Kick 2 × 75 yards. Rest 2 minutes after each.
Pull 2 × 50 yards. Rest 2 minutes after each.
Swim 100 yards.
Total: 500 yards

Workout 5

Swim 100 yards easy warm-up.
Kick 2 × 75 yards. Rest 2 minutes after each.
Swim 200 yards. Rest 2 minutes.
Pull 2 × 75 yards. Rest 2 minutes after each.
Swim 100 yards.
Total: 700 yards

Workout 6

Swim 100 yards easy warm-up.
Kick 2 × 100 yards. Rest 2 minutes after each.
Swim 300 yards. Rest 3 minutes.
Kick 2 × 50 yards. Rest 1 1/2 minutes after each.
Pull 150 yards.
Swim 50 yards easy warm-down.
Total: 900 yards

Workout 7

Swim 100 yards easy warm-up.
Kick 2 × 100 yards. Rest 1 1/2 minutes.
Swim 400 yards. Rest 3 minutes.
Kick 4 × 50 yards. Rest 1 minute after each.
Pull 200 yards.
Swim 100 yards easy warm-down
Total: 1,200 yards

Workout 8

Swim 100 yards easy warm-up.
Kick 2 × 100 yards. Rest 1 1/2 minutes.
Swim 500 yards. Rest 3 minutes.
Kick 4 × 50 yards. Rest 1 minute after each.
Pull 2 × 125 yards.
Swim 100 yards easy warm-down.
Total: 1,350 yards

Workout 9
Swim 100 yards easy warm-up.
Kick 3 × 100 yards. Rest 1 1/2 minutes.
Swim 500 yards. Rest 2 minutes.
Kick 4 × 75 yards. Rest 1 minute after each.
Pull 2 × 150 yards.
Swim 150 yards easy warm-down.
Total: 1,650 yards

You now are ready to do the fitness/lap swimmer level of the following workouts. These are harder than the beginner workouts you've just completed. Again, I recommend that you swim only three times a week until your body becomes acclimated to your new regime. After that, try to build up to five times a week. At a minimum, you should swim two to three times every week.

NINE DYNAMITE WORKOUTS

An Early Season Workout

Just as the leaves begin to fall and nature takes on a different style and appearance, Masters and fitness swimmers may also be going through a seasonal transition from summer to fall. Long course season has ended, perhaps with a regional or national championship meet. Those fortunate to have trained in fifty-meter pools are returning to twenty-five-yard courses. The kids are back in school, and adjustments are made in daily schedules. With your hectic schedule, you may have decided to take a short break from training before diving into your short course season.

The fall is a great time to "start over." Establish your goals for the coming months, get back to the basics of technique and training, and build an aerobic base to carry you through the winter and spring competitions. With these thoughts in mind, the following workouts should send you on your way to a successful season of swimming.

About This Workout

1. Warm-up. Do some light stretching before entering the pool. Swimmers often develop sore muscles when returning to the water after

Coach's Chalkboard

	Fitness/Lap	*Intermediate*	*Advanced*
1. Warm-up (deck) (pool)	Light stretching 200 swim	Light stretching 250 swim	Light stretching 300 swim
2. Variety set	12 × 25/:10 rest	12 × 25/:10 rest	12 × 25/:10 rest
3. Push-off drill	8 push-offs/:45	8 push-offs/:45	8 push-offs/:45
4. Conditioning set	100-200-300—300-200-100	100-200-300-400—300-200-100	100-200-300-400—400-300-200-100
	:10 rest per 100 swum	:10 rest per 100 swum	:10 rest per 100 swum
5. "Know the clock"	12 × 25/:40, :35, :30	15 × 25/:35, :30, :25	18 × 25/:30, :25, :20
6. Cool-down	100 swim	125 swim	150 swim
TOTAL	2,300 yards	2,850 yards	3,400 yards

prolonged layoffs. Keep yourself loose and limber with a few arm swings, tricep stretches, toe touches, and thigh extensions.

After stretching, spend about 5 minutes becoming accustomed to the water with a moderate effort warm-up swim.

2. Variety set. An important aspect of swimming is training the mind as well as the body! This "variety set" is an extension of your warm-up and keeps you thinking as well.

The set may be also called double rotation. Rotate through the strokes in IM order: 25 yards of butterfly, backstroke, breaststroke, and freestyle. Simultaneously, rotate a length swim, a length kick, and a length pull. The result is

1. fly swim	5. fly kick	9. fly pull
2. back kick	6. back pull	10. back swim
3. breast pull	7. breast swim	11. breast kick
4. free swim	8. free kick	12. free pull

By the twelfth twenty-five, you will have swum, kicked, and pulled 25 yards of each of the four strokes. Tricky, but effective.

If you wish to use a kick board and a pull buoy, place your board at the opposite end of the pool before you start the set. The equipment will be in the proper place as you swim, kick, and pull through the set.

3. Push-off drill. Virtually every length begins with a push off, so why not start the season with a technique drill designed to maximize your distance on push offs? Keep in mind that in a short course pool, a good push off can account for 20 to 25 percent of the distance covered on each length—all without taking a stroke! See the following section for complete details on how to do the push-off drill.

4. Conditioning set. This main set is designed to improve your aerobic capacity. Commonly known as a ladder set, its distances increase through the first half of the set, then decrease during the second half. The rest between swims is relatively short, and the effort should be in the moderate to high range.

For example, the advanced swimmer will begin with a one hundred and increase 100 yards each swim until having completed a 400. Then, the "ladder" is descended by beginning with a four hundred and finishing with a one hundred. The total of the advanced set is 2,000 yards.

The rest interval between swims is 10 seconds per 100 yards swum. So, rest 10 seconds after a 100, 20 after a 200, 30 after a 300, and so on.

For an added challenge, attempt to swim faster on the second half of the set.

5. "Know the Clock." In order to measure your progress throughout the season, it is imperative to use the pace clock in a number of ways. Some Masters and fitness swimmers have better math skills than oth-

ers, but, with a little practice, all can become more effective with the numbers. Those who "know the clock" are able to create additional possibilities for more challenging sets. In contrast, swimmers who only know what the "top" means are a bit limited.

This set requires a bit of mathematical skill. The beginner, for example, will swim 12 × 25 on rotating intervals of 40, 35, and 30 seconds. To further explain, the first 25 yards is on an interval of 40 seconds (swim time plus rest). The next 25 is on 35, and the third is on 30.

On the pace clock, the swimmer will begin the set on the "top," the next twenty-five will begin with the clock on :40, the following on the :15, and the next on the :45. After the third twenty-five, continue to rotate throughout the intervals of 40, 35, and 30 seconds until the set is completed.

6. Cool-down. Swim easy for 2 to 3 minutes at a moderate to easy pace.

Push-off Drill

How does the push-off drill work? Do one underwater push off, gliding until coming to a complete stop. Mark the spot by removing your goggles and placing them securely on the lane rope where you came to a stop. Return to the wall and try again. The key is to try to increase your distance on each succeeding push off. Leave approximately every 45 seconds. Some helpful hints about push offs:

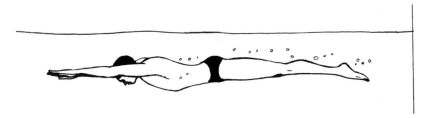

Figure A.1A. By streamlining your push off, you will maximize distance and speed

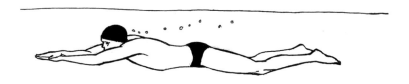

Figure A.1B. By *not* streamlining, you increase resistance, reducing distance and speed.

1. Place one hand on the wall and the other at your side. Face sideways, perpendicular to the wall. This is the proper push-off position.
2. Allow the hand that is on the wall to move forward just above your ear. Your arm should be bent at about a ninety-degree angle. Take a deep breath as your hand moves forward.
3. Submerge your entire body as both feet are placed on the wall.
4. As you submerge and push off the wall, move your underneath arm forward to join your upper arm in a stretched and streamlined position.
5. Use great leg force for the push off and place your entire body in a streamlined, straight position (see Figure A.1A). Avoid lifting your head to look forward.

The Value of Rest in Your Training

Coach's Chalkboard

	Fitness/Lap	*Intermediate*	*Advanced*
1. Warm-up free, breast, back (10-second rest)	3 × 50	3 × 75	3 × 100
2. Warm-up drill (10-second rest)	4 × 50	5 × 50	6 × 50
3. Pull (45-second rest)	2 × 150	2 × 200	2 × 300
4. Broken pull (5-second rest break halfway)	2 × 150	2 × 200	2 × 300
5. Kick set (Progressive 20-second rest) easy 50 swim	6 × 75	6 × 75	6 × 75
6. Broken swim 10-second rest break halfway and 45 between each swim	2 × 150	2 × 200	2 × 300
7. Broken swim 20-second rest break halfway and 45 between each swim Easy 50 swim	2 × 150	2 × 200	2 × 300
8. Quality swim sprints (30-second rest)	6 × 25	6 × 50	6 × 50
9. Warm-down and Drill	150	200	300
Total yards	2,300	3,025	4,050

About This Workout

1. Relaxed and casual warm-up with one each of the three strokes: free, back, and breast.
2. Set of warm-up fifties using the drills described in the Tech Drill.
3 and 4. These four swims are all done pulling and can be viewed as one set. Swim the first two without stopping. Break the second two in the middle with 5 seconds rest. Breaking a swim aids psychologically in increasing speed. And it works! The extra rest should help you improve your pace. Try to swim the second half the same speed as the first—it will take a little extra effort to do so. Make sure that the two broken swims are faster than the two first straight pulls.

   If you don't use paddles, remember the thumb stroke tip (see Tech Drill). *If you specialize in a stroke other than freestyle, use it for this set.*
5. Kick set. If you are a poor kicker, wear fins or reduce the distance to

a fifty. The first one is easy; on the second and third, work the last lap; on the fourth and fifth, work the last fifty; and, finally, the last seventy-five is an all-out effort.

6 and 7. Big swim set: Do these broken swims taking a little more rest than you did in the earlier pull set (3 and 4). Try to go faster. On the first two, break for 10 seconds rest at the halfway point. On the final two, take 20 seconds rest at the midpoint. Using your legs should assist you in swimming faster than you did in the pulls.

8. Quality swim sprints will finish off the workout with a good balance. You want to go home (or to work) with your muscles knowing you really did a workout. Do the first easy; the second half easy, half fast; the third all fast; repeat.

9. Easy swim to get the heart rate down.

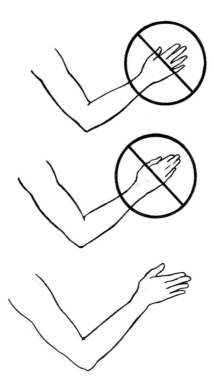

Figure A.2. TECHNIQUE THEORY: All Thumbs. Thumbs are overlooked by many coaches. *Thumbs should be separate from the hand during the underwater pull for all of the four strokes (see following diagrams).* The top two figures illustrate poor technique: Either all the fingers are separated (top) or all are held tightly together (middle). The bottom figure illustrates proper technique: The thumb is held apart from the rest of the hand.

Thumbing It Drill

During the recovery stage (when the hand is out of the water) the thumb and all the fingers are relaxed. Once underwater the fingers should be lightly closed, not clamped tightly, during the pull cycle. The thumb separates as shown in Figure A.3 as the pull begins. It remains separated during the full underwater stroke. Finally, the thumb again closes in (relaxed) as the hand exits the water.

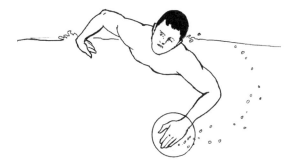

Figure A.3. The correct thumb position in the freestyle. During the stroke it remains separated from the other fingers. As the hand exits the water, the thumb and all the fingers are relaxed and held together.

Here is why:

1. Corrects wrist/hand distortions. (Many swimmers have bent wrists.)
2. Relaxation. (Many swimmers have too much tension in their hands.)
3. Gives you a better feel of the water. Your sensitivity is enhanced more than with the "clamped" hand.
4. Stability. The thumb acts as a stabilizer or as a minifin.

TIDBIT FACTS

Top Olympic swimmers take about twelve strokes per length of a twenty-five-yard pool.

Advanced swimmers take thirteen to seventeen strokes per length.

Intermediate swimmers take eighteen to twenty-four strokes.

Beginning, uncoached, or poor technical form swimmers take twenty-five and over.

If you are not reaching/extending forward, not rolling your shoulders, or not getting the correct "feel," you will be taking more strokes and being less efficient.

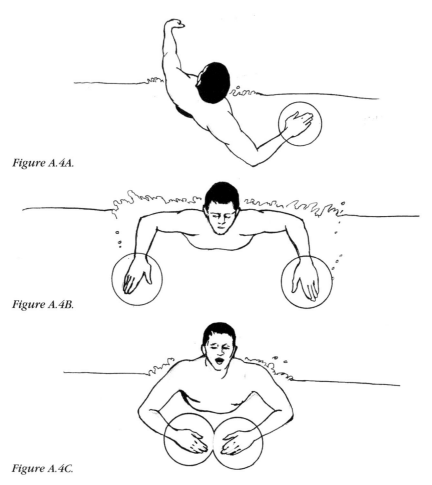

Figure A.4A.

Figure A.4B.

Figure A.4C.

The correct thumb position is illustrated for the backstroke (fig. A.4A), butterfly (fig. A.4B), and breaststroke (fig. A.4C).

Tech Drill

Here are some interesting drills for the fifties in set 2. Swim the first lap with an open thumb on one hand and a closed thumb on the other hand. Then alternate for the second length. You should feel the difference.

Learn to "feel" the water as well as to relax. The separated thumb will make a great difference in this ability. When you feel, you will of course be attempting to maximize the amount of water you are catching. You will become more efficient each arm stroke. (Yes, that does mean more work underwater; but that is what coaches want. More feel, more water grabbed, means more push out of each cycle.)

New Year's Workout

By now you probably have made your swimming resolutions and fitness goals for the new year. If not, there's still time. Here are some possible resolutions: to learn a new stroke, work on your weaknesses (you improve the most here), work out with a group (it's good for motivation and camaraderie), try entering your first Masters swim meet or open water swim.

Choose a resolution and stick with it!

Coach's Chalkboard

	Fitness/lap	*Intermediate*	*Advanced*
1. Warm-up free	200	250	300
2. Warm-up drill 1/2 drills/ 1/2 swim	4 × 50	4 × 75	4 × 100
3. Harder warm-up drill 20-second rest	3 × 50	3 × 75	3 × 100
4. Drill and get faster	2 × 50	2 × 75	2 × 100
5. Drill	1 × 50	1 × 75	1 × 100
6. IM commitment set (2-minute rest before you swim):	400 IM	600 IM	800 IM
New Year's Challenge	400 Free	600 Free	800 Free
7. Fin kick	300	300	300
8. Quality swim with Zoomers	4 × 50	4 × 50	4 × 50
9. Warm-down	200	200	200
Total yards	2,200	2,900	3,600

About This Workout

1. Easy warm-up.
2–5. Drills and swims in all the strokes. Do the first drill (2) in your worst stroke, the next (3) in your second worst, and so on. For all four sets, advanced and intermediate swimmers should do the first 50 yards as a drill and the remaining yardage swimming; fitness/lap swimmers should do 25 drill, 25 swim.
6. Year's goal achievement set. This is tough, but try your best to make it through the long individual medley thinking about all the stroke tips on which you've worked. The butterfly probably will be hardest. It may take every ounce of energy and courage you possess, but you'll

be very proud of your accomplishment. Get your time at the end of the IM. Subtract 1 minute. That will be your goal time for the long freestyle swim. Two-minute rest between the two swims.

7. Fin kick. Kick an easy 300 yards freestyle or backstroke with Zoomers.
8. Quality swim with Zoomers. Zoomers are great for swimming as well as kicking. They will help you maintain a high body position for these last four fifties. Swim these at 90 percent, accentuating a strong six-beat kick and a long arm reach for each stroke cycle.
9. Warm-down. Easy 200-yard swim.

DRILLS REFRESHER

Freestyle: Long glide freestyle. Stretch at the front and the back end of your stroke and try to take the least number of strokes you can to do a length of the pool. Overglide.

Breaststroke: Do two kicks to every pull cycle, making sure that your index fingers are together and arms fully extended before starting the next kick. Glide!

Butterfly: Concentrate on a shoulder-width entry with your thumbs turned down and palms facing outward. Do not enter or extend within the shoulder line.

Backstroke: Switch sides drill: Kick on your side. See stroke drill and Figures A.5A and B.

Stroke Drill

See Figures A.5A–C. The swimmer is entirely on his side facing right. Show how much your shoulders should roll when you are swimming, from facing the right wall to facing the left wall! Start the drill kicking on your right side with the right arm extended and the left arm at your side pointing backward. The left shoulder will be protruding out of the water near your chin. Your head position is looking straight up. *It does not move.*

After 12 kicks switch to the other side. Avoid the temptation to throw your head about. Again, it never moves in this drill, just as it never moves in backstroke! This pattern, switching sides every 12 kicks, is kept up the whole length of the pool. This is the best drill for learning the shoulder roll.

A top backstroker rolls his shoulder up against his chin with a circular shoulder shrug. At the same time, the other shoulder is extended down, pulling deep in the water. Why? Because this position gives the body, the shoulder, and the arm greater leverage in the entire underwater stroke, thus attaining more power (Figure A.5C). Break the habit of leaving your shoulders flat on the surface and making your aching arms do all the work. A great swimmer, like a great quarterback or pitcher, will roll the shoulder, getting his entire body into a more advantageous position.

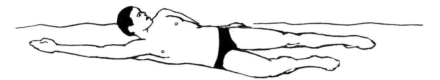

Figure A.5A. Notice the stationary head position and the high left shoulder almost touching the chin as the body is rolled to the right side with the right shoulder below the surface of the water. Notice the little finger's entry at eleven o'clock.

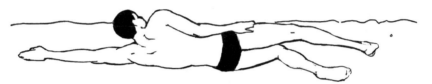

Figure A.5B. Again the head is stationary. The high right shoulder is almost touching the chin as the body is rolled to the left side, with the left shoulder below the surface of the water. Notice the little finger's entry at one o'clock.

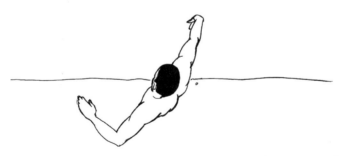

Figure A.5C. The body is rolled to the left side, giving greater leverage to a deep left shoulder that emphasizes a more powerful pull. Again, see the stationary head position.

All swimmers—competitive and fitness swimmers alike—should warm up carefully before starting to swim breaststroke intensely or vigorously. Because the breaststroke kick is an explosive and powerful movement, it puts much stress on the knee, groin, and lower back. These areas are very susceptible to injury. Start off your breaststroke with narrow, low-intensity kicks; gradually build up to wider, more powerful kicks.

Workout Theory

This workout was designed with many drills to keep you thinking about and practicing proper technique. The correlation between improving technique and enhancing performance is very high in swimming—perhaps more than in any other sport. You have to get into the habit of thinking about your technique with every stroke. Work hard, but remember to use good form!

TIDBIT FACTS

Health magazine reports 91 million Americans make New Year's resolutions and 71 million fail them by the end of the first week in January. *I hope these suggestions will help you stay with your swimming resolutions.*

A Breaststroke Workout (It works for other strokes too)

Coach's Chalkboard

	Fitness/Lap Swimmer	Intermediate	Advanced
1. Warm-up	100 Free	150 Free	200 Free
2. Warm-up	100 IM reverse order	200 IM reverse order	200 IM reverse order
3. Warm-up drill	100 2K-1P and LGB*	150 2K-1P and LGB*	200 2K-1P and LGB*
4. Pre-main set	4 × 50 (25-second rest)	3 × 75 (25-second rest)	4 × 75 (25-second rest)
5. Main set	6 × (2 × 25 AR; 1 × 50 H) (20-second rest)	5 × (12 × 50 AR; 1 × 100 H) (20-second rest)	6 × (2 × 50 AR; 1 × 100 H) (20-second rest)
6. Kick	100-75-50-25	150-100-50-25	150-100-75-50-25
7. Pull	4 × 100	5 × 100	6 × 100
8. Warm-down	100 2K-1P & LGB	150 2K-1P and LGB	200 2K-1P and LGB
Total	1,850 yards	2,700 yards	3,300 yards

* LGB = Long glide breaststroke. The objective is to accomplish one length of breaststroke in the least number of strokes. Try to reduce your stroke count (number of arm strokes per length) by 30 to 40 percent. Here you are working on all aspects of the stroke; the last 18 inches of the kick, the fully extended arms, and the glide. Wait until the legs smash together and the body almost comes to a complete stop before starting the next pull.

About This Workout

1. Easy warm-up.
2. An easy individual medley to stretch all the muscle groups.
3. This is the first drill: LGB for the even twenty-fives; 2K-1P (2 kicks per one pull) for the odd twenty-fives. Long glide breaststroke means that you should swim the entire length with as few strokes as possible. Remember to glide almost to a complete stop before initiating the next stroke, as emphasized by the stroke tips (see drill).
4. This finishes the warm-up. Kick, without a board, the first 25 yards with the hands extended, fingertips touching or thumbs interlocked, emphasizing the kick tip—snap the legs together by trying to crash

the ankles into each other. On the last 50 or 25 yards, use a complete stroke. Here you will build to an 85 percent effort by the end of each repeat.

5. Take some rest, then get ready for a great breaststroke workout. Note that AR = active rest; H = hard or 100 percent efforts. In this set, emphasize the hundreds with 100 percent performance. The two fifties are rest periods termed active rest. Here you swim breaststroke at a lower intensity (60 percent) but concentrate on good form, thinking about those stroke tips while preparing for the next all-out one hundred. Take 20 seconds rest between each effort. Keep a log of all your times. Remember, you can do this set with any stroke.

6. Kicking is next. By this point in the workout, the adductor muscles (the large muscles on the inside of the thigh) are fatigued. Take this opportunity to concentrate on the kick stroke tip while working at a lower intensity. Alternate one length freestyle kick as recovery, then one length breaststroke kick. Take 20 seconds rest between each kick distance.

7. It's always good to balance out the muscle groups and, at the same time, get in some additional yardage. Pull the next set freestyle using a pull buoy and hand paddles. Do the same stroke drill you did in set 3, but here it's long glide *freestyle*. Do this for the first two one hundreds as you begin increasing your intensity and building up your speed throughout the set. Pull the remaining one hundreds with a normal stroke, using the pull buoy and paddles.

8. Finish off the workout with a loosen-down of LGB.

Stroke Tips Drill

To achieve all the potential power in the kick, make sure that your heels are drawn up close to the buttocks with the toes pointing outward to the side walls of the pool. Then uncoil this potential energy in an explosive manner with special emphasis on the last 18 inches of the kick, trying to smash the ankles together. There is no specific drill for this, but it is important to think about the correct movement every time you kick.

Drill

Try doing the breaststroke with two kicks to each pull. As you finish with the first kick, lock your thumbs together as your arms are fully extended, then kick again. At that kick's completion, start the outward skull to begin the next pull. This will help alleviate that squished bug look and introduce the glide portion of the stroke at the right time. See Figures A.6A and B.

Workout Theory

The long warm-up is for injury prevention. Since breaststroke is an

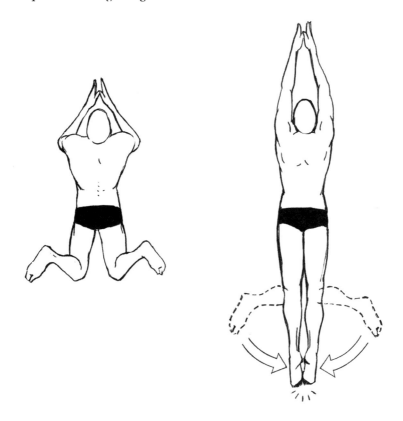

Figure A.6A. (Left) Hands extended out front with thumbs interlocked, knees bent, heels drawn up toward buttocks, toes pointing outward.

Figure A.6B. (Right) Hands extended out front with thumbs interlocked, legs are uncoiled in a straight position 18 inches apart. Note that the arrows show the movement the foot just went through, and the spot where the ankles smash together.

explosive or ballistic stroke, the workout should have intensity swims to prepare the body for these movements. Thus the all-out hundreds.

Some fitness swimmers may feel that since they are not training or preparing for a race, there's no reason to swim at 100 percent effort. The answer is that it is easy to swim at 50 percent output in breaststroke. But easy breaststroke is more like a stretching routine that can be done without getting chlorine in your hair. These sets were designed to put some life and effort into your workouts.

The long glide breaststrokes and the 2K-1P at the beginning and ending of the workout are to remind and familiarize you with the long, extended reach and streamlined body position at the end of the stroke. Breaststroke swimmers who don't streamline and coordinate the finish of the kick before the start of the next stroke look like squished, squirming bugs. You must concentrate on having a long, streamlined body position at the completion of the stroke. The workout finishes off with a freestyle pull to add to the total distance and balance out usage of the muscle groups.

TIDBIT FACTS

The fastest ever 100-yard breaststroke is 52.48 for a man and 1:00.46 for a woman.

The fastest 100-yard breaststroke in the fifty to fifty-four age-group is 1:05.29 for a man and 1:17.72 for a woman.

After a month, most beginner adults can swim a 100-yard breast in 2:25; an intermediate swimmer is at 1:40.

"Lactic Acid" Workouts

If you compete, April to May means the end of short course season, in other words, *taper time!* It's time to rest the ol' bod, fine-tune the engine, blast a few twenty-fives, and shave down for the big meet.

Well, there may be some bad news for those of you who have just started your taper—it may be too late!

It takes more than a few weeks of rest and sprinting to achieve a peak performance at the big meet. The months of long mileage and short rest interval training get you in shape, but they do not prepare you physically or mentally for the 100 percent effort you need to achieve a personal best at the big meet. That's why many swimmers begin a weekly "lactic acid" workout if they are training for a championship meet in April–May.

Lactic acid is a by-product of short-term, high-intensity exercise. As lactic acid builds up, it prevents the muscles from contracting. Improvement in higher-intensity swimming—swimming faster—can only be obtained by adapting your body to the increased stresses by overloading the metabolic and physiological systems involved. What all this means is that training at or near race speed is the only way to prepare for and adapt to the stresses placed on the body during peak competitions.

I do not recommend these workouts for the lap swimmer or part-time (two workouts per week or less) Masters swimmer. However, for those of you training regularly, athletes training for triathlons or ocean competitions, an occasional lactic acid workout may just be what the coach ordered to break up the monotony and prompt you to a new level of performance.

Rotate four sets of all-out swims each month as described. In addition to enhancing high-quality performances, these workouts promote team enthusiasm and camaraderie.

Coach's Chalkboard

Week 1	*Week 2*	*Week 3*	*Week 4*
1. Meet warm-up	1. Meet warm-up	1. Meet warm-up	1. Meet warm-up
2. 6 × 100 @ 10 minutes	2. 12 × 50 @ 5 minutes	3. 4 × 200 "broken" [10-second rest each 50 @ 12 minutes]	2. 8 × 75 @ 6 minutes
4. 400-yard cooldown	4. 400-yard cooldown	4. 400-yard cooldown	4. 400-yard cooldown

---

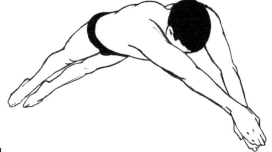

Figure A.7A

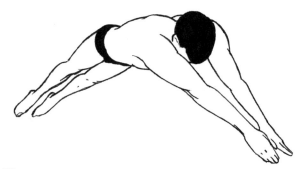

Figure A.7B

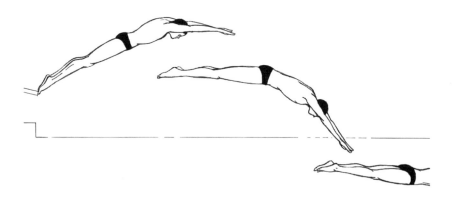

Figure A.7C

Lactic acid workouts should be discontinued two weeks before your big meet and replaced with the conventional taper: a long warm-up, some build/pace fifties and hundreds, and a few all-out sprints from the blocks.

About This Workout

1. Always begin with a complete meet warm-up to be ready for an all-out effort on the first swim. Most Masters swimmers need a minimum of 1,000 to 1,400 yards warm-up.
2. These rotating sets add up to only 600 yards, but they are "all-out" efforts—hold nothing back. Simulate meet conditions by starting from the blocks. Record your times on a log sheet to compare with the next month, when the set will be done again. If the set is done correctly, your times on the first three swims will be fairly consistent and close to meet performance times. Then it happens: lactic acid invades the body. Your times start dropping off. You tighten. You shake. You fatigue. But keep fighting! Think "technique" to battle the fatigue. Keep your stroke long. Streamline off the wall. Head down on your finish. When the big meet comes, the pain and fatigue will be familiar friends that you will face without fear or intimidation.
3. The "broken" two hundreds in week 3 are approached somewhat differently than the other three sets. The goal here is to achieve your meet 200 time *and splits*. (Remember you are getting 10 seconds rest after each fifty, which you won't get in the big meet.) By repeating this set over the course of the season, you will learn how to pace a meet performance 200-yard swim.
4. The 400-yard loosen-down. This is a *minimum* and a must!
   You worked hard. Let your body cool down gradually.

Technique Tip
Let's discuss dives.

Most coaches encourage their swimmers to have their hands on top of each other during the start (Figure A.7A). But it is equally acceptable to have the fingers just lightly touch, thumbs together (Figure A.7B). This is really up to the individual swimmer, depending on flexibility.

Notice the pointed toes (Figure A.7C). It is essential to concentrate on extending to a complete toe point. The foot flex is dramatic and powerful right from the push off the block. Keep your toes pointed throughout the dive. Your knees will stay together and won't bend if your toes remain pointed. Your entry into the water will have a better chance of being streamlined if your toes stay in this extended pointed position.

Dive Drill
The best drill for improving your dive: practice!

WARNING:
DO NOT DIVE UNLESS YOUR
POOL IS OVER SIX FEET DEEP
AND PERMITS DIVING—
CHECK WITH YOUR COACH OR
POOL MANAGER!

TIDBIT FACTS

The fastest swimmers (under 20 seconds for the fifty) hit the water at just about 8 miles per hour (11.9 feet per second). If these swimmers could continue at this speed, they would complete 50 yards in 12.5 seconds.

The typical 25 seconds per 50 yards Masters swimmer hits the water at around 5.7 miles per hour. For a fifty, this would be 16.7 seconds.

The typical 30 seconds per 50 yards Masters swimmer hits the water at around 4.7 miles per hour. For a fifty, this would be 21.4 seconds.

Sprint Workout

Coach's Chalkboard

	Fitness/Lap Swimmer	*Intermediate*	*Advanced*
1. Warm-up	200 free	250 free	300 free
2. Warm-up	100 IM reverse order	200 IM reverse order	300 IM reverse order
3. Warm-up	100 IM kick	200 IM kick	200 IM kick
4. Warm-up	4 × 50 (10–15-second rest)	4 × 75 (10–15-second rest)	4 × 100 (10–15-second rest)
5. Warm-up	4 × 25 easy/fast (15 seconds)	6 × 25 easy/fast (10 seconds)	8 × 25 easy/fast (10 seconds)
6. Warm-up	100 easy stroke drill	100 easy stroke drill	100 easy stroke drill
7. Warm-up Sprint	100 "simulation"	100 "simulation"	100 "simulation"
8. Main set	5 × 75 sprint + 50 easy @ 5 minutes	6 × 75 sprint + 75 easy @ 5 minutes	7 × 75 sprint + 75 easy @ 5 minutes
9. Pull	300	400	500
TOTAL	1,825 yards	2,600 yards	3,150 yards

About This Workout

There are two objectives for giving this workout: (1) to teach you how the Olympians do it while training for competition, but tapered down for adult recreation training; and (2) to get you to do it and enjoy it.

The first part of the workout is an extensive warm-up. Yes, it's long! You need to swim this far if you are going to reach your physical potential. It usually takes over 15 minutes before you start swimming your best in workout. So make sure that you warm up for at least that period. You may even be a little tired, but your muscles are now ready to perform at their peak.

1. Start with easy freestyle or the stroke with which you are most comfortable.
2. The individual medley is used to warm up and stretch all the muscles. It's done in reverse so that you are a little loosened up before the butterfly leg. You may kick part of the fly leg, but do try to swim at least half.

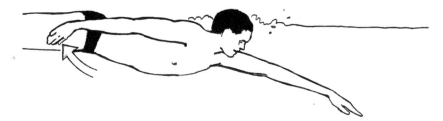

Figure A.8. A helpful tip while sprinting is to focus on the legs. Fast feet will help increase the arm rate. Push the hands all the way back at the end of every stroke cycle. The tendency, especially exaggerated when sprinting, is to now allow the follow-through in the push-back phase of the stroke cycle. Push all the way back until you lock your elbows out (as above), making sure that the palm of your hand is parallel to the wall you are swimming away from. That extended hand should finish its underwater stroke cycle with the thumb being close to (almost touching) the outer thigh.

3. The kick is to really get your legs going again. Again, the IM helps stretch and loosen all the leg muscle groups.
4. A short interval set to raise the heart rate and nourish the muscles with full blood flow. This should be performed at 70 to 80 percent of maximum heart rate.
5. These twenty-fives are easy/fast with 10 to 25-second rest periods between. This completes the warm-up. Your body should now be ready to perform at peak performance for the main set—*sprinting!*
6. Do 100 yards easy. See stroke drill.
7. Simulation is for gearing up. It's an easy hundred, thinking about the necessary ingredients for optimal performance. In this case, you are getting ready to sprint. Think about the head position and the finish through. This is your psyche-up swim.
8. Main set: These seventy-fives are done at 100 percent effort from the beginning, no saving up for the last one. They are on a 5-minute interval with an easy seventy-five swim-down after each sprint. You will be getting almost 4 minutes rest. Don't hold anything back! This is the type of set that helps every level of swimmer improve upon strength, power, and speed. An all-quality set. This is an essential part of training, developing power, speed, and strength conditioning. Remember that every exercise program should be balanced, and these three elements are essential for a balanced exercise routine.
9. Finally, finish off with a long pull to warm down. Use hand paddles if you have them. They will help because your arms will be like noodles after the seventy-fives. Make sure that you do this pull set; it will help alleviate some of the lactate acid buildup in your muscles. Have a good workout, and congratulations on doing it.

Stroke Drill

Because this is a quality workout, concentrate on the desired body and head position for sprinting. Swim the easy hundred with 15-second rest periods after each length.

Workout Theory

This is the hardest workout you will ever do! It is a high-quality, demanding, 60 percent anaerobic/40 percent aerobic workout. You are going to sprint! This workout is especially good for those swimmers competing at the nationals and for those who wish to develop swimming power.

The base facts are these: If you want to get fast you must train fast. Fast swimming helps recruit and develop fast-twitch muscle fibers because of the increase in muscle tension requirements. These muscle fibers play a very significant role in swims between 50 and 200 yards/meters. This workout is therefore designed to help recruit fast-twitch fibers, develop power, and increase swimming strength—all three of which ultimately result in faster swimming at all levels.

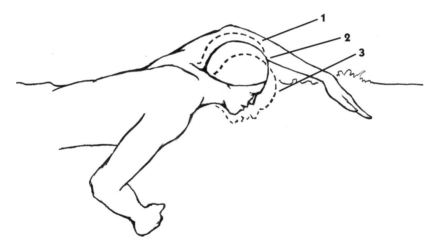

Figure A.9A. 1. Swim the first length with your head above the water and your eyes looking straight ahead at your fingertips entering the water, palms facing outward, thumbs pointing down (water level below mouth). You will need to kick hard to prevent your legs from dropping to the bottom.

2. The second length is swum with water level slightly above eyes. Your head is still held high, eyes looking ahead. You are checking to see that your hands are not crossing over the body's center line at entry. You do need to kick. Remember, palms facing outward and thumbs down.

3. The third length is with your head in its regular swimming position for normal, relaxed swimming (i.e., above your swim cap or at the hairline). Swim the last length easy, thinking about these head positions and gearing up to sprint with water level above eyes as in length 2.

A Summer Workout

	Fitness/Lap	*Intermediate*	*Advanced*
Workout *1*			
1. Warm-up	4 × 100 free	5 × 100 free	6 × 100 free
2. Warm-up	2 × 50 drill	2 × 75 drill	2 × 100 drill
3. Kick	100	150	200
4. Main set 1	4 × 200	4 × 250	4 × 300
5. Kick	100	150	200
6. Main set 2	4 × 150	4 × 200	4 × 250
7. Kick	100	150	200
8. Main set 3	4 × 100	4 × 150	4 × 200
9. Warm-down	100 easy	150 easy	200 easy
Total	2,700 yards	3,650 yards	4,600 yards
Workout *2*			
10. Straight swim	25-minute swim	25-minute swim	25-minute swim
11. Skill acquisition	6 × 4-minute swims	6 × 4-minute swims	6 × 4-minute swims
Total	49 minutes	49 minutes	49 minutes

No, this is not Summer Sanders's workout routine. But if you apply it, you will improve your summer's swimming.

About Workout 1

1. Easy hundreds warm-up, 10 to 20 seconds rest.
2. See drills for pool and open-water swimmers.
3, 5, 7. Easy kicking to loosen up the legs. These kicks are mainly social opportunities and to break up the swimming, so grab a partner to kick and socialize.
4, 6, 8. Three descending series, each becoming faster, the last being at race pace. With descending intervals on each set (1:20/100, 1:15/100, 1:10/100—advanced), this builds you into the workout leading to that last set at race pace.

Workout 2
(for those doing—or considering—an open-water swim in the summer)

10. A straight 25-minute swim for distance. Start slowly, then increase your pace, finishing off with your fastest at the end.

11. Besides building muscular strength and endurance, these short swims are to practice and acquire the skills of navigation, water entry and exit, and drafting. Land-start each time with 2 minutes rest after each swim.

Workout Theory

This workout has one goal: to increase the distance swum over a set period time. Essentially this means increasing your speed over an established distance, leaving you time to increase the distance of the workout within its time frame.

Example

Within a one-hour workout, you may accomplish 2,400 yards in July, 2,700 by August, and 3,000 by September. The advanced swimmer or triathlete should be able to cover 4,500 yards. Although the total 49 minutes of open-water swimming remains the same in workout 2, the distance you cover should be greater as you round into shape.

One-Arm Drill

The one-arm drill helps teach good body roll for breathing. With the nonbreathing arm extended out front in a stationary position (the arm-in-front position), swim with the breathing arm only (see Figure A.10). Alternate the extended arm each length of the pool. Drill also with the arm extended back (arm-behind position), the palm touching the thigh. With the right arm extended back, you would be swimming with the left arm only while breathing to the right. Alternate sides each length.

Open-Water Drill

For open-water swimmers. The look-and-breathe swimming style is incorporated with your breathing cycle. Lift the head forward and out of the water by pressing down deeper with the breathing side's arm, then turn to the side to breathe. This press occurs after arm entry into the water and continues throughout the beginning of the catch phase of the

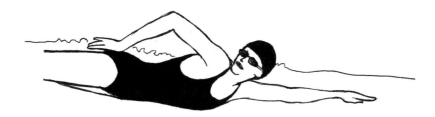

Figure A.10.

stroke, with the goal being to lift the eyes out of the water (see Figure A.11). When pool practicing, swim one length taking two looks eight strokes apart, then swim the alternate length taking three looks in succession. Successive looks provide you with a good fix on your position.

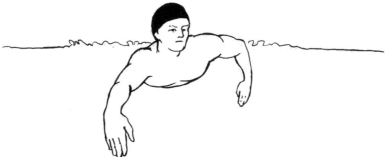

Figure A.11.

Technique Tips

All swimmers, distance or sprint specialists, should key on good form. Proper breathing rhythm can help this. Distance swimmers need to have a *consistent* rhythmic breathing pattern. Choose any one of the following three: (1) every right side or left side; (2) bilateral/alternate breathing, i.e., breathing to the right on the first stroke cycle, no breath on the second stroke cycle, and breathe to the left on the third stroke cycle, thus giving two breaths every three stroke cycles; (3) two right sides, two left sides: take two breaths to the right, one stroke cycle without a breath, then two breaths to the left.

TIDBIT FACTS

How much speed do great distance swimmers really have?

Mark Spitz, known mainly as a sprinter, missed the 1,500-meter world record by four tenths of a second.

Rick DeMont, a former distance swimmer and world record holder, switched to the 100-meter freestyle and became one of the world's top sprinters.

At the Olympics, Australia's Shane Gould, a middle-distance swimmer, won both the 200- and 400-meter freestyle. She showed her versatility by taking second in the 800 meters and third in the 100-meter sprint.

Long Distance

Coach's Chalkboard

	Fitness/Lap	*Intermediate*	*Advanced*
1. Warm-up	100 free	150 free	200 free
2. Warm-up	2 × 100 drill	2 × 150 drill	2 × 200 drill
3. Kick	100	150	200
4. Main set 1	Straight (20 minutes)	Straight (20 minutes)	Straight (20 minutes)
5. Kick	100	150	200
6. Main set 2	Straight (15 minutes)	Straight (15 minutes)	Straight (15 minutes)
7. Kick	100	150	200
8. Main set 3	Straight (10 minutes)	Straight (10 minutes)	Straight (10 minutes)
9. Warm-down	100 easy	150 easy	200 easy
Total	1,800 yards	2,450 yards	3,000 yards

About This Workout

This workout is designed for all adult summer swimmers—both those who swim in pools and those who swim in open water. It is long and it is aerobic. It's geared for building an aerobic base that will assist all swimmers, from recreational to Masters national competitors, and from open-water aerobic swimmers to drop-dead anaerobic sprinters. Distance swimmers must maximize aerobic capacity—that means yardage.

Summer open-water competitions have arrived and can be found all over the country in lakes, reservoirs, rivers, the gulf, and our two oceans. Try one this summer. Remember, when doing any exercise program, balance is critical. You may like sprints, but you should do some long-distance swimming to build your aerobic base.

1. Easy warm-up.
2. See the drill, as well as the open-water tip, which will correct your stroke as you warm up. Do the drill on the even laps, and regular swim on the odd laps. Practice your technique from these warm-up drills through the end of the long sets.
3. A kick set will finish off your warm-up and prepare you for the first long swim. If you are in the open water, roll onto your back and kick

this casually with your hands extended above your head. Go for 3 minutes.

4. Here is the work: 20 minutes straight swim. Count your laps.
5. Kick again to space the long swims. This should be medium effort. If you are trying this in the open water, try it again where you can keep kicking as you kick backstroke.
6. Back to work: 15 minutes—this time of straight crawl. Your goal is to go farther than three fourths of the 20-minute set.
7. Another kick to give you a breather, physically and mentally, and get you ready for that last long swim.
8. Last, but best effort: 10 minutes. The goal is to go farther than at the 10-minute average of the 20- or 15-minute swim. If you want to make this a pull set, go ahead and put on the pull buoy and paddles.
9. Loosen down.

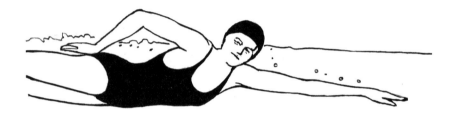

Figure A.12. With long distance, the swimmer should concentrate on lengthening the stroke. At the entry of the water by the fingers, stretch, slide the arm forward, and glide, then glide, and then glide some more. People invariably don't glide enough, jumping into the next stroke before completing the underwater stroke. As you are entering, and then gliding, you are not doing any work. It should be only smooth, relaxed extension as you reach and stretch forward. Don't forget to roll/stretch your shoulder forward as well. It is the underwater stroke that has to work. The over-the-water recovery is just relaxed, then glide at the surface.

Catch-up Freestyle Drill

Just about the oldest swim drill is the catch-up freestyle drill. It is used by every coach to some extent because it is so effective. The catch-up will teach you how to glide at the entry of your stroke.

The catch-up can be on one side or alternating arms after each stroke. Start with one side; you can try alternating later. The idea is that you swim with only one hand, while the other hand sits stretched out in front of your head on the centerline of your body like Superman. This stationary hand acts as a target. It does not move. Your other arm does the

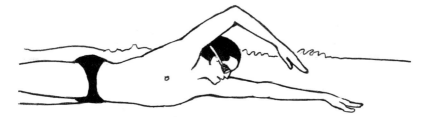

Figure A.13A. Right arm recovery, notice the high elbow

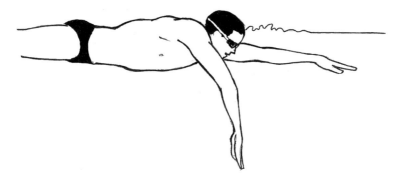

Figure A.13B. Right arm stretching to its full extension

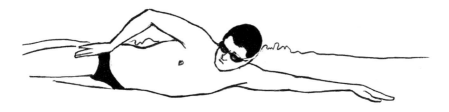

Figure A.13C. Right arm pulling the length of the body, notice again the high elbow

stroke cycle alone, recovering over the water to meet it. Since it is stretched out, you are forced to stretch out to meet it with the moving arm. Glide, glide, glide. The elbows lock completely out as you stretch that hand forward; don't cross over the centerline with either hand. Ever! The best part about this drill is with only one hand swimming, the movements are slowed down to a pace that is easier to visualize and feel. Your single arm stroke improves greatly without the asymmetrical alternating. Even the underwater *S* or scull improves.

Open-water Strategy

The number-one key is navigation. Without a line and lane lines corralling you in, you will definitely deviate off course. You have to sight your path regularly using some marker either on- or offshore. I suggest looking every eight to twelve strokes for your target, less if drafting off experienced swimmers. The frequency of lifting depends on the conditions of the water, your familiarity with the course, your ability to swim straight, and the number of experienced swimmers around you. The idea is when you have to raise your head, to be as efficient as possible. The "look-and-breathe" style first has you lifting your head forward to sight your course, then turning your head to the side to breathe. The "breathe-and-look" style has you take a breath to the side, then turn your head forward to look. Minimize this extra burden of turning your head by practicing these tips.

Workout Theory

The kick is stuck in between the long swims for two reasons: to give you a physical as well as a mental break to prepare for the next hard swim.

TIDBIT FACTS

The fastest ever "mile" (1,650 yards—sixty-six lengths, swimming's official competitive mile) is about 14:35. For a 20-minute swim that converts to 90 lengths of a twenty-five-yard pool (2,250 yards). That is 1.85 yards per second or 112 yards a minute.

The fastest ever mile by a Masters thirty-five-year-old man is 16:21. For a 20-minute swim that would be 2,018 yards.

The fastest ever mile in the fifty age-group is 18:53. For a 20-minute swim that would be 1,745 yards.

The fastest ever mile in the eighty-five age-group is 31:02. For a 20-minute swim that would be 1,063 yards.

After a month, most adult swimmers can complete approximately 30 to 40 lengths (750 to 1000 yards) in 20 minutes. An intermediate swimmer can do about forty-six to fifty-six lengths (average 1:25–1:45 speed per 100 yards).

Also, with this distance you need a little kicking since the legs are not worked as hard as the yardage increases.

For motivation, keep track of your distance (or pace if you can see a wall clock). The 10-minute swim should be faster (more lengths on average) than the 15, which is faster than the 20-minute swim. Keep a record of your distances.

For a little competitive fun to plug into your workout, bring a buddy close to the same speed and try an old coaches' swim gimmick: alternate leading. Every 100 yards switch your positions. The leader goes all out. The second place drafts behind.

This gimmick is good training, especially for open-water racing. Not only is the hard-medium-hard-medium, great cardiovascular training but it heightens concentration and gives you the edge for those spurts in an open-water race that you need to pass someone, go around a buoy, catch a wave, lose a shark, or finish off with any race's necessary sprint at the end. And it is fun working with a swim buddy.

Coach's Chalkboard

	Fitness/Lap	*Intermediate*	*Advanced*
1. Warm-up	150 free drill/think!	150	200
	(If you have an extra 5 minutes, work on your turns with someone.)		
2. Warm-up	2 × 100 free flip turn drill	2 × 150	2 × 200
3. Development	10 × 50	10 × 50	14 × 50 strokes
4. Hard	3 × 100 mixed up IM	5 × 100	6 × 100
5. Kick	125, 100, 75, 50 Dolphin on your back	150, 125, 100, 50	200, 150, 100, 50
6. Quality	1 × 100 IM all out	1 × 100	1 × 100
7. Pull	3 × 150 every third lap 1, 2, or 3 breaths	3 × 200	3 × 300
8. Sprint	3 × 50 fly/back, back/breast, breast/free	3 × 50	3 × 50
	(Alternative: relays with a group of four or more)		
9. Warm-down	100	150	200
Total	2,300 yards	2,875 yards	3,750 yards

About This Workout

The workouts here have been "serious." The main goal was for you to accomplish something. For this workout, the orientation is fun! Fun is especially important during the "off season."

Fall is the off season, the hardest time to stay motivated. You have finished a summer of vigorous swimming and/or other aerobic sports, days are getting shorter, and the temperature is dropping. Whatever "high" you had after nationals, triathlon season, or just the sunny swim weather, is subsiding. Other areas of life are getting your attention, making it hard to get back in the water.

Read up on swim literature, see swim videos, practice stroke drills, try new strokes in workouts, work on your turns, find friends for relays, start a supplemental weight workout, surgical tube resistance training, perhaps do some running, and *definitely* start planning your next year's sea-

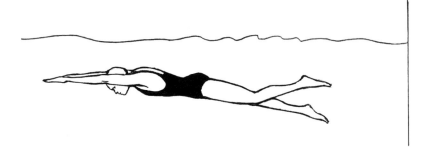

Figure A.14A. After the flip, glide, stretch, and kick under the turbulence.

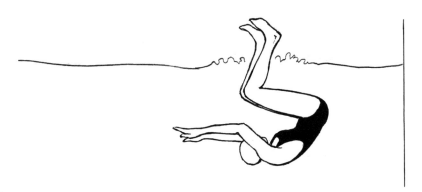

Figure A.14B. Relaxed pike flip

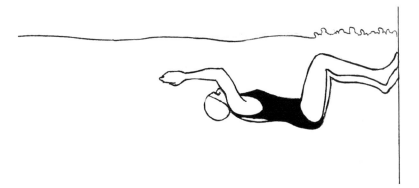

Figure A.14C. Stay mainly on your back.

son and goals. No matter what, plan on swimming at least twice a week—OK, I'll settle for just once. This workout is designed to keep you wet and aerobic during the cold months.

The off season is a time to experiment: time to change your strokes and concentrate on technique. Go over Chapters 7 through 10 or use any *SWIM Magazine* technical articles to help clean up your strokes. Establish good habits now, before next season. Read your swim literature, listen to your coach (or seek some coaching), and go at that stroke problem you have had for too long.

1. Warm-up. Pick some drills for the odd twenty-fives and swim for even twenty-fives. See next section for technique drills you can use.
2. More warm-up. Do 2 × 200 (2 × 150) with 45 seconds rest. Do the flip turn drills (see next section). If you have extra time, do some flips under the guidance of a friend or coach.
3. Development set for all levels. Do 10 × 50—four of your worst stroke, three of second worst stroke, two of your third worst stroke, and one of your fourth worst stroke (your best stroke?). Take about 20 seconds rest. Starting with your worst stroke is a way to encourage you to focus on your weaknesses.
4. Hard set individual medley, but never do the same order. Examples: fly, back, breast, free; then back, breast, fly, free; breast, fly, back . . . Great fun motivator! Interesting to see how the different strokes feel as they are placed differently in the 100-yard swim. See how your times fare when you change the order. The regular IM order should generally be the fastest. Take about 20 seconds rest.
5. Kick set. Start easy and gradually build your effort. You should be able to descend your times. This kick set is challenging: dolphin kicking on your back is like doing sit-ups as you kick. (Note: *any time* during workout, swim an easy fifty if you have the time. This is a great relaxer and psychologically builds you into the next set.
6. One last IM here. Go for your best time of the day! You'll be surprised how fast you can go—even if you're out of shape. Reason: you're relaxed and say, "What the heck, I'll just do it." There is no pressure to perform.
7. Pull 3 × 300 (or 200, 150). Try breathing less often every third lap. The off season is time to try pulling some other strokes. If you are a serious IMer, or backstroker, you should pull 40 percent of your pull back. If your shoulders can take it, do it with paddles. Paddles probably aid backstroke more than any other stroke.
8. Sprint 3 × 50 mixing up strokes. The first one is fly/back, second is back/breast, third is breast/free. These also should be high-quality sprints. If you have friends with you, do these in relays.
9. Warm-down. Finish up the way you started out.

Flip Drill

During the 2 × 200 (or 2 × 150), concentrate on the walls. Go very easy in the middle of the pool, between the flags. The extra effort and concentration come as you pass the flags, to the turn and back to the flags.

From the flags to the wall, kick only, keeping your arms to your sides. Do not let your arms leave your sides; glue your elbows to your ribs until you bring your legs out of the water for the turn.

On the flip, concentrate on the tips here. As you push off, kick below the surface under the turbulence until you pass the flags (see Figure A.14A).

Stretch your arms ahead of you, Superman-style. Unlike the Man of Steel, you have limited power, so keep your head tucked, glide, conserve the thrust, and start kicking. Stay streamlined!

Start your first arm pull after you kick past the flags, then don't breathe until your third stroke. Go easy swim until the next flags—you will need the time to catch your breath.

Tips

BEGINNER'S FLIP TIP:

Don't take that extra stroke before the wall. Relax, skip that last stroke, glide in. Flip turns can be easy. They don't need to be a huge acrobatic effort. You don't need to lift your head up to look at the wall just as you start turning. That is called the Bunny Hop. A slow, relaxed, tucking pike will be faster than a huge effort (See Fig. A.14B). Keep both elbows glued to your sides.

TIDBIT FACTS

Fastest swimming human over 50 yards
19.05 seconds   5.37 miles per hour

Fastest Masters swimmer over 50 yards
19.83 seconds   5.16 miles per hour

Average beginning Masters swimmer over 50 yards
1 minute   1.7 miles per hour

Average intermediate Masters swimmer over 50 yards
40 seconds   2.56 miles per hour

Average advanced Masters swimmer over 50 yards
30 seconds   3.41 miles per hour

Do not twist! Flip over and then, after you leave the wall, roll onto your front. Twisting during the flip is old style. It takes time and effort. Instead, push off while mainly still on your back (see Figure A.14C). It is during the stretch and glide off the wall that you roll over completely to your stomach.

ADVANCED FLIP TIP:

Retain your air during the flip. Most swimmers blow it all out as they tuck. If you can learn to keep your air, you won't have to surface right away for a big gulp. This allows for a longer stretch and glide and a delay of your first breath to the second stroke. This push off should extend past the flags (five yards) under the incoming turbulence that you brought behind you (see Figure A.14A).

DRILLS

One of the major keys to success in swimming is improving your technique. Stroke drills help you focus on one aspect of your swimming, so you can emphasize proper technique. Try to do one drill set in every workout. Even Olympic swimmers use drills daily to improve their technique.

Here is a variety of drills used by top swim coaches to help improve technique in each of the four strokes. Many of these drills have been adapted from *Swimming Technique* magazine.

Freestyle

Arm Recovery Drills

CATCH-UP

Pull with one arm while the other arm remains outstretched in front of you. Recover with a high elbow until hands touch out in front. Then repeat, using the other arm.

FINGERTIP DRAG

Drag the tips of your fingers through the water with a high elbow and your hand close to your body.

Pulling Drills

PULLING DRILL 1

Five × 50 yards. Pull one length (25 yards) with your right arm while the left arm is stretched out in front of you. Then swim the next length using the left arm with your right arm outstretched. Concentrate on your underwater pull and on getting a good body roll to each side.

PULLING DRILL 2

Pull one length (25 yards) with one arm while the other arm remains at your side. Concentrate on rotating your shoulders out of the water during the recovery and the opposite shoulder out during the pulling phase. Keep a good head position. Then swim another length using the other arm.

Body Roll Drill

SIX- OR TWELVE-KICK SWITCH

Kick on your side with the bottom arm out and the top arm on your hip.

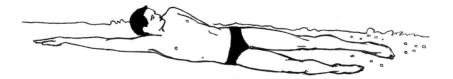

Figure A.15

After every twelve or six kicks, take a good freestyle pull, then switch sides (see Figure A.15).

Hand Entry Drill

SPLASHLESS DRILL
Emphasize entering the water without making a splash and then run your hand forward. Repeat for 4 × 50 yards.

Stroke Finishing Drill

WEIGHT THROW
Pretend that you have a weight in your hand. As you lift your hand at the end of each stroke, throw the weight out of the water.

Stroke Rate/Breathing/Timing Drills

FIST DRILL
Instead of holding your hand flat, make it into a fist while you swim 4 × 25 yards freestyle. This will feel very awkward, but it can add speed to your arm pull.

DISTANCE PER STROKE DRILL
Swim 5 × 50 yards. For each fifty try to decrease the number of strokes you take by one to two. Use a six-beat kick.

ALTERNATE BREATHING DRILL
Swim 8 × 50 yards. On the odd fifties (1, 3, 5, 7), breathe to the right on the first lap and to the left on the second. On the evens, breathe to the left on the first lap and to the right on the second.

Streamlining Drill

TURN DRILL
Starting at the center of the pool, swim to the wall and do a flip turn. Hold the streamline position past the flags (5 yards). Still holding that position, kick back to the center of the pool. Repeat six times.

Breath Control/Sprinting Drill

SHOOTERS

Wearing Zoomers, push off the wall and kick one length (25 yards) underwater as fast as you can. Try to go the entire length without breathing. Wait one minute, then do another length. Swim 6 × 25 yards. As these become easier, gradually reduce your recovery time.

My Favorite Freestyle Drill

ALL-PURPOSE DRILL

Swim 100 yards as follows:

1. 25 yards right arm only;
2. 25 yards left arm only;
3. 25 yards kick, with arms in front;
4. 25 yards swim, stretching out the stroke, emphasizing body roll, correct underwater pull, and breathing every third or fifth stroke.

Do 4 × 100 yards.

This drill combines elements of many other drills, allowing you to focus successively on the correct underwater pull with each arm and the body roll, the leg kick, streamlining, and alternate breathing.

Backstroke

Arm Recovery Drills

KICK WITH HALF RECOVERY

Lift your thumb out of the water and recover to the midpoint. Stop your arm and slowly lower it to your hip. Repeat with the other arm. Do 6 × 25 yards.

THUMB-PINKIE DRILL

Exit the water with your thumb up, bring your arm straight up and stop. Turn your hand to palm out so that your pinkie will enter the water first, then finish the recovery.

Hand Entry Drills

ONE-ARM BACKSTROKE DRILL

Swim 6 × 50 yards. Swim backstroke for 25 yards using your right arm while keeping the left arm at your side. Then swim another length using only your left arm, keeping your right arm at your side. Concentrate on the roll and slicing down in the water so that the catch is deep.

BACK CATCH-UP DRILL

Start on your back with both arms over your head. Pull with one arm while the other remains outstretched. Complete the stroke until your hands touch. Then swim a stroke with the other arm.

DOUBLE-ARM BACKSTROKE

Swim with both arms recovering together while concentrating on entering with your pinkie. Swim 2 × 100 yards. This drill is good for correcting overreaching—a common error.

Pulling Drills

PULLING DRILL 1

Swim 5 × 50 yards. Pull one length (25 yards) with your right arm while the left arm is stretched out. Then swim the next length using the left arm with your right arm outstretched. Concentrate on your underwater pull and on getting a good body roll to each side (see Figure A.16).

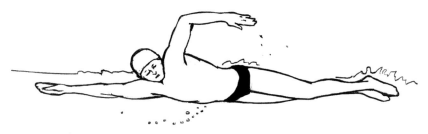

Figure A.16

PULLING DRILL 2

Pull one length (25 yards) with one arm while the other arm remains at your side. Concentrate on rotating your shoulders without moving your head. Then swim another length using the other arm.

Streamlining Drills

BELLY BUTTON DRILL

Kick 25 yards with your hands locked overhead, concentrating on keeping a streamlined position. Your belly button should be out of the water; kick just below the surface.

FLAGS DRILL

After each turn, maintain a streamlined position and kick (at least) until you pass the backstroke flags.

Body Roll Drills

KICK AND ROLL DRILL

Kick with your arms at your sides and roll your body from one side to the other every twelve kicks for one length. Kick the second length rolling every six kicks. Repeat 6 × 50 yards. Keep your head very still.

HESITATION DRILL

Take twelve kicks on one side, take a stroke, then roll to the other side for one length. Repeat the second length, stroking every six kicks. Repeat 6 × 50 yards.

Stroke Rate/Breathing/Timing Drills

DISTANCE PER STROKE DRILL

Swim 5 × 50 yards. For each fifty try to decrease the number of strokes you take by one or two.

INHALE/EXHALE DRILL

Inhale on one arm recovery, exhale on the other. Swim 5 × 50 yards.

Breath Control/Sprinting Drill

SHOOTERS

Wearing Zoomers, push off the wall on your back and kick one length (25 yards) underwater as fast as you can using the reverse dolphin kick. Try to go the entire length without breathing. Wait one minute, then do another length. Do 6 × 25 yards. As these become easier, gradually reduce your recovery time.

My Favorite Backstroke Drill

ALL-PURPOSE DRILL

Swim 100 yards as follows:

1. 25 yards right arm only
2. 25 yards left arm only
3. 25 yards kick, with arms stretched back in a streamlined position
4. 25 yards swim, stretching out the stroke, emphasizing body roll and the correct underwater pull

Do 4 × 100 yards.

This drill combines elements of many other drills, allowing you to focus successively on the correct underwater pull with each arm and the body roll, the leg kick, streamlining, and putting it all together.

Breaststroke

Arm Recovery Drills

ELBOW SQUEEZE DRILL

Swim 6 × 25 yards concentrating on squeezing your elbows together in front of your chest. Shrug your shoulders to lift your body higher out of the water and to speed up the recovery (see Figure A.17).

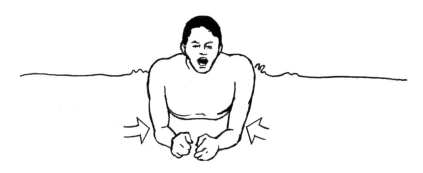

Figure A.17

HALF PULL BREASTSTROKE

Swim breaststroke using only half a pull. Your arms should stay in front, and the motion should be fast from the end of the out sweep to the end of the recovery.

DISTANCE PER STROKE DRILL

Swim 5 × 50 yards counting strokes. For each fifty try to keep your stroke count the same or decrease the number of strokes you take by one. This drill helps you concentrate on reaching and making a full recovery before starting the next stroke.

Sculling Drill

COORDINATION DRILL

For one length of the pool, pull with your right arm and kick with your left leg, while your left arm holds your right leg. Reverse the procedure for the next lap.

Underwater Pulling Drills

ALTERNATE ARM PULLS

Swim 25 yards, pulling with one hand only while the other is outstretched. Then repeat with the other hand. Glide as much as possible, stretch, catch, and accelerate through the pull. Do 6 × 25 yards.

DOUBLE ARM PULLS

Take two right-hand-only pulls, leaving your left arm straight out. Take two regular breaststroke pulls. Then take two left-hand-only pulls (right arm straight out). Do 6 × 25 yards.

Kicking Drills

OUT-OF-WATER KICK

Kick 25 yards with your head out of the water and your arms at your side. Do 8 × 25 yards.

HANDS LOCKED DRILL

Kick breaststroke with your hands locked behind your back. Concentrate on lifting your heels together all the way to the buttocks, until they touch your hands. Keep your knees inside the width of your hips during recovery. Repeat using a kick board (but without having your hands locked behind your back). Do 8 × 50 yards.

BACK KICK DRILL

Kick breaststroke on your back 2 × 100 yards. You will quickly realize whether you are pulling your knees up under instead of pulling your feet to your buttocks.

Streamlining Drills

TWO KICKS, ONE PULL DRILL

Keep a streamlined position and take two kicks before each pull. During the kicks your head should be underwater. Do 2 × 100 yards.

THREE KICKS, ONE PULL DRILL

This is the same as the preceding drill, except you take three kicks per pull.

NO ARMS DRILL

Kick breaststroke without a board, keeping a streamlined position with your arms in front of you. At each turn, take three underwater kicks before coming to the surface. Do 2 × 100 yards.

Pull-Out Drills

PULL-OUT PROGRESSION

1. Push off the wall in a streamlined position and glide to the surface.
2. Push off wall, pull, and glide to surface.
3. Push off wall, pull, kick, and glide to surface.

4. Push off wall, pull, kick, then take a second pull, exploding out of the water as high as you can.

Repeat the sequence four times.

DOUBLE PULL-OUTS

Push off the wall, pull, kick, and glide. Then pull, kick, and glide again before popping to the surface. Swim the rest of the way to the end of the pool. Repeat six times. After you build up your lung capacity, you may want to try triple pull-outs.

Stroke Rate/Breathing/Timing Drills

STRETCH-OUT DRILL

Swim 25 yards and try to stretch out your glide as much as possible, maintaining a streamlined position. It is important to understand how crucial distance per stroke is in breaststroke. If you do this drill correctly, you will take about half as many strokes per length as you normally do.

TIMING DRILL

Swim the full breaststroke cycle, then take a two- to three-second glide in a streamlined position. Do 2 × 50 yards. Repeat, reducing your glide to one to two seconds. Do 2 × 50 yards. Then repeat using your normal stroke. Do 2 × 50 yards.

My Favorite Breaststroke Drill

ALL-PURPOSE DRILL
Swim 100 yards as follows:

1. 25 yards arms only (let legs move naturally in an undulating pattern)
2. 25 yards kick with arms in front
3. 25 yards of two kicks, one pull
4. 25 yards swim, stretching out the stroke. Do 4 × 100 yards.

This drill combines elements of many other drills, allowing you to focus successively on your arm pull, leg kick, streamlining, and putting it all together.

Butterfly

Stroke Rate/Breathing/Timing Drills

TIMING DRILL
Dolphin kick with your arms at your sides, emphasizing constant undulating head motion coordinated with breathing (see Figure A.18).

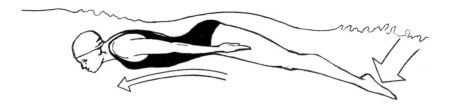

Figure A.18

HALF FLY

Swim 100 yards. For each lap, take one stroke butterfly, then swim easy freestyle. As this gets easier, take two strokes of fly, then three, and so on.

Arm Recovery Drills

ONE-ARM DRILL

Using a dolphin kick, swim 25 yards butterfly with your right arm, left arm out front. Breathe to the side. Then swim 25 yards using just your left arm, right arm out front. Concentrate on straight-arm recovery. Swim 4 × 50 yards.

COMBINATION DRILL

Swim one length as follows:

1. Two right-arm fly pulls
2. Two full fly pulls (do not breathe)
3. Two left-arm fly pulls
4. Repeat.

Swim 6 × 25 yards.

Underwater Pulling Drill

FIN SWIM

Swim 25 yards fly using fins. Concentrate on the pull, as you feel the lift from each kick. Swim 4 × 25 yards.

Streamlining Drills

UNDERWATER DRILL

Dolphin kick the width of the pool underwater without a board. Maintain a streamlined position. Repeat ten times.

FLAGS DRILL

Push off the wall and begin dolphin kicking, maintaining a streamlined position. Kick until you pass the backstroke flags.

Kicking Drills

REVERSE FLY KICK

Dolphin kick on your back for 25 yards. Rest. Do 6 × 25 yards.

BACK KICKS

Kick on your back, concentrating on keeping your shoulders above the water and making sure your knees do not break the surface. Do 4 × 50 yards. This drill can also be done wearing Zoomers.

Hand Entry Drill

HEAD UP DRILL

Swim four strokes of butterfly with your head out of the water, using a flutter kick, then four strokes of regular butterfly. Do 4 × 25 yards. This is a difficult drill, but it is good for correcting an entry that is too narrow.

My Favorite Butterfly Drill

ALL-PURPOSE DRILL

Swim 100 yards as follows:

1. 25 yards right arm only
2. 25 yards left arm only
3. 25 yards kick, with arms stretched in front in a streamlined position
4. 25 yards swim, stretching out the stroke and the correct underwater pull

Do 4 × 100 yards.

This drill combines elements of many other drills, allowing you to focus successively on the correct underwater pull with each arm, the strong dolphin kick, streamlining, and putting it all together.

My All-time Favorite Combined Drill

MEDLEY DRILL

Swim 400 yards individual medley, combining 100 yards of my favorite drills in butterfly, backstroke, breaststroke, and freestyle:

1. 100 yards butterfly: 25 yards right arm, 25 yards left arm, 25 yards kick, 25 yards swim

2. 100 yards backstroke: 25 yards right arm, 25 yards left arm, 25 yards kick, 25 yards swim
3. 100 yards breaststroke: 25 yards arms only, 25 yards legs only, 25 yards of two kicks to one pull, 25 yards swim
4. 100 yards freestyle: 25 yards right arm, 25 yards left arm, 25 yards kick, 25 yards swim

Do 2 × 400 yards. This is my favorite and most challenging drill, because it allows me to work on technique in all four strokes.

THE SWIMMER'S MARKETPLACE

SWIMMING MAGAZINES

SWIM Magazine, leading magazine for fitness and Masters swimmers. 6 issues/year. Newsstand: $2.95/issue. One-year subscription: $15.00. P.O. Box 91870, Pasadena, CA 91109-9769. Tel.: 800-538-9787 throughout North America except California (in CA: 800-345-SWIM). Ask for Operator 4.

Swimming World, the bible of competitive swimming, for competitive swimmers from age eight through college. 12 issues/year. Newsstand: $2.50/issue. One-year subscription: $19.00. P.O. Box 91870, Pasadena, CA 91109-9769. Tel.: 800-538-9787 throughout North America except California (in CA: 800-345-SWIM). Ask for Operator 4.

Swimming Technique, for swim coaches, trainers, and exercise physiologists. 4 issues/year. Newsstand: $3.50/issue. One-year subscription: $13.00. P.O. Box 91870, Pasadena, CA 91109-9769. Tel.: 800-538-9787 throughout North America except California (in CA: 800-345-SWIM). Ask for Operator 4.

SWIM Canada, for Canadian age-group through college competitive swimmers. 12 issues/year. One-year subscription: $30.00 Canadian. 402 King Street East, Toronto, Ontario M5A 1L3

SWIM CAMPS FOR ADULTS

Billabong Aquatics, Judy Bonning, director, c/o Coral Springs Aquatic Complex, 12441 Royal Palm Boulevard, Coral Springs, FL 33065. Tel.: 305-345-5370.

Custom Swim Clinics, Debbie Meyer, director, Palmer Swim Center, 4840 Marconi Ave., Carmichael, CA 95608. Tel.: 916-962-0807.

Jack Nelson Swim Camp, Nick Baker, director, 503 Seabreeze Boulevard, Fort Lauderdale, FL 33316. Tel.: 305-764-4822.

Crowder Swim Camps (held at Lagunamar Resort, Margarita Island, Venezuela), Bob and Barbara Crowder, directors, 100 High Meadow Lane, Wakefield, RI 02879. Tel.: 401-783-0917.

Total Immersion Swim Camps (held at various vacation resorts in the United States and Barbados), Terry Laughlin, director, 381 Main Street, Goshen, NY 10924. Tel.: 914-294-3510.

Stern Swimming Clinics (held at various locations in the Caribbean), Doug Stern, director, 700 Columbus Ave., New York, N.Y. 10025. Tel.: 212-222-0720.

Stanford Swim Camp, Judy Heller, director, Stanford University, Stanford, CA 94305-6150. Tel.: 415-591-0946.

University of San Diego Masters Swimming and Family Camp, Bill Morgan, director, 5998 Alcala Park, San Diego, CA 92110-2492. Tel.: 800-248-4873, ext. 4593.

SWIM EQUIPMENT

Basic swim equipment is available at most sporting goods stores throughout North America. However, if you are unable to find the equipment you need locally, or you would like to order directly from a mail-order catalog, manufacturer, or distributor, consult this list:

Swim Catalogs

Arena North America	800-925-4286
The Finals	800-345-3485
Kast-A-Way Swimwear	800-543-2763
Recreonics	800-428-3254
Speedo America	800-547-8770
truWest Inc.	800-322-3669
TYR Sport	800-934-6907
The Victor	800-356-5132

Swimsuits

Manufacturers/Distributors

Adolph Kiefer & Associates	800-323-4071
Arena North America	800-925-4286
Dolfin, International	800-441-8818
The Finals	800-345-3485
Hind-Wells	800-235-4150
Jantzen	800-626-0215
Ocean Pool Co.	800-645-5316
Rothhammer International	805-943-5129
truWest Inc.	800-322-3669
USA Aquatics	800-882-8721
The Victor	800-356-5132
Waterwear	800-321-7848

Manufacturers

Speedo America	800-547-8770
TYR Sport	800-934-6907

Distributors

Aardvark Swim & Sport	800-729-1577
Action Accents	800-338-0231
Circle City Swim & Sportswear	800-669-SWIM
Competitive Aquatic Supply	800-421-5192
4 Seasons Swimwear	800-934-6907
Kast-A-Way Swimwear	800-543-2763
NorCal Swim Shop	800-752-7946
Swimmer's Connection	800-545-7999
Swimmers Edge	800-441-SWIM
Swim Plus	800-437-5666
Swim T's	800-541-8060
Swim Zone	813-822-SWIM
Water Safety Products	800-987-7238
World Wide Aquatics	800-726-1530

Drag Suits

Manufacturers/Distributors

Adolph Kiefer & Associates	800-323-4071
KYTEC Innovative Sport Equipment	612-884-3424
USA Aquatics, Inc.	800-882-8721

Manufacturers

Speedo America	800-547-8770

Distributors

Competitive Aquatic Supply	800-421-5192
4 Seasons Swimwear	800-934-6907
Swimmer's Connection	800-545-7999
Swimmers Edge	800-441-SWIM
Swim Zone	813-822-SWIM
Water Safety Products	800-987-7238

Swim Gear (goggles, caps, nose clips, earplugs, and so on)

Manufacturers/Distributors

Adolph Kiefer & Associates	800-323-4071
Arena North America	800-925-4286
Competitor Swim Products	800-888-SWIM
The Finals	800-345-3485
Leader Sport Products	518-562-1653
INNOVAUDIO	800-426-4428
Ocean Pool Co.	800-645-5316
Recreonics	800-428-3254
truWest Inc.	800-322-3669
USA Aquatics	800-882-8721
The Victor	800-356-5132

Manufacturers

Speedo America	800-547-8770
TYR Sport	714-897-0799

Distributors

Aardvark Swim & Sport	800-729-1577
Action Accents	800-338-0231
Circle City Swim & Sportswear	800-669-SWIM
Competitive Aquatic Supply	800-421-5192
4 Seasons Swimwear	800-934-6907
Kast-A-Way Swimwear	800-543-2763
NorCal Swim Shop	800-752-7946
Recreonics	800-428-3254
See Below	516-868-3672
Swimmer's Connection	800-545-7999
Swimmers Edge	800-441-SWIM
Swim Plus	800-437-5666
Swim T's	800-541-8060
Swim Zone	813-822-SWIM
USA Aquatics	800-882-8721
The Victor	800-356-5132
World Wide Aquatics	800-726-1530

Corrective Lens Goggles

Manufacturers/Distributors

Adolph Kiefer & Associates	800-323-4071
Arena North America	800-925-4286
Leader Sport Products	518-562-1653
See Below	516-868-3672
USA Aquatics	800-882-8721

Manufacturer

Speedo America	800-547-8770

Swim Training Equipment (swim fins, kick boards, hand paddles, pull buoys, parachutes, and so on)

Manufacturers/Distributors

Adolph Kiefer & Associates	800-323-4071
Arena North America	800-925-4286
Competitor Swim Products	800-888-SWIM

Force Fin/Slim Fin	800-FIN-SWIM
Hyperfin	800-343-FINS
KYTEC Innovative Sport Equipment	612-884-3424
Leader Sport Products	518-562-1653
Natare Corp.	800-336-7946
Ocean Pool Co.	800-645-5316
Recreonics	800-428-3254
Streamliners	805-373-1473
truWest Inc.	800-322-3669
USA Aquatics	800-882-8721
The Victor	800-356-5132
Zoomers	800-852-2909

Manufacturers

Speedo America	800-547-8770
TYR Sport	800-934-6907

Distributors

Aardvark Swim & Sport	800-729-1577
Action Accents	800-338-0231
Circle City Swim & Sportswear	800-669-SWIM
Competitive Aquatic Supply	800-421-5192
4 Seasons Swimwear	800-934-6907
Kast-A-Way Swimwear	800-543-2763
NorCal Swim Shop	800-752-7946
Swimmer's Connection	800-545-7999
Swimmers Edge	800-441-SWIM
Swim Plus	800-437-5666
Swim T's	800-541-8060
Swim Zone	813-822-SWIM
World Wide Aquatics	800-726-1530

Ear and Eye Care

Manufacturers/Distributors

Adolph Kiefer & Associates	800-323-4071
Arena North America	800-925-4286
See Below	516-868-3672
Stellar Pharmacal Corp.	800-845-7827
USA Aquatics	800-882-8721

Distributors

Aardvark Swim & Sport	800-729-1577
Action Accents	800-338-0231
Circle City Swim & Sportswear	800-669-SWIM
Competitive Aquatic Supply	800-421-5192
4 Seasons Swimwear	800-934-6907
NorCal Swim Shop	800-752-7946
Swimmer's Connection	800-545-7999
Swimmers Edge	800-441-SWIM
Swim Plus	800-437-5666
Swim T's	800-541-8060
Swim Zone	813-822-SWIM
World Wide Aquatics	800-726-1530

Resistance and Dry Land Training Equipment

Manufacturers/Distributors

Adolph Kiefer & Associates	800-323-4071
KYTEC Innovative Sport Equipment	612-884-3424
Recreonics	800-428-3254
Vasa Swim Trainer	800-862-VASA
Zoomers	800-852-2909

Manufacturer

NZ Manufacturing	800-886-6621

Distributors

Aardvark Swim & Sport	800-729-1577
Action Accents	800-338-0231
Circle City Swim & Sportswear	800-669-SWIM
Competitive Aquatic Supply	800-421-5192
4 Seasons Swimwear	800-934-6907
Swimmers Edge	800-441-SWIM
Swim Zone	813-822-SWIM
World Wide Aquatics	800-726-1530

The Swimmer's Marketplace

Nutrition Bars

| Eicotec Foods (formerly Bio/Syn) | 800-223-EICO |
| PowerBar | 800-444-5154 |

Underwater Audio Equipment (Swimman, and so on)

Manufacturer/Distributor

| INNOVAUDIO | 800-426-4428 |

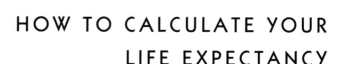

HOW TO CALCULATE YOUR
LIFE EXPECTANCY

THE LIFE-EXPECTANCY TEST described in Chapter 5 consists of thirty-two items in four broad categories: Heredity and Family, Education and Occupation, Life-style, and Health:

  I. *Heredity and Family*
      1. Longevity of grandparents
      2. Longevity of parents
      3. Cardiovascular disease of close relatives
      4. Other hereditable diseases of close relatives
      5. Childbearing
      6. Mother's age at your birth
      7. Birth order
      8. Intelligence

  II. *Education and Occupation*
      9. Years of education
     10. Occupational level
     11. Family income
     12. Activity on the job
     13. Age and work

III. *Life-style*
   14. Urban vs. rural living
   15. Marital status
   16. Living status if single
   17. Life changes
   18. Friendship
   19. Aggressive personality
   20. Flexible personality
   21. Risk-taking personality
   22. Depressive personality
   23. Happy personality

IV. *Health*
   24. Percent body fat
   25. Dietary habits
   26. Smoking
   27. Drinking
   28. Exercise
   29. Sleep
   30. Sexual activity
   31. Regular physical examinations
   32. Health status

HOW THE TEST WORKS

Begin by finding your life expectancy from an actuarial table. This figure shows how many years the "average" American of your age and sex can expect to live. The most recent actuarial table, produced by the U.S. Department of Health and Human Services, appears on page 304.

Then, by keeping a running score based on your personal attributes, you will end up with a personalized life expectancy.

As mentioned in Chapter 5, there's no guarantee that you actually will live the precise number of years predicted by the test. These figures are based on a large pool of people and only predict what is *likely* to happen to the majority of people in your age, sex, and racial category. But the results of this test should be taken seriously. Based on the best scientific evidence now available, the test points out those aspects of your life-style that may shorten your life.

TAKING THE LIFE-EXPECTANCY TEST

1. Find your life expectancy from the actuarial table on page 304. Enter this figure on the score sheet.
2. Next, add and subtract years according to how you answer the questions on pages 70 to 76 in Chapter 5.
3. Enter your scores on the score sheet and tally up the years you gain or lose.
4. Add this number to or subtract it from your life expectancy taken from the actuarial table. This is your *personalized* life expectancy.

   Three score sheets have been provided. After you begin swimming on a regular basis, take the life-expectancy test at six-month intervals to see how your swimming may be affecting your life expectancy.

Life-Expectancy Test

Score Sheet

Your Average Life Expectancy (from actuarial table)　　　_____

PART I. Heredity and Family
　1.　Longevity of grandparents　　　_____
　2.　Longevity of parents　　　_____
　3.　Cardiovascular disease of close relatives　　　_____
　4.　Other hereditable diseases of close relatives　　　_____
　5.　Childbearing　　　_____
　6.　Mother's age at birth　　　_____
　7.　Birth order　　　_____
　8.　Intelligence　　　_____

PART II. Education and Occupation
　9.　Years of education　　　_____
　10.　Occupational level　　　_____
　11.　Family income　　　_____
　12.　Activity on the job　　　_____
　13.　Age and work　　　_____

PART III. Life-style
　14.　Urban vs. rural living　　　_____
　15.　Marital status　　　_____
　16.　Living status if single　　　_____
　17.　Life changes　　　_____
　18.　Friendship　　　_____
　19.　Aggressive personality　　　_____
　20.　Flexible personality　　　_____
　21.　Risk-taking personality　　　_____
　22.　Depressive personality　　　_____
　23.　Happy personality　　　_____

PART IV. Health
　24.　Percent body fat　　　_____
　25.　Dietary habits　　　_____
　26.　Smoking　　　_____
　27.　Drinking　　　_____
　28.　Exercise　　　_____
　29.　Sleep　　　_____
　30.　Sexual activity　　　_____
　31.　Regular physical examinations　　　_____
　32.　Health status　　　_____

Total years gained or lost　　　_____

YOUR PERSONALIZED LIFE EXPECTANCY　　　_____

Life-Expectancy Test 2 (after six months of swimming)

Score Sheet

Your Average Life Expectancy (from actuarial table)   _____

PART I. Heredity and Family
1. Longevity of grandparents   _____
2. Longevity of parents   _____
3. Cardiovascular disease of close relatives   _____
4. Other hereditable diseases of close relatives   _____
5. Childbearing   _____
6. Mother's age at birth   _____
7. Birth order   _____
8. Intelligence   _____

PART II. Education and Occupation
9. Years of education   _____
10. Occupational level   _____
11. Family income   _____
12. Activity on the job   _____
13. Age and work   _____

PART III. Life-style
14. Urban vs. rural living   _____
15. Marital status   _____
16. Living status if single   _____
17. Life changes   _____
18. Friendship   _____
19. Aggressive personality   _____
20. Flexible personality   _____
21. Risk-taking personality   _____
22. Depressive personality   _____
23. Happy personality   _____

PART IV. Health
24. Percent body fat   _____
25. Dietary habits   _____
26. Smoking   _____
27. Drinking   _____
28. Exercise   _____
29. Sleep   _____
30. Sexual activity   _____
31. Regular physical examinations   _____
32. Health status   _____

Total years gained or lost   _____

YOUR PERSONALIZED LIFE EXPECTANCY   _____

Life-Expectancy Test 3 (after twelve months of swimming)

Score Sheet

Your Average Life Expectancy (from actuarial table)   _____

PART I. *Heredity and Family*
1. Longevity of grandparents   _____
2. Longevity of parents   _____
3. Cardiovascular disease of close relatives   _____
4. Other hereditable diseases of close relatives   _____
5. Childbearing   _____
6. Mother's age at birth   _____
7. Birth order   _____
8. Intelligence   _____

PART II. *Education and Occupation*
9. Years of education   _____
10. Occupational level   _____
11. Family income   _____
12. Activity on the job   _____
13. Age and work   _____

PART III. *Life-style*
14. Urban vs. rural living   _____
15. Marital status   _____
16. Living status if single   _____
17. Life changes   _____
18. Friendship   _____
19. Aggressive personality
20. Flexible personality   _____
21. Risk-taking personality   _____
22. Depressive personality   _____
23. Happy personality   _____

PART IV. *Health*
24. Percent body fat   _____
25. Dietary habits   _____
26. Smoking   _____
27. Drinking   _____
28. Exercise   _____
29. Sleep   _____
30. Sexual activity   _____
31. Regular physical examinations   _____
32. Health status   _____

Total years gained or lost   _____

YOUR PERSONALIZED LIFE EXPECTANCY   _____

| At Age | Life Expectancy | |
	Men	Women
0	72.0	78.9
20	73.5	80.0
25	73.9	80.2
30	74.3	80.4
35	74.8	80.6
40	75.3	80.8
45	75.8	81.0
50	76.5	81.5
55	77.5	82.2
60	78.7	83.1
65	80.4	84.2
70	82.3	85.6
75	84.6	87.3
80	87.4	89.3
85	90.6	91.9

Adapted from Table 6.3, "Expectation of Life at Single Years of Age by Sex," *Vital Statistics of the United States, Life Tables,* vol. 2, sec. 6, U.S. Dept. of Health and Human Services, 1991. Revised to include data in "Advance Report of Final Mortality Statistics, 1991," *Monthly Vital Statistics Report,* vol. 42, no. 2, supplement, U.S. Dept. of Health and Human Services, August 31, 1993.

HOW TO CALCULATE
YOUR PERCENT BODY FAT

WOMEN

To measure your percent of body fat, follow these five steps:

1. Measure your hips at their widest point and your waist at your belly button.
2. Measure your height without shoes.
3. Record your height, hips, and waist measurements on the work sheet on page 306.
4. Find each of these measurements in the appropriate column in the tables on pages 308–9 and record the constants on the work sheet.
5. Add constants A and B, then subtract constant C from this sum. Round to the nearest whole number. The figure is your percent of body fat.

Work Sheet for Women
to Calculate Their Percent Body Fat

Hip measurement: _____ (for constant A)
Waist measurement: _____ (for constant B)
Height: _____ (for constant C)

Look up each of the measurements in the appropriate column of the table on pages 308–9. Enter these constants here:

Constant A = _____
Constant B = _____
Constant C = _____

To determine your approximate percent body fat, add constant A and constant B. Then subtract constant C:

Constant A: _____
plus Constant B: +_____
Subtotal: _____
minus Constant C: −_____
% Body Fat: _____

Work Sheet 2 for Women
to Calculate Their Percent Body Fat

Hip measurement: _____ inches (for constant A)
Waist measurement: _____ inches (for constant B)
Height: _____ inches (for constant C)

Look up each of the measurements in the appropriate column of the table on pages 308–9. Enter these constants here:

Constant A = _____
Constant B = _____
Constant C = _____

To determine your approximate percent body fat, add constant A and constant B. Then subtract constant C:

Constant A: _____
plus Constant B: +_____
Subtotal: _____
minus Constant C: −_____
% Body Fat: _____

Conversion Constants to Predict Percent Body Fat in Women

Hips		Waist		Height	
Inches	*Constant A*	*Inches*	*Constant B*	*Inches*	*Constant C*
30	33.48	20	14.22	55	33.52
30.5	33.83	20.5	14.40	55.5	33.67
31	34.87	21	14.93	56	34.13
31.5	35.22	21.5	15.11	56.5	34.28
32	36.27	22	15.64	57	34.74
32.5	36.62	22.5	15.82	57.5	34.89
33	37.67	23	16.35	58	35.35
33.5	38.02	23.5	16.53	58.5	35.50
34	39.06	24	17.06	59	35.96
34.5	39.41	24.5	17.24	59.5	36.11
35	40.46	25	17.78	60	36.57
35.5	40.81	25.5	17.96	60.5	36.72
36	41.86	26	18.49	61	37.18
36.5	42.21	26.5	18.67	61.5	37.33
37	43.25	27	19.20	62	37.79
37.5	43.60	27.5	19.38	62.5	37.94
38	44.65	28	19.91	63	38.40
38.5	45.00	28.5	20.09	63.5	38.55
39	46.05	29	20.62	64	39.01
39.5	46.40	29.5	20.80	64.5	39.16
40	47.44	30	21.33	65	39.62
40.5	47.79	30.5	21.51	65.5	39.77
41	48.84	31	22.04	66	40.23
41.5	49.19	31.5	22.22	66.5	40.38
42	50.24	32	22.75	67	40.84
42.5	50.59	32.5	22.93	67.5	40.99
43	51.64	33	23.46	68	41.45
43.5	51.99	33.5	23.64	68.5	41.60
44	53.03	34	24.18	69	42.06
44.5	53.41	34.5	24.36	69.5	42.21
45	54.53	35	24.89	70	42.67
45.5	54.86	35.5	25.07	70.5	42.82
46	55.83	36	25.60	71	43.28
46.5	56.18	36.5	25.78	71.5	43.43
47	57.22	37	26.31	72	43.89
47.5	57.57	37.5	26.49	72.5	44.04
48	58.62	38	27.02	73	44.50
48.5	58.97	38.5	27.20	73.5	44.65

	Hips		Waist		Height
Inches	*Constant A*	*Inches*	*Constant B*	*Inches*	*Constant C*
49	60.02	39	27.73	74	45.11
49.5	60.37	39.5	27.91	74.5	45.26
50	61.42	40	28.44	75	45.72
50.5	61.77	40.5	28.62	75.5	45.87
51	62.81	41	29.15	76	46.32
51.5	63.16	41.5	29.33	76.5	46.47
52	64.21	42	29.87	77	46.93
52.5	64.56	42.5	30.05	77.5	47.08
53	65.61	43	30.58	78	47.54
53.5	65.96	43.5	30.76	78.5	47.69
54	67.00	44	31.29	79	48.15
54.5	67.35	44.5	31.47	79.5	48.30
55	68.40	45	32.00	80	48.76
55.5	68.75	45.5	32.18	80.5	48.91
56	69.80	46	32.71	81	49.37
56.5	70.15	46.5	32.89	81.5	49.52
57	71.19	47	33.42	82	49.98
57.5	71.54	47.5	33.60	82.5	50.13
58	72.59	48	34.13	83	50.59
58.5	72.94	48.5	34.31	83.5	50.74
59	73.99	49	34.84	84	51.20
59.5	74.34	49.5	35.02	84.5	51.35
60	75.39	50	35.56	85	51.81

MEN

To measure your percent body fat, follow these five steps:

1. Measure your waist at your belly button.
2. Measure your wrist where it bends, at the space between your hand and wrist bone.
3. Record these measurements on the work sheet on page 310.
4. Subtract your wrist measurement from your waist measurement and find the resulting value in the table on pages 312–17.
5. Find your weight on the left-hand side of the table. Then, move right to your waist-minus-wrist figure. At the point where these two intersect is your body-fat percentage.

Work Sheet for Men
to Calculate Their Percent Body Fat

Waist measurement: _____ inches
Wrist measurement: _____ inches
Subtract your wrist measurement from your waist measurement:

Waist measurement: _____
minus Wrist measurement: −_____
Subtotal: _____

Using the table on pages 312–17, find your weight in the left-hand column. Then find your waist-minus-wrist number. Your body-fat percentage can be found where the two columns intersect.

% Body Fat: _____

Work Sheet 2 for Men to Calculate Their Percent Body Fat

Waist measurement: _____ inches
Wrist measurement: _____ inches
Subtract your wrist measurement from your waist measurement:

Waist measurement: _____
minus Wrist measurement: –_____
Subtotal: _____

Using the table on pages 312–17, find your weight in the left-hand column. Then find your waist-minus-wrist number. Your body-fat percentage can be found where the two columns intersect.

% Body Fat: _____

Waist-Minus-Wrist to Calculate Body Fat in Men

Waist Minus Wrist

Weight in lbs. (in inches) :	22	22.5	23	23.5	24	24.5	25	25.5	26	26.5	27	27.5	28	28.5	29	29.5	30	30.5	31
120 :	4	6	8	10	12	14	16	18	20	21	23	25	27	29	31	33	35	37	39
125 :	4	6	7	9	11	13	15	17	19	20	22	24	26	28	30	32	33	35	37
130 :	3	5	7	9	11	12	14	16	18	20	21	23	25	27	28	30	32	34	36
135 :	3	5	7	8	10	12	13	15	17	19	20	22	24	26	27	29	31	32	34
140 :	3	5	6	8	10	11	13	15	16	18	19	21	23	24	26	28	29	31	33
145 :	3	4	6	7	9	11	12	14	15	17	19	20	22	23	25	27	28	30	31
150 :	2	4	6	7	9	10	12	13	15	16	19	19	21	23	24	26	27	29	30
155 :	2	4	5	6	8	10	11	13	15	16	18	19	20	22	23	25	26	28	29
160 :	2	4	5	6	8	9	11	12	14	15	17	18	19	21	22	24	25	27	28
165 :	2	3	5	6	8	9	10	12	13	15	16	17	19	20	22	23	24	26	27
170 :	2	3	4	6	7	9	10	11	13	14	15	17	18	19	21	22	24	25	26
175 :	2	3	4	6	7	8	10	11	12	13	15	16	17	19	20	21	23	24	25
180 :	1	3	4	5	7	8	9	10	12	13	14	16	17	18	19	21	22	23	25
185 :	1	3	4	5	6	8	9	10	11	13	14	15	16	18	19	20	21	23	24
190 :	1	2	4	5	6	7	8	10	11	12	13	15	16	17	18	19	21	22	23
195 :	1	2	3	5	6	7	8	9	11	12	13	14	15	16	18	19	20	21	22
200 :	1	2	3	4	6	7	8	9	10	11	12	14	15	16	17	18	19	21	22
205 :	1	2	3	4	6	7	8	9	10	11	12	13	14	15	17	18	19	20	21
210 :	1	2	3	4	6	6	7	8	9	11	12	13	14	15	16	17	18	19	21
215 :	1	2	3	4	5	6	7	8	9	10	11	12	13	15	16	17	18	19	20
220 :	0	2	3	4	5	6	7	8	9	10	11	12	13	14	15	16	17	18	19

Waist Minus Wrist (in inches)

Weight in lbs.	22	22.5	23	23.5	24	24.5	25	25.5	26	26.5	27	27.5	28	28.5	29	29.5	30	30.5	31
225 :	0	1	2	3	4	6	7	8	9	10	11	12	13	14	15	16	17	18	19
230 :	0	1	2	3	4	5	6	7	8	9	10	11	12	13	14	15	16	17	18
235 :	0	1	2	3	4	5	6	7	8	9	10	11	12	13	14	15	16	17	18
240 :	0	1	2	3	4	5	6	7	8	9	10	11	12	13	14	15	16	17	17
245 :	0	1	2	3	4	5	6	7	8	9	9	10	11	12	13	14	15	16	17
250 :	0	1	2	3	4	5	6	6	7	8	9	10	11	12	13	14	15	16	17
255 :	0	1	2	3	3	4	5	6	7	8	9	10	11	12	13	14	14	15	17
260 :	0	1	2	2	3	4	5	6	7	8	9	10	10	11	12	13	14	15	16
265 :	0	1	1	2	3	4	5	6	7	8	8	9	10	11	12	13	14	15	16
270 :	0	1	1	2	3	4	5	6	7	7	8	9	10	11	12	13	13	14	15
275 :	0	1	1	2	3	4	5	5	6	7	8	9	10	11	11	12	13	14	15
280 :	0	0	1	2	3	4	4	5	6	7	8	9	9	10	11	12	13	14	15
285 :	0	0	1	2	3	4	4	5	6	7	8	8	9	10	11	12	12	13	14
290 :	0	0	1	2	3	3	4	5	6	7	7	8	9	10	11	11	12	13	14
295 :	0	0	1	2	2	3	4	5	6	6	7	8	9	10	10	11	12	13	14
300 :	0	0	1	2	2	3	4	5	5	6	7	8	9	9	10	11	12	12	13

Waist Minus Wrist
(in inches)

Weight in lbs.	31.5	32	32.5	33	33.5	34	34.5	35	35.5	36	36.5	37	37.5	38	38.5	39	39.5	40	40.5
120	41	43	45	47	49	50	52	54	56	58	60	62	64	66	68	70	70	74	76
125	39	41	43	45	46	48	50	52	54	56	58	59	61	63	65	67	69	71	72
130	37	39	41	43	44	46	48	50	52	53	55	57	59	61	62	64	66	68	69
135	36	38	39	41	43	44	46	48	50	51	53	55	56	58	60	62	63	67	68
140	34	36	38	39	41	43	44	46	48	49	51	53	54	56	58	59	61	63	64
145	33	35	36	38	39	41	43	44	46	47	49	51	52	54	55	57	59	60	62
150	32	33	35	36	38	40	41	43	44	46	47	49	50	52	53	55	57	58	60
155	31	32	34	35	37	38	40	41	43	44	46	47	49	50	52	53	55	56	58
160	30	31	33	34	35	37	38	40	41	43	44	46	47	48	50	51	53	54	56
165	29	30	31	33	34	36	37	38	40	41	43	44	45	47	48	50	51	52	54
170	28	29	30	32	33	34	36	37	39	40	41	43	44	45	47	48	49	51	52
175	27	28	29	31	32	33	35	36	37	39	40	41	43	44	45	47	48	49	51
180	26	27	28	30	31	32	34	35	36	38	39	40	41	43	44	45	47	48	49
185	25	26	28	29	30	31	33	34	35	37	38	39	40	41	43	44	45	46	48
190	24	26	27	28	29	30	32	33	34	35	37	38	39	40	41	43	44	45	46
195	24	25	26	27	28	30	31	32	33	34	35	37	38	39	40	41	43	44	45
200	23	24	25	26	28	29	30	31	32	33	35	36	37	38	39	40	41	43	44
205	22	23	25	26	27	28	29	30	31	32	34	35	36	37	38	39	40	41	43
210	22	23	24	25	26	27	28	29	30	32	33	34	35	36	37	38	39	40	42
215	21	22	23	24	25	26	28	29	30	31	32	33	34	35	36	37	38	39	40
220	20	22	23	24	25	26	27	28	29	30	31	32	33	34	35	36	37	38	39
225	20	21	22	23	24	25	26	27	28	29	30	31	32	33	34	35	36	37	38
230	19	20	21	22	23	24	25	26	27	28	30	31	32	33	34	35	36	37	38
235	19	20	21	22	23	24	25	26	27	28	29	30	31	32	33	34	35	36	37

Waist Minus Wrist (in inches)

Weight in lbs.	31.5	32	32.5	33	33.5	34	34.5	35	35.5	36	36.5	37	37.5	38	38.5	39	39.5	40	40.5
240	18	19	20	21	22	23	24	25	26	27	28	29	30	31	32	33	34	35	36
245	18	19	20	21	22	23	24	25	26	27	27	28	29	30	31	32	33	34	35
250	18	18	19	20	21	22	23	24	25	26	27	28	29	30	31	31	32	33	34
255	17	18	19	20	21	22	23	24	24	25	26	27	28	29	30	31	32	33	34
260	17	18	19	19	20	21	22	23	24	25	26	27	27	28	29	30	31	32	33
265	16	17	18	19	20	21	22	22	23	24	25	26	27	28	29	29	30	31	32
270	16	17	18	19	19	20	21	22	23	24	25	25	26	27	28	29	30	31	31
275	16	16	17	18	19	20	21	22	22	23	24	25	26	27	27	28	29	30	31
280	15	16	17	18	19	19	20	21	22	23	23	24	25	26	27	28	29	29	30
285	15	16	17	17	18	19	20	21	21	22	23	24	25	26	26	27	28	29	30
290	15	15	16	17	18	19	19	20	21	22	23	23	24	25	26	27	27	28	29
295	14	15	16	17	17	18	19	20	21	21	22	23	24	25	25	26	27	28	28
300	14	15	16	16	17	18	19	19	20	21	22	22	23	24	25	26	26	27	28

Waist Minus Wrist
(in inches)

Weight in lbs.	:	41	41.5	42	42.5	43	43.5	44	44.5	45	45.5	46	46.5	47	47.5	48	48.5	49	49.5	50
120	:	77	79	81	83	85	87	89	91	93	95	97	99	99	99	99	99	99	99	99
125	:	74	76	78	80	82	84	85	87	89	91	93	95	96	98	99	99	99	99	99
130	:	71	73	75	77	78	80	82	84	86	87	89	91	93	94	96	98	99	99	99
135	:	68	70	72	74	75	77	79	80	82	84	86	87	89	91	92	94	96	98	99
140	:	66	68	69	71	72	74	76	77	79	81	82	84	86	87	89	91	92	94	96
145	:	63	65	67	68	70	71	73	75	76	78	79	81	83	84	86	87	89	91	92
150	:	61	63	64	66	67	69	70	72	74	75	77	78	80	81	83	84	86	87	89
155	:	59	61	62	64	65	67	68	70	71	73	74	76	77	79	80	82	83	85	86
160	:	57	59	60	61	63	64	66	67	69	70	72	73	75	76	77	79	80	82	83
165	:	55	57	58	60	61	62	64	65	67	68	69	71	72	74	75	76	78	79	81
170	:	54	55	56	58	59	60	62	63	64	66	67	69	70	71	73	74	75	77	78
175	:	52	53	55	56	57	59	60	61	63	64	65	66	68	69	70	72	73	74	76
180	:	50	52	53	54	56	57	58	59	61	62	63	65	66	67	68	70	71	72	74
185	:	49	50	51	53	54	55	56	58	59	60	61	63	64	65	66	68	69	70	71
190	:	48	49	50	51	52	54	55	56	57	58	60	61	62	63	65	66	67	68	69
195	:	46	47	49	50	51	52	53	55	56	57	58	59	60	62	63	64	65	66	68
200	:	45	46	47	48	50	51	52	53	54	55	57	58	59	60	61	62	63	65	66
205	:	44	45	46	47	48	49	51	52	53	54	55	56	57	58	60	61	62	63	64
210	:	43	44	45	46	47	48	49	50	51	53	54	55	56	57	58	59	60	61	62
215	:	42	43	44	45	46	47	48	49	50	51	52	53	54	56	57	58	59	60	61
220	:	41	42	43	44	45	46	47	48	49	50	51	52	53	54	55	56	57	58	59
225	:	40	41	42	43	44	45	46	47	48	49	50	51	52	53	54	55	56	57	58
230	:	39	40	41	42	43	44	45	46	47	48	49	50	51	52	53	54	55	56	57
235	:	38	39	40	41	42	43	44	45	46	47	48	49	50	51	52	53	54	55	55

Waist Minus Wrist
(in inches)

Weight in lbs.	41	41.5	42	42.5	43	43.5	44	44.5	45	45.5	46	46.5	47	47.5	48	48.5	49	49.5	50
240 :	37	38	39	40	41	42	43	44	45	46	46	47	48	49	50	51	52	53	54
245 :	36	37	38	39	40	41	42	43	44	44	45	46	47	48	49	50	51	52	53
250 :	35	36	37	38	39	40	41	42	43	44	44	45	46	47	48	49	50	51	52
255 :	34	35	36	37	38	39	40	41	42	43	44	44	45	46	47	48	49	50	51
260 :	34	35	35	36	37	38	39	40	41	42	43	43	44	45	46	47	48	49	50
265 :	33	34	35	36	36	37	38	39	40	41	42	43	43	44	45	46	47	48	49
270 :	32	33	34	35	36	37	37	38	39	40	41	42	43	43	44	45	46	47	48
275 :	32	32	33	34	35	36	37	38	38	39	40	41	42	43	43	44	45	46	47
280 :	31	32	33	33	34	35	36	37	38	38	39	40	41	42	43	43	44	45	46
285 :	30	31	32	33	34	34	35	36	37	38	39	39	40	41	42	43	44	44	45
290 :	30	31	31	32	33	34	35	35	36	37	38	39	39	40	41	42	43	43	44
295 :	29	30	31	32	32	33	34	35	36	36	37	38	39	39	40	41	42	43	43
300 :	29	29	30	31	32	33	33	34	35	36	36	37	38	39	39	40	41	42	43

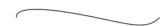

FOR THE RECORD

This appendix contains records for three categories of swimmers:

1. *Senior swimmers:*
   - World and American records (long course) for men and women
   - American records (short course) for men and women
2. *Masters swimmers:*
   - World and American records (long course) for men and women
   - American records (short course) for men and women
3. *Age-group swimmers:*
   - American records (short course) for boys and girls

Note: Long course refers to pools that are fifty meters in length, sometimes called "Olympic size." Virtually all international competition is held in long course pools.

Short course refers to pools that are twenty-five yards or twenty-five meters in length. The United States is the only country that conducts competition in twenty-five-yard pools. The short course records listed here are American records set in pools twenty-five *yards* in length.

WORLD AND AMERICAN RECORDS: LONG COURSE METERS (AS OF 1994)

	Men		Event	Women	
	World	American		World	American
	21.81, Tom Jager, USA, 1990	21.81, Tom Jager, 1990	50 free	24.79, Yang Wenyi, CHN, 1992	25.20, Jenny Thompson, 1992
	48.42, Matt Biondi, USA, 1988	48.42, Matt Biondi, 1988	100 free	54.48, Jenny Thompson, USA, 1992	54.48, Jenny Thompson, 1992
	1:46.69, Giorgio Lamberti, ITA 1989	1:47.72, Matt Biondi, 1988	200 free	1:57.55, Heike Freidrich, GDR, 1986	1:57.90, Nicole Haislett, 1992
	3:45.00, Evgueni Sadovyi, RUS, 1992	3:48.06, Matt Cettlinski, 1988	400 free	4:03.85, Janet Evans, USA, 1988	4:03.85, Janet Evans, 1988
	7:46.60, Kieren Perkins, AUS, 1992	7:52.45, Sean Killion, 1987	800 free	8:16.22, Janet Evans, USA, 1989	8:16.22, Janet Evans, 1989
	14:43.48, Kieren Perkins, AUS, 1992	15:01.51, George DiCarlo, 1984	1,500 free	15:52.10, Janet Evans, USA, 1988	15:52.10, Janet Evans, 1988
	53.86, Jeff Rouse, USA, 1992	53.86, Jeff Rouse, 1992	100 back	1:00.31, Kristina Egerszegl, HUN, 1991	1:00.82, Lea Loveless, 1992
	1:56.57, Martin Zubero, ESP, 1991	1:58.66, Royce Sharp, 1992	200 back	2:06.62, Kristina Egerszegl, HUN, 1991	2:08.60, Betsy Mitchell, 1986
	1:00.95, Karolyi Guttler, HUN, 1993	1:01.40, Nelson Diebel, 1992	100 breast	1:07.91, Silke Horner, GDR, 1987	1:08.17, Anita Nall, 1992
	2:10.16, Mike Barrowman, USA, 1992	2:10.16, Mike Barrowman, 1992	200 breast	2:24.76, Rebecca Brown, AUS, 1994	2:25.35, Anita Nall, 1992

Event	Men		Women	
	World	American	World	American
100 fly	52.84, Pablo Morales, USA, 1986	52.84, Pablo Morales, 1986	57.93, Mary T. Meagher, USA, 1981	57.93, Mary T. Meagher, 1981
200 fly	1:55.69, Melvin Stewart, USA, 1991	1:55.69, Melvin Stewart, 1991	2:05.97 Mary T. Meagher, USA, 1981	2:05.97, Mary T. Meagher, 1981
200 IM	1:59.36, Tamas Darnyl, HUN, 1991	2:00.11, David Wharton, 1989	2:11.65, Lin Li, CHN, 1992	2:11.91, Summer Sanders, 1992
400 IM	4:12.36, Tamas Darnyl, HUN, 1991	4:13.52, Tom Dolan, 1994	4:36.10, Petra Schneider, GDR, 1982	4:37.58, Summer Sanders, 1992
400 medley relay	3:36.93, USA Olympic Team, 1988, 1992	3:36.93, USA Olympic Team, 1988, 1992	4:02.54, USA Olympic Team, 1992	4:02.54, USA Olympic Team, 1992
400 free relay	3:16.53, USA Olympic Team, 1988	3:16.53, USA Olympic Team, 1988	3:39.46, USA Olympic Team, 1992	3:39.46, USA Olympic Team, 1992
800 free relay	7:11.95, EUN Olympic Team, 1992	7:12.51; USA Olympic Team, 1988	7:55.47, GDR National Team, 1987	8:02.12, USA World Championship Team, 1986

AMERICAN RECORDS: SHORT COURSE YARDS (AS OF 1994)

Women	Event	Men
21.77, Amy Van Dyken, 1994	50 free	19.05, Tom Jager, 1990
47.61, Jenny Thompson, 1992	100 free	41.80, Matt Biondi, 1987
1:43.28, Nicole Haislett, 1992	200 free	1:33.03, Matt Biondi, 1987
4:34.39, Janet Evans, 1990	500 free	4:11.59, Chad Carvin, 1994
9:25.49, Janet Evans, 1989	1,000 free	8:47.38, Mike O'Brien, 1985
15:39.14, Janet Evans, 1990	1,650 free	14:34.91, Chad Carvin, 1994
52.79, Lea Loveless, 1992	100 back	45.74, Brian Retterer, 1994
1:52.98, Whitney Hedgepath, 1992	200 back	1:40.64, Jeff Rouse, 1992
1:00.66, Mary Ellen Blanchard, 1989	100 breast	52.48, Steve Lundquist, 1983
2:09.06, Mary Ellen Blanchard, 1989	200 breast	1:53.77, Mike Barrowman, 1990
51.75, Crissy Ahmann-Leighton, 1992	100 fly	46.26, Pablo Morales, 1986
1:52.99, Mary T. Meagher, 1981	200 fly	1:41.78, Melvin Stewart, 1991
1:55.54, Summer Sanders, 1992	200 IM	1:43.52, Greg Burgess, 1993
4:02.28, Summer Sanders, 1992	400 IM	3:40.64, Greg Burgess, 1994
1:38.68, Stanford Univ. team, 1992	200 medley relay	1:25.88, Stanford Univ. team, 1992
1:28.90, Univ of Texas team, 1989	200 free relay	1:16.93, Stanford Univ. team, 1994
3:35.64 Stanford Univ. team, 1992	400 medley relay	3:08.39, Stanford Univ. team, 1992
3:14.97, Univ of Florida team, 1993	400 free relay	2:51.07, Univ of Texas team, 1994
7:04.06, Stanford Univ. team, 1992	800 free relay	6:21.39, Univ of Texas team, 1990

FINA WORLD RECORDS LONG COURSE METERS (as of 1994)

Men

25–29

Event		Name	Country	Year	Time
50	Free	Kevin DeForrest	USA	1983	22.59
100	Free	Jim Montgomery	USA	1981	51.25
200	Free	John Keppeler	USA	1992	1:52.17
400	Free	Marcus Mattioli	BRA	1988	4:06.99
800	Free	Jeff Erwin	USA	1992	8:36.83
1500	Free	Cameron Reid	USA	1987	16:28.69
50	Back	Romulo Arantes	BRA	1986	27.39
100	Back	John Keppeler	USA	1992	58.24
200	Back	John Keppeler	USA	1992	2:07.57
50	Brst	Dewey Wyatt	USA	1993	29.77
100	Brst	David Lundberg	USA	1989	1:04.60
200	Brst	Thomas Ligl	GER	1987	2:26.73
50	Fly	DeForrest/Bottom	USA	1984	25.16
100	Fly	Michael Bottom	USA	1984	56.34
200	Fly	Miloslav Lukasek	TCH	1984	2:05.25
200	IM	Cameron Reid	USA	1987	2:09.21
400	IM	Cameron Reid	USA	1987	4:34.08

30–34

Event		Name	Country	Year	Time
50	Free	Rowdy Gaines	USA	1990	23.21
100	Free	Rowdy Gaines	USA	1991	51.50
200	Free	Rowdy Gaines	USA	1990	1:54.04
400	Free	Jim Montgomery	USA	1986	4:08.70

Women

25–29

Event		Name	Country	Year	Time
50	Free	Sara Shand	USA	1991	26.68
100	Free	Sara Shand	USA	1991	58.23
200	Free	Sara Shand	USA	1989	2:07.11
400	Free	Sara Shand	USA	1989	4:27.53
800	Free	Sara Shand	USA	1989	9:18.43
1500	Free	Amy Pope	USA	1988	17:38.78
50	Back	Diane Graner	USA	1989	30.80
100	Back	Monique Rodahl	NZL	1989	1:06.46
200	Back	Diane Graner	USA	1989	2:19.97
50	Brst	Sabrina Seminatore	ITA	1989	32.01
100	Brst	Sabrina Seminatore	ITA	1990	1:16.05
200	Brst	Sharon Davies	GBR	1990	2:42.02
50	Fly	Rosemarie Seaman	USA	1987	28.79
100	Fly	Rosemarie Seaman	USA	1987	1:03.91
200	Fly	Susan Palmer-White	AUS	1992	2:18.69
200	IM	Sharon Davies	GBR	1990	2:22.00
400	IM	Sharon Davies	GBR	1990	5:05.29

30–34

Event		Name	Country	Year	Time
50	Free	Sandy Neilson-Bell	USA	1988	26.37
100	Free	Sandy Neilson-Bell	USA	1988	58.09
200	Free	Beth Knight	USA	1989	2:07.84
400	Free	Beth Knight	USA	1991	4:30.38

30–34

Men

Time	Year	Country	Name	Distance	Stroke
8:46.99	1986	USA	Jim Montgomery	800	Free
16:36.06	1993	USA	Bobby Patten	1500	Free
27.32	1988	USA	Dix Ozier	50	Back
1:00.03	1993	USA	Jay Yarid	100	Back
2:09.84	1993	USA	Jay Yarid	200	Back
29.42	1992	USA	David Guthrie	50	Brst
1:05.65	1991	USA	David Lundberg	100	Brst
2:24.06	1991	USA	David Lundberg	200	Brst
25.31	1988	USA	Mike Bottom	50	Fly
56.64	1988	USA	Mike Bottom	100	Fly
2:07.43	1993	USA	Bobby Patten	200	Fly
2:09.69	1991	USA	David Lundberg	200	IM
4:40.44	1992	USA	David Lundberg	400	IM

Women

Distance	Stroke	Name	Country	Year	Time
800	Free	Lynn Marshall	CAN	1992	9:16.82
1500	Free	Karen Burton	USA	1992	17:40.50
50	Back	Beth Mauer	USA	1988	32.11
100	Back	Zena Herrmann	USA	1992	1:09.07
200	Back	Daphne Fuchs	GER	1993	2:23.47
50	Brst	Mary Hohmann	GBR	1988	34.56
100	Brst	Mary Hohmann	GBR	1988	1:14.52
200	Brst	Dagmar Hilbig	GER	1989	2:48.41
50	Fly	Beth Harrell	USA	1992	29.22
100	Fly	Beth Harrell	USA	1992	1:06.08
200	Fly	Karen Burton	USA	1992	2:27.54
200	IM	Sandy Neilson-Bell	USA	1988	2:29.22
400	IM	Karen Burton	USA	1992	5:11.39

35–39

Men

Time	Year	Country	Name	Distance	Stroke
24.56	1992	RUS	Alexei Markovsky	50	Free
54.28	1992	USA	James Montgomery	100	Free
1:57.95	1992	USA	Dan Stephenson	200	Free
4:15.49	1992	USA	Dan Stephenson	400	Free
8:52.22	1992	USA	Dan Stephenson	800	Free
17:26.29	1989	USA	Jim McConica	1500	Free
28.04	1978	USA	Thompson Mann	50	Back
1:00.95	1993	USA	William Specht	100	Back
2:13.83	1990	USA	Tom Wolf	200	Back
30.79	1992	USA	Doug Malcolm	50	Brst
1:07.90	1992	USA	Mark Schuman	100	Brst
2:33.05	1992	USA	Mark Schuman	200	Brst
25.93	1993	USA	Michael Bottom	50	Fly

Women

Distance	Stroke	Name	Country	Year	Time
50	Free	Sandy Neilson-Bell	USA	1993	26.89
100	Free	Susan Halfacre	USA	1988	1:00.25
200	Free	Susan Halfacre	USA	1988	2:09.33
400	Free	Susan Halfacre	USA	1988	4:33.08
800	Free	Susan Halfacre	USA	1988	9:24.54
1500	Free	Susan Pamelia	USA	1987	18:12.11
50	Back	Laura Val	USA	1990	32.39
100	Back	Laura Val	USA	1989	1:10.94
200	Back	Karen Farnsworth	USA	1992	2:35.44
50	Brst	Leslie Wetzel-Osborne	USA	1989	34.41
100	Brst	Leslie Wetzel-Osborne	USA	1990	1:17.44
200	Brst	Dagmar Hilbig	GER	1993	2:51.75
50	Fly	Susan Halfacre	USA	1988	29.27

Women

35–39

100	Fly	Susan Halfacre	USA	1988	1:05.39
200	Fly	Laura Val	USA	1989	2:26.38
200	IM	Sandy Neilson-Bell	USA	1993	2:36.67
400	IM	Karen Farnsworth	USA	1992	5:34.47

40–44

50	Free	Laura Val	USA	1992	28.05
100	Free	Laura Val	USA	1992	1:02.99
200	Free	Laura Val	USA	1993	2:17.01
400	Free	Barbara Dunbar	USA	1990	4:54.49
800	Free	Laura Val	USA	1993	9:57.69
1500	Free	Barbara Dunbar	USA	1992	19:00.40
50	Back	Laura Val	USA	1992	32.42
100	Back	Laura Val	USA	1992	1:11.03
200	Back	Brigitte Bazureau	FRA	1992	2:43.23
50	Brst	Alice Wright-Belknap	USA	1992	37.02
100	Brst	Debra Walker	USA	1991	1:21.73
200	Brst	Gayle Benty	USA	1993	2:59.24
50	Fly	Laura Val	USA	1992	30.13
100	Fly	Laura Val	USA	1992	1:06.27
200	Fly	Barbara Dunbar	USA	1989	2:33.51
200	IM	Laura Val	USA	1993	2:38.20
400	IM	Laura Val	USA	1993	5:39.70

45–49

50	Free	Ardeth Mueller	USA	1987	29.08
100	Free	Ardeth Mueller	USA	1987	1:05.44
200	Free	Ardeth Mueller	USA	1987	2:24.24

Men

35–39

100	Fly	William Specht	USA	1993	57.44
200	Fly	James Belardi	USA	1992	2:09.18
200	IM	Mark Schuman	USA	1992	2:16.49
400	IM	James Belardi	USA	1992	4:55.13

40–44

50	Free	Tom Whatley	USA	1992	24.93
100	Free	Terence Downes	RSA	1993	56.00
200	Free	Tim Broderick	USA	1993	2:03.28
400	Free	Tim Broderick	USA	1993	4:24.26
800	Free	Kevin Polansky	USA	1990	9:19.37
1500	Free	Kevin Polansky	USA	1990	17:30.13
50	Back	Peter O'Keeffe	USA	1990	29.38
100	Back	Peter O'Keeffe	USA	1990	1:03.39
200	Back	Peter O'Keeffe	USA	1990	2:18.17
50	Brst	Peder Dahlberg	USA	1992	30.82
100	Brst	Peder Dahlberg	USA	1992	1:09.95
200	Brst	Rick Colella	USA	1992	2:32.17
50	Fly	John Foote	USA	1991	27.04
100	Fly	Lance Larson	USA	1980	1:02.05
200	Fly	Edward Brown	USA	1993	2:20.81
200	IM	Rick Colella	USA	1992	2:18.92
400	IM	Rick Colella	USA	1992	4:57.46

45–49

50	Free	Richard Abrahams	USA	1990	25.30
100	Free	Andrew McPherson	USA	1992	57.04
200	Free	Tim Garton	USA	1990	2:07.18

45–49

Event		Men				Women		
		Time	Year	Country	Name	Name	Country	Year	Time
400	Free	4:27.70	1992	USA	Bob Momsen	Ardeth Mueller	USA	1987	5:08.67
800	Free	9:31.38	1992	USA	Bob Momsen	Ardeth Mueller	USA	1987	10:48.41
1500	Free	18:34.73	1983	USA	Ed Hinshaw	Ardeth Mueller	USA	1987	21:08.30
50	Back	30.42	1993	USA	Hugh Wilder	Satoko Takeuji	JPN	1988	34.51
100	Back	1:06.00	1992	USA	Hugh Wilder	Satoko Takeuji	JPN	1989	1:17.06
200	Back	2:26.91	1992	USA	John Calvert	Sandra O'Neil	GBR	1992	2:50.27
50	Brst	32.76	1991	USA	Rick Nesbit	Jane MacLeod	AUS	1991	37.77
100	Brst	1:12.98	1992	USA	Robert Strand	Carolyn Boak	USA	1992	1:26.28
200	Brst	2:41.88	1992	USA	Peter Wisner	Carolyn Boak	USA	1992	3:09.19
50	Fly	27.12	1992	USA	Dan Thompson	Ardeth Mueller	USA	1987	30.74
100	Fly	1:02.84	1992	USA	Andrew McPherson	Ardeth Mueller	USA	1987	1:12.67
200	Fly	2:27.56	1993	AUS	John Covacevich	Ardeth Mueller	USA	1987	2:44.10
200	IM	2:24.39	1992	USA	Bob Momsen	Ardeth Mueller	USA	1987	2:46.91
400	IM	5:12.03	1992	USA	Bob Momsen	Ardeth Mueller	USA	1987	5:54.98

50–54

Event		Men				Women		
		Time	Year	Country	Name	Name	Country	Year	Time
50	Free	26.16	1983	USA	Don Hill	Ardeth Mueller	USA	1993	29.33
100	Free	58.62	1993	USA	Timothy Garton	Ardeth Mueller	USA	1992	1:07.42
200	Free	2:09.74	1993	USA	Timothy Garton	Ardeth Mueller	USA	1993	2:29.22
400	Free	4:43.72	1992	USA	Timothy Garton	Ardeth Mueller	USA	1991	5:16.62
800	Free	9:55.59	1992	USA	Timothy Garton	Ardeth Mueller	USA	1991	10:58.47
1500	Free	18:49.43	1993	GBR	Sandy Galletly	Ardeth Mueller	USA	1991	21:02.46
50	Back	30.93	1988	USA	John Smith	Satoko Takeuji	JPN	1992	34.87
100	Back	1:09.82	1993	USA	Richard Burns	Satoko Takeuji	JPN	1993	1:19.45
200	Back	2:32.81	1993	USA	Richard Burns	Satoko Takeuji	JPN	1992	2:51.11
50	Brst	33.38	1986	JPN	Hiroshi Kotegawa	Monika Senftleben	GER	1992	39.52
100	Brst	1:15.60	1983	USA	Manuel Sanguily	Joann Leilich	USA	1990	1:28.83
200	Brst	2:51.68	1992	AUS	Michael Moloney	Diane Ford	GBR	1993	3:13.64

50–54

Men Time	Year	Country	Name	Event	Stroke	Name	Country	Year	Women Time
28.19	1993	USA	Keefe Lodwig	50	Fly	Ardeth Mueller	USA	1993	31.69
1:05.83	1992	USA	Timothy Garton	100	Fly	Ardeth Mueller	USA	1993	1:13.86
2:32.65	1993	AUS	Peter Gilmore	200	Fly	Ardeth Mueller	USA	1991	2:49.53
2:28.70	1993	USA	Timothy Garton	200	IM	Ardeth Mueller	USA	1991	2:54.57
5:25.32	1993	USA	Timothy Garton	400	IM	Ardeth Mueller	USA	1992	6:12.08

55–59

Men Time	Year	Country	Name	Event	Stroke	Name	Country	Year	Women Time
27.42	1988	USA	Michael Muckleroy	50	Free	Jayne Bruner	USA	1991	32.59
1:01.95	1991	USA	Bob Bailie	100	Free	Yoshiko Osaki	JPN	1993	1:11.01
2:21.33	1992	JPN	Kazuya Nishino	200	Free	Yoshiko Osaki	JPN	1993	2:36.58
4:58.41	1988	USA	Burwell Jones	400	Free	Yoshiko Osaki	JPN	1993	5:26.57
10:27.08	1988	USA	Burwell Jones	800	Free	Lavelle Stoinoff	USA	1988	11:30.97
19:54.72	1990	USA	Burwell Jones	1500	Free	Lavelle Stoinoff	USA	1988	22:18.91
32.94	1992	USA	Yoshi Oyawaka	50	Back	Betsy Jordan	USA	1992	37.30
1:13.15	1990	USA	Jack Beattie	100	Back	Betsy Jordan	USA	1992	1:21.42
2:42.37	1988	USA	Don Brown	200	Back	Betsy Jordan	USA	1992	2:59.18
33.03	1993	JPN	Hiroshi Kotegawa	50	Brst	Jayne Bruner	USA	1991	39.91
1:17.87	1988	USA	John Kortheuer	100	Brst	Jayne Bruner	USA	1992	1:29.88
2:56.20	1990	GBR	Thomas Walker	200	Brst	Flora Connolly	GBR	1989	3:18.11
30.17	1992	USA	Robert Proebsting	50	Fly	Gail Roper	USA	1985	35.29
1:10.28	1992	USA	Robert Proebsting	100	Fly	Gail Roper	USA	1985	1:27.49
2:48.42	1993	USA	Robert Proebsting	200	Fly	Flora Connolly	GBR	1989	3:17.68
2:43.57	1990	USA	Burwell Jones	200	IM	Jayne Bruner	USA	1992	3:06.11
5:53.53	1990	USA	Burwell Jones	400	IM	Gail Roper	USA	1985	6:42.05

60–64

Men Time	Year	Country	Name	Event	Stroke	Name	Country	Year	Women Time
27.86	1992	USA	Donald Hill	50	Free	Jane Asher	GBR	1992	33.60
1:02.80	1992	USA	Donald Hill	100	Free	Jane Asher	GBR	1991	1:14.25

60–64

		Men				Women			
200	Free	Donald Hill	USA	1992	2:23.11	Lavelle Stoinoff	USA	1993	2:43.83
400	Free	Graham Johnston	USA	1991	5:05.54	Lavelle Stoinoff	USA	1993	5:47.52
800	Free	Graham Johnston	USA	1991	10:36.09	Lavelle Stoinoff	USA	1993	12:04.16
1500	Free	Graham Johnston	USA	1991	20:06.80	Lavelle Stoinoff	USA	1993	23:17.39
50	Back	Yoshi Oyakawa	USA	1993	33.74	Doris Steadman	USA	1989	40.35
100	Back	Donald Brown	USA	1993	1:15.66	Grethe Bendtsen	DEN	1992	1:30.22
200	Back	Donald Brown	USA	1993	2:45.93	Lavelle Stoinoff	USA	1993	3:14.11
50	Brst	John Kortheuer	USA	1991	35.91	Edith Boehm	GER	1988	42.49
100	Brst	John Kortheuer	USA	1991	1:21.58	Flora Connolly	GBR	1993	1:35.86
200	Brst	John Kortheuer	USA	1991	3:08.59	Flora Connolly	GBR	1993	3:27.50
50	Fly	Jean-Louis Ledall	FRA	1993	31.52	Jane Asher	GBR	1991	38.54
100	Fly	Jean-Louis Ledall	FRA	1993	1:16.39	Judie Oliver	CAN	1992	1:31.52
200	Fly	John Masters	USA	1990	3:00.99	Judie Oliver	CAN	1992	3:28.58
200	IM	Graham Johnston	USA	1993	2:50.08	Flora Connolly	GBR	1993	3:15.30
400	IM	Graham Johnston	USA	1991	6:04.99	Flora Connolly	GBR	1993	6:59.08

65–69

		Men				Women			
50	Free	B. Schlurike	GER	1991	28.94	Clara Walker	USA	1992	34.75
100	Free	James Welch	USA	1983	1:08.15	Clara Walker	USA	1992	1:16.84
200	Free	Peter Powlison	USA	1987	2:32.90	Clara Walker	USA	1992	2:48.51
400	Free	James Welch	USA	1983	5:38.79	Clara Walker	USA	1991	6:05.22
800	Free	Randall Hartley	AUS	1991	11:35.97	Clara Walker	USA	1992	12:27.60
1500	Free	Win Wilson	USA	1992	22:29.32	Clara Walker	USA	1992	24:07.05
50	Back	George Gandsey	USA	1989	35.47	Clara Walker	USA	1992	39.85
100	Back	Roger Franks	USA	1992	1:20.74	Doris Steadman	USA	1990	1:31.58
200	Back	Roger Franks	USA	1992	2:55.46	Doris Steadman	USA	1990	3:17.12
50	Brst	Joseph Kurtzman	USA	1991	38.28	Erika Lange	GER	1993	45.61
100	Brst	Joseph Kurtzman	USA	1991	1:28.91	Clara Walker	USA	1991	1:42.841

65–69

Time	Year	Country	Men Name	Dist	Stroke	Women Name	Country	Year	Time
3:16.90	1990	GER	Karl Heinz Knops	200	Brst	Margaret Evans	GBR	1989	3:45.7
33.34	1987	GBR	Jack Hale	50	Fly	Florence Carr	USA	1990	43.35
1:20.59	1992	USA	Joseph Kurtzman	100	Fly	June Krauser	USA	1991	1:40.35
3:08.79	1991	USA	Joseph Kurtzman	200	Fly	June Krauser	USA	1992	3:42.61
2:57.61	1993	USA	Charles Moss	200	IM	Clara Walker	USA	1992	3:20.58
6:25.02	1993	USA	Charles Moss	400	IM	Clara Walker	USA	1992	7:09.69

70–74

Time	Year	Country	Men Name	Dist	Stroke	Women Name	Country	Year	Time
29.35	1984	USA	Kelley Lemmon	50	Free	Olga Johnson	NZL	1992	37.61
1:11.61	1983	USA	Kelley Lemmon	100	Free	Catherine Kerr	CAN	1992	1:28.07
2:44.86	1983	USA	Kelley Lemmon	200	Free	Catherine Kerr	CAN	1992	3:21.01
5:57.45	1991	JPN	Domei Suzuki	400	Free	Margery Meyer	USA	1993	7:07.58
12:34.22	1991	JPN	Domei Suzuki	800	Free	Margery Meyer	USA	1993	15:00.12
23:59.01	1991	JPN	Domei Suzuki	1500	Free	Margery Meyer	USA	1993	28:39.46
37.49	1989	USA	Ray Taft	50	Back	Bunny Cederlund	USA	1992	44.53
1:25.35	1989	USA	Ray Taft	100	Back	Beryl Anderson	AUS	1987	1:39.85
3:13.25	1989	USA	Ray Taft	200	Back	Beryl Anderson	AUS	1987	3:47.59
40.56	1990	GER	Walter Minnich	50	Brst	Ingeborg Fritze	GER	1992	49.57
1:33.20	1984	USA	Bennett Allen	100	Brst	Betty Christian	USA	1992	1:52.88
3:32.90	1988	USA	Aldo Da Rosa	200	Brst	Betty Christian	USA	1992	4:06.80
35.65	1989	USA	Ray Taft	50	Fly	Catherine Kerr	CAN	1992	46.55
1:32.85	1990	USA	Andrew Holden	100	Fly	Maria Lenk	BRA	1985	2:02.61
3:38.48	1987	AUS	Donald Jeffrey	200	Fly	Maxine Merlino	USA	1982	4:37.05
3:11.42	1989	USA	Ray Taft	200	IM	Catherine Kerr	CAN	1992	3:51.91
6:59.24	1989	USA	Ray Taft	400	IM	Eva Rauner	GER	1990	8:33.57

75–79

Time	Year	Country	Men Name	Dist	Stroke	Women Name	Country	Year	Time
32.50	1983	USA	Lyle Collet	50	Free	Hatsuho Sugaya	JPN	1991	40.85

75–79

Men

Distance	Stroke	Name	Country	Year	Time
100	Free	Kelley Lemmon	USA	1987	1:14.86
200	Free	Kelley Lemmon	USA	1987	2:53.73
400	Free	Arthur Rule	USA	1981	6:27.76
800	Free	Herbert Howe	USA	1987	13:35.96
1500	Free	Herbert Howe	USA	1987	25:41.55
50	Back	Arthur Hargrave	USA	1982	40.47
100	Back	Arthur Hargrave	USA	1982	1:32.92
200	Back	Edward Shea	USA	1991	3:25.93
50	Brst	Hiromu Yoshimoto	JPN	1990	42.58
100	Brst	Augusto Romano	ITA	1993	1:37.55
200	Brst	Augusto Romano	ITA	1993	3:39.00
50	Fly	Yoshi Miyamoto	JPN	1993	39.65
100	Fly	Anton Cerer	USA	1992	1:39.80
200	Fly	Anton Cerer	USA	1992	3:43.56
200	IM	Kelley Lemmon	USA	1987	3:30.50
400	IM	Anton Cerer	USA	1992	7:33.32

Women

Distance	Stroke	Name	Country	Year	Time
100	Free	Louise Donovan	USA	1993	1:38.28
200	Free	Rita Simonton	USA	1993	3:37.64
400	Free	Rita Simonton	USA	1993	7:38.77
800	Free	Rita Simonton	USA	1993	15:42.58
1500	Free	Rita Simonton	USA	1993	29:45.90
50	Back	Willy Van Rysel	GBR	1991	46.64
100	Back	Willy Van Rysel	GBR	1991	1:49.73
200	Back	Marie Wicklun	USA	1989	4:07.44
50	Brst	Emmi Pauli	GER	1989	52.90
100	Brst	Gertrud Zint	USA	1993	2:05.99
200	Brst	Marlene Butzbach	GER	1986	4:36.72
50	Fly	Gertrud Zint	USA	1993	55.38
100	Fly	Kay Schimpf	USA	1992	2:19.44
200	Fly	Maxine Merlino	USA	1988	4:54.79
200	IM	Maria Lenk	BRA	1990	4:20.42
400	IM	Maxine Merlino	USA	1987	9:11.23

80–84

Men

Distance	Stroke	Name	Country	Year	Time
50	Free	Woodrow Bowersock	USA	1993	34.00
100	Free	Woodrow Bowersock	USA	1993	1:23.56
200	Free	Gus Langner	USA	1983	3:31.79
400	Free	Gus Langner	USA	1983	7:23.09
800	Free	Toshio Terao	JPN	1990	15:48.62
1500	Free	Gus Langner	USA	1983	28:54.95
50	Back	Art Hargrave	USA	1987	45.69
100	Back	Rolf Reinstadtler	GER	1992	1:45.37
200	Back	Rolf Reinstadtler	GER	1993	3:47.46
50	Brst	Karl Wittenberg	GER	1991	46.59

Women

Distance	Stroke	Name	Country	Year	Time
50	Free	Ume Wada	JPN	1991	44.25
100	Free	Ume Wada	JPN	1991	1:39.30
200	Free	Ume Wada	JPN	1992	3:44.00
400	Free	Ume Wada	JPN	1991	8:23.50
800	Free	Ume Wada	JPN	1991	17:21.19
1500	Free	Ume Wada	JPN	1992	33:59.65
50	Back	Marian Wright	AUS	1989	53.73
100	Back	Marian Wright	AUS	1989	2:01.87
200	Back	Marian Wright	AUS	1989	4:22.89
50	Brst	Dorothy Weston	GBR	1993	59.60

Men

80–84

Time	Year	Country	Name	Distance	Stroke
1:51.25	1991	GER	Karl Wittenberg	100	Brst
4:25.69	1992	USA	Harold Perry	200	Brst
52.05	1991	USA	Jesse Coon	50	Fly
2:21.06	1991	USA	Jesse Coon	100	Fly
5:11.48	1989	AUS	Frank Griffiths	200	Fly
4:20.05	1993	GER	Rolf Reinstadtler	200	IM
9:47.72	1988	AUS	Frank Griffiths	400	IM

85–89

Time	Year	Country	Name	Distance	Stroke
41.53	1993	AUS	Frank Griffiths	50	Free
1:43.03	1988	USA	Gus Langner	100	Free
3:48.91	1988	USA	Gus Langner	200	Free
8:14.50	1988	USA	Gus Langner	400	Free
17:11.21	1988	USA	Gus Langner	800	Free
33:08.42	1989	USA	Gus Langner	1500	Free
58.07	1993	USA	Jim Penfield	50	Back
2:07.06	1993	USA	Jim Penfield	100	Back
4:43.49	1993	USA	Jim Penfield	200	Back
58.96	1992	GER	Franck Meerwald	50	Brst
2:18.92	1991	JPN	Shohei Yoshida	100	Brst
5:09.86	1991	JPN	Shohei Yoshida	200	Brst
59.50	1991	JPN	Shohei Yoshida	50	Fly
2:33.63	1993	AUS	Frank Griffiths	100	Fly
5:24.28	1993	AUS	Frank Griffiths	200	Fly
4:40.15	1993	AUS	Frank Griffiths	200	IM
12:27.27	1991	USA	Abe Olanoff	400	IM

90+

Time	Year	Country	Name	Distance	Stroke
49.51	1993	USA	Gus Langner	50	Free

Women

80–84

Distance	Stroke	Name	Country	Year	Time
100	Brst	Dorothy Weston	GBR	1993	2:17.08
200	Brst	Dorothy Weston	GBR	1993	5:01.36
50	Fly	Vivienne Cherriman	GBR	1988	1:13.71
100	Fly	Maxine Merlino	USA	1992	2:37.32
200	Fly	Maxine Merlino	USA	1992	5:29.93
200	IM	Maxine Merlino	USA	1992	4:47.02
400	IM	Maxine Merlino	USA	1992	10:05.13

85–89

Distance	Stroke	Name	Country	Year	Time
50	Free	Aileen Soule	USA	1991	51.48
100	Free	Aileen Soule	USA	1991	2:07.61
200	Free	Aileen Soule	USA	1991	4:49.52
400	Free	Ella Peckham	USA	1984	13:22.48
800	Free	Anna Bauscher	USA	1988	24:23.38
1500	Free	Anna Bauscher	USA	1991	52:15.77
50	Back	Aileen Soule	USA	1991	58.42
100	Back	Aileen Soule	USA	1991	2:13.13
200	Back	Aileen Soule	USA	1991	4:47.82
50	Brst	Yoshi Kuchiba	JPN	1993	1:26.13
100	Brst	Yoshi Kuchiba	JPN	1993	3:06.40
200	Brst	Yoshi Kuchiba	JPN	1993	7:15.13
50	Fly	Ella Peckham	USA	1985	1:27.77
100	Fly	Katherine Pelton	USA	1991	3:01.14
200	Fly	Katherine Pelton	USA	1990	7:18.41
200	IM	Katherine Pelton	USA	1991	6:44.53
400	IM	Katherine Pelton	USA	1990	14:02.65

90+

Distance	Stroke	Name	Country	Year	Time
50	Free	Pearl Miller	USA	1988	2:02.38

	Men						Women		
1:57.91	1993	USA	Gus Langner	100	Free	Pearl Miller	USA	1988	4:08.22
4:28.34	1993	USA	Gus Langner	200	Free				
9:44.11	1993	USA	Gus Langner	400	Free				
23:15.77	1993	USA	Gus Langner	800	Free				
36:47.02	1993	USA	Gus Langner	1500	Free				
1:16.30	1989	USA	Tom Lane	50	Back	Vera Fernance	AUS	1988	2:01.70
3:19.14	1992	USA	Tom Lane	100	Back	Vera Fernance	AUS	1988	3:59.89
8:59.53	1990	USA	Tony Lopez	200	Back	Pearl Miller	USA	1989	10:47.76
1:36.87	1989	USA	Tom Lane	50	Brst				
5:16.03	1982	USA	Ludwig Magener	100	Brst				

90+

25-29

		Men			Women		
Dist.	Stroke	Name	Year	Time	Name	Year	Time
50	Free	Robert Peel	1991	0:19.83	Anna Pettis-Scott	1992	0:23.20
100	Free	Robert Peel	1991	0:44.39	Sara Shand	1993	0:51.07
200	Free	Franz Mortensen	1993	1:39.38	Sara Shand	1993	1:51.53
500	Free	Franz Mortensen	1993	4:31.90	Karen Burton	1991	4:56.18
1,000	Free	Franz Mortensen	1993	9:26.80	Karen Burton	1991	10:17.82
1,650	Free	Bobby Patten	1990	15:46.91	Karen Burton	1991	16:50.17
50	Back	Mook Rodenbaugh	1991	0:23.23	Diane Graner	1989	0:26.76
100	Back	Andrew Gill	1992	0:49.83	Diane Graner	1991	0:56.70
200	Back	Robert Hauck	1993	1:50.32	Diane Graner	1991	2:01.29
50	Breast	Greg Rodenbaugh	1991	0:25.34	Sharon McIntyre-Woods	1991	0:30.60
100	Breast	David Lundberg	1990	0:56.21	Sharon McIntyre-Woods	1991	1:06.50
200	Breast	Douglas Soltis	1988	2:03.69	Bethanne Lambert	1993	2:24.87
50	Fly	Coy Cobb	1991	0:22.27	Linda Lanini	1987	0:25.68
100	Fly	Stuart Knowles	1991	0:49.71	Diane Graner	1991	0:57.01
200	Fly	Bobby Patten	1990	1:49.21	June Ford	1987	2:03.38
100	IM	Mook Rodenbaugh	1991	0:50.47	Sara Shand	1993	0:58.84
200	IM	Cameron Reid	1988	1:52.55	Sara Shand	1993	2:05.98
400	IM	Cameron Reid	1988	3:59.73	Sara Shand	1991	4:28.40

30-34

		Men			Women		
Dist.	Stroke	Name	Year	Time	Name	Year	Time
50	Free	John Smith	1992	0:20.90	Sandy Neilson-Bell	1988	0:23.04
100	Free	Jim Montgomery	1985	0:45.29	Sandy Neilson	1987	0:50.83
200	Free	Jim Montgomery	1988	1:39.97	Sandy Neilson	1987	1:52.57
500	Free	Steven Fisher	1992	4:39.38	June Ford	1993	5:05.06
1,000	Free	Cameron Reid	1991	9:38.13	Beth Knight	1990	10:31.89

Men

Distance	Stroke	Name	Year	Time
1,650	Free	James Kegley	1988	16:06.55
50	Back	Clay Britt	1992	0:23.39
100	Back	Clay Britt	1992	0:50.21
200	Back	Jay Yarid	1993	1:50.57
50	Breast	David Lundberg	1991	0:25.88
100	Breast	David Lundberg	1991	0:56.58
200	Breast	David Lundberg	1991	2:02.32
50	Fly	Robert Placak	1989	0:22.66
100	Fly	William Specht	1989	0:49.84
200	Fly	Bobby Patten	1993	1:50.32
100	IM	David Lundberg	1991	0:50.98
200	IM	David Lundberg	1991	1:50.45
400	IM	Tom Fristoe	1991	4:00.04

35–39

Distance	Stroke	Name	Year	Time
50	Free	Stu Marvin	1991	0:21.19
100	Free	Stu Marvin	1991	0:46.43
200	Free	James Montgomery	1990	1:42.78
500	Free	Hess Yntema	1991	4:41.53
1,000	Free	Jim McConica	1989	10:05.99
1,650	Free	Hess Yntema	1991	16:21.14
50	Back	William Specht	1993	0:24.16
100	Back	William Specht	1993	0:51.96
200	Back	William Specht	1993	1:53.46
50	Breast	Bruce Howell	1992	0:26.63
100	Breast	Mark Schuman	1991	0:59.07
200	Breast	Mark Schuman	1991	2:10.41
50	Fly	William Specht	1993	0:22.93

Women

Distance	Stroke	Name	Year	Time
1,650	Free	Karen Burton	1993	17:07.52
50	Back	Sue Walsh-Stankavage	1992	0:27.36
100	Back	Zena Herrmann	1993	0:59.47
200	Back	Zena Herrmann	1993	2:06.26
50	Breast	Rosemarie Seaman	1989	0:29.84
100	Breast	Rosemarie Seaman	1989	1:05.05
200	Breast	Karen Melick	1990	2:29.75
50	Fly	Rosemarie Seaman	1989	0:25.62
100	Fly	Rosemarie Seaman	1989	0:55.68
200	Fly	June Ford	1993	2:07.94
100	IM	Rosemarie Seaman	1989	0:58.78
200	IM	Sandy Neilson	1987	2:09.99
400	IM	Karen Burton	1993	4:34.29

35–39

Distance	Stroke	Name	Year	Time
50	Free	Sandy Neilson-Bell	1993	0:24.21
100	Free	Susan Halfacre	1988	0:52.24
200	Free	Susan Halfacre	1988	1:52.79
500	Free	Susan Halfacre	1988	5:01.04
1,000	Free	Susan Halfacre	1988	10:39.87
1,650	Free	Susan Halfacre	1988	17:15.23
50	Back	Laura Val	1991	0:27.82
100	Back	Laura Val	1991	1:01.68
200	Back	Karen Farnsworth	1992	2:15.44
50	Breast	Leslie Osborne	1989	0:30.85
100	Breast	Leslie Osborne	1989	1:07.58
200	Breast	Karen Melick	1992	2:30.53
50	Fly	Laura Val	1987	0:26.86

Time	Year	Name	Stroke	Distance	Name	Year	Time
0:50.50	1993	William Specht	Fly	100	Susan Halfacre	1988	0:56.90
1:52.17	1993	William Specht	Fly	200	Laura Val	1987	2:10.80
0:54.11	1991	Mark Schuman	IM	100	Susan Halfacre	1988	1:00.22
1:57.44	1991	Mike Drews	IM	200	Sandy Neilson-Bell	1992	2:13.88
4:15.20	1991	Hess Yntema	IM	400	Sandy Neilson-Bell	1992	4:46.69

		Men		**40–44**			**Women**

Time	Year	Name	Stroke	Distance	Name	Year	Time
0:21.72	1992	Tom Whatley	Free	50	Laura Val	1992	0:24.95
	1993	Lawrence Shulman					
0:48.52	1993	James Griffith	Free	100	Laura Val	1992	0:54.48
1:47.17	1993	Tim Broderick	Free	200	Barbara Dunbar	1990	2:04.00
4:50.80	1987	David Gray	Free	500	Barbara Dunbar	1989	5:30.58
10:17.35	1992	Kevin Polansky	Free	1,000	Barbara Dunbar	1990	11:20.18
17:02.40	1990	Kevin Polansky	Free	1,650	Barbara Dunbar	1989	18:58.23
0:25.61	1991	Jerry Heidenreich	Back	50	Laura Val	1992	0:27.91
0:54.15	1991	Peter O'Keeffe	Back	100	Laura Val	1992	1:02.22
2:01.54	1991	Peter O'Keeffe	Back	200	Janet Pesavento	1992	2:23.47
0:27.45	1992	Chet Miltenberger	Breast	50	Deborah Walker	1993	0:32.84
0:59.40	1993	Chet Miltenberger	Breast	100	Dot Munger	1992	1:11.73
2:12.85	1992	Rick Colella	Breast	200	Gayle Benty	1993	2:37.37
0:23.63	1991	Dan Thompson	Fly	50	Laura Val	1993	0:26.92
0:53.77	1993	James Griffith	Fly	100	Laura Val	1992	0:59.22
2:02.09	1990	Boo Gallas	Fly	200	Laura Val	1992	2:11.08
0:55.69	1992	Tom Whatley	IM	100	Bonnie Adair	1993	1:03.82
2:03.31	1991	Peter O'Keefe	IM	200	Bonnie Adair	1993	2:20.57
4:27.29	1993	Bruce Mallette	IM	400	Catherine Kohn	1993	5:02.59

45–49

Men

Distance	Stroke	Name	Year	Time
50	Free	Richard Abrahams	1990	0:21.87
100	Free	Andrew McPherson	1992	0:48.13
200	Free	Andrew McPherson	1992	1:49.27
500	Free	Bob Momsen	1992	5:03.69
1,000	Free	Edward Crossmore	1993	10:43.60
1,650	Free	William Steuart	1983	17:59.11
50	Back	Robert Smith	1988	0:25.65
100	Back	Robert Smith	1988	0:56.14
200	Back	John Calvert	1992	2:05.50
50	Breast	Richard Nesbit	1991	0:28.32
100	Breast	Martin Hull	1989	1:02.48
200	Breast	Robert Strand	1993	2:18.37
50	Fly	Martin Hull	1989	0:24.24
100	Fly	Martin Hull	1989	0:54.27
200	Fly	Boo Graner-Gallas	1993	2:03.96
100	IM	Robert Smith	1988	0:56.23
200	IM	Andrew McPherson	1992	2:03.82
400	IM	Timothy Garton	1988	4:31.40

Women

Distance	Stroke	Name	Year	Time
50	Free	Ardeth Mueller	1988	0:25.98
100	Free	Ardeth Mueller	1987	0:57.91
200	Free	Ardeth Mueller	1988	2:05.71
500	Free	Ardeth Mueller	1988	5:40.37
1,000	Free	Ardeth Mueller	1991	11:54.44
1,650	Free	Ardeth Mueller	1986	20:12.73
50	Back	Betty Bennett	1988	0:32.57
100	Back	Betty Bennett	1988	1:11.07
200	Back	Carol Chidester	1991	2:30.46
50	Breast	Diana Todd	1989	0:34.46
100	Breast	Ginger Pierson	1991	1:14.11
200	Breast	Carolyn Boak	1993	2:44.46
50	Fly	Ardeth Mueller	1988	0:28.26
100	Fly	Ardeth Mueller	1988	1:03.08
200	Fly	Ardeth Mueller	1988	2:20.14
100	IM	Diana Todd	1990	1:07.38
200	IM	Ardeth Mueller	1988	2:24.53
400	IM	Ardeth Mueller	1987	5:10.24

50–54

Men

Distance	Stroke	Name	Year	Time
50	Free	Robert Smith	1993	0:22.84
100	Free	Timothy Garton	1993	0:51.32
200	Free	Timothy Garton	1993	1:53.42
500	Free	Edward Hinshaw	1990	5:13.80
1,000	Free	Edward Hinshaw	1987	11:00.03
1,650	Free	Sandy Galletly	1993	18:28.45
50	Back	Robert Smith	1993	0:26.24
100	Back	Robert Smith	1993	0:59.49

Women

Distance	Stroke	Name	Year	Time
50	Free	Nancy Ridout	1992	0:27.29
100	Free	Ardeth Mueller	1993	0:59.05
200	Free	Ardeth Mueller	1992	2:12.11
500	Free	Ardeth Mueller	1992	5:53.05
1,000	Free	Ardeth Mueller	1992	12:04.75
1,650	Free	Ardeth Mueller	1992	20:08.79
50	Back	Betsy Jordan	1990	0:32.72
100	Back	Betsy Jordan	1990	1:11.96

Men

Time	Year	Name	Distance	Stroke
2:12.97	1993	Edward Cazalet	200	Back
0:29.70	1984	Manuel Sanguily	50	Breast
1:05.29	1984	Manuel Sanguily	100	Breast
2:28.78	1989	Drury Gallagher	200	Breast
0:25.50	1991	Michael Mealiffe	50	Fly
0:57.34	1993	Timothy Garton	100	Fly
2:13.71	1992	Jack Geoghegan	200	Fly
0:58.15	1993	Timothy Garton	100	IM
2:08.36	1993	Timothy Garton	200	IM
4:39.70	1993	Timothy Garton	400	IM

55–59

Time	Year	Name	Distance	Stroke
0:23.41	1987	Donald Hill	50	Free
0:52.59	1987	Donald Hill	100	Free
2:01.67	1993	Jeff Farrell	200	Free
5:32.17	1988	Burwell Jones	500	Free
11:26.99	1988	Burwell Jones	1,000	Free
19:02.45	1988	Burwell Jones	1,650	Free
0:28.15	1991	Yoshi Oyakawa	50	Back
1:02.56	1991	Yoshi Oyakawa	100	Back
2:20.56	1991	Don Brown	200	Back
0:30.18	1989	Manuel Sanguily	50	Breast
1:06.93	1989	Manuel Sanguily	100	Breast
2:34.15	1989	Manuel Sanguily	200	Breast
0:26.58	1993	Robert Proebsting	50	Fly
1:00.88	1989	Wally Dobler	100	Fly
2:21.48	1993	Robert Proebsting	200	Fly
1:01.70	1993	Jeff Farrell	100	IM

Women

Time	Year	Name	Distance	Stroke
2:38.09	1991	Betsy Jordan	200	Back
0:35.55	1985	Jayne Bruner	50	Breast
1:17.72	1989	Joann Leilich	100	Breast
2:50.93	1990	Joann Leilich	200	Breast
0:28.91	1993	Ardeth Mueller	50	Fly
1:05.69	1992	Ardeth Mueller	100	Fly
2:25.73	1992	Ardeth Mueller	200	Fly
1:09.66	1993	Ardeth Mueller	100	IM
2:32.89	1992	Ardeth Mueller	200	IM
5:22.42	1992	Ardeth Mueller	400	IM

55–59

Time	Year	Name	Distance	Stroke
0:28.03	1990	Jayne Bruner	50	Free
1:02.38	1990	Jayne Bruner	100	Free
2:22.66	1988	Lavelle Stoinoff	200	Free
6:09.83	1988	Lavelle Stoinoff	500	Free
12:45.02	1988	Lavelle Stoinoff	1,000	Free
21:22.63	1989	Lavelle Stoinoff	1,650	Free
0:32.97	1993	Betsy Jordan	50	Back
1:11.11	1992	Betsy Jordan	100	Back
2:34.80	1992	Betsy Jordan	200	Back
0:35.16	1991	Jayne Bruner	50	Breast
1:18.52	1991	Jayne Bruner	100	Breast
3:00.46	1991	Jayne Bruner	200	Breast
0:31.76	1985	Gail Roper	50	Fly
1:15.18	1991	Jayne Bruner	100	Fly
2:51.18	1986	Gail Roper	200	Fly
1:12.56	1992	Jayne Bruner	100	IM

Men Time	Year	Name	Distance	Stroke	Women Name	Year	Women Time
2:17.88	1988	Burwell Jones	200	IM	Betsy Jordan	1992	2:44.30
5:03.44	1990	Burwell Jones	400	IM	Nancy Brown	1991	5:54.24

Men — 60–64 — Women

Men Time	Year	Name	Distance	Stroke	Women Name	Year	Women Time
0:24.52	1993	Donald Hill	50	Free	Dorothy Donnelly	1982	0:30.67
0:54.49	1993	Donald Hill	100	Free	Lavelle Stoinoff	1993	1:08.08
2:07.53	1985	Peter Powlison	200	Free	Lavelle Stoinoff	1993	2:26.09
5:38.17	1991	Graham Johnston	500	Free	Lavelle Stoinoff	1993	6:22.62
11:51.48	1991	Graham Johnston	1,000	Free	Lavelle Stoinoff	1993	13:12.73
19:41.57	1991	Graham Johnston	1,650	Free	Lavelle Stoinoff	1993	22:13.13
0:30.65	1985	Paul Hutinger	50	Back	Clara Walker	1991	0:35.27
1:07.47	1985	Paul Hutinger	100	Back	Clara Walker	1991	1:17.94
2:28.48	1991	Richard Bennett	200	Back	Lavelle Stoinoff	1993	2:54.33
0:31.34	1993	Manuel Sanguily	50	Breast	Carol Taylor	1990	0:39.74
1:10.08	1993	Manuel Sanguily	100	Breast	Ann Pisciotta	1991	1:27.13
2:39.95	1993	Manuel Sanguily	200	Breast	Ann Pisciotta	1991	3:11.24
0:28.50	1986	Paul Hutinger	50	Fly	Roxanne Motter	1993	0:34.63
1:06.31	1991	John Kortheuer	100	Fly	Jeannette Eppley	1980	1:23.43
2:38.59	1991	John Masters	200	Fly	June Krauser	1988	3:10.64
1:06.39	1986	Paul Hutinger	100	IM	Clara Walker	1989	1:18.93
2:29.46	1993	Graham Johnston	200	IM	Clara Walker	1991	2:52.50
5:21.45	1993	Graham Johnston	400	IM	Clara Walker	1991	6:14.72

Men — 65–69 — Women

Men Time	Year	Name	Distance	Stroke	Women Name	Year	Women Time
0:25.62	1987	Peter Powlison	50	Free	Clara Walker	1992	0:31.01
0:56.24	1987	Peter Powlison	100	Free	Clara Walker	1992	1:09.04
2:10.80	1987	Peter Powlison	200	Free	Clara Walker	1992	2:35.44
6:15.85	1991	Frank Piemme	500	Free	Clara Walker	1992	6:49.80

Men

Distance	Stroke	Name	Year	Time
1,000	Free	Roger Franks	1993	13:00.78
1,650	Free	Roger Franks	1993	21:39.42
50	Back	Paul Hutinger	1993	0:31.26
100	Back	Roger Franks	1993	1:10.07
200	Back	Roger Franks	1993	2:30.53
50	Breast	Joseph Kurtzman	1991	0:33.24
100	Breast	Joseph Kurtzman	1991	1:17.34
200	Breast	Ted Haartz	1993	2:53.27
50	Fly	Frank Piemme	1991	0:29.42
100	Fly	Joseph Kurtzman	1991	1:09.77
200	Fly	Charles Moss	1993	2:41.99
100	IM	Peter Powlison	1987	1:06.74
200	IM	Charles Moss	1993	2:35.07
400	IM	Charles Moss	1993	5:34.61

70–74 (Men)

Distance	Stroke	Name	Year	Time
50	Free	Kelley Lemmon	1982	0:27.45
100	Free	Kelley Lemmon	1984	1:01.22
200	Free	Kelley Lemmon	1982	2:24.72
500	Free	Fred Taioli	1991	6:52.21
1,000	Free	Fred Taioli	1991	14:15.81
1,650	Free	Aldo DaRosa	1988	23:44.48
50	Back	Ray Taft	1993	0:34.13
100	Back	John Dilley	1991	1:15.70
200	Back	Ray Taft	1993	2:50.06
50	Breast	Paul Krup	1989	0:36.17
100	Breast	Aldo DaRosa	1988	1:21.03
200	Breast	Aldo DaRosa	1988	3:03.29

Women

Distance	Stroke	Name	Year	Time
1,000	Free	Clara Walker	1993	14:04.18
1,650	Free	Clara Walker	1993	23:46.31
50	Back	Clara Walker	1992	0:36.03
100	Back	Clara Walker	1993	1:21.48
200	Back	Clara Walker	1992	2:58.87
50	Breast	Clara Walker	1993	0:40.79
100	Breast	Clara Walker	1993	1:29.00
200	Breast	Clara Walker	1993	3:14.79
50	Fly	Jeannette Eppley	1985	0:38.39
100	Fly	June Krauser	1991	1:28.14
200	Fly	June Krauser	1991	3:13.72
100	IM	Clara Walker	1992	1:19.84
200	IM	Clara Walker	1992	2:54.51
400	IM	Clara Walker	1993	6:24.09

70–74 (Women)

Distance	Stroke	Name	Year	Time
50	Free	Dorothy Donnelly	1993	0:33.79
100	Free	Dorothy Donnelly	1992	1:15.98
200	Free	Margery Meyer	1993	2:51.42
500	Free	Margery Meyer	1993	7:51.53
1,000	Free	Margery Meyer	1993	16:23.35
1,650	Free	Margery Meyer	1993	27:15.78
50	Back	Margery Meyer	1993	0:40.87
100	Back	Jeanne Merryman	1993	1:33.65
200	Back	Margery Meyer	1993	3:19.98
50	Breast	Betty Christian	1993	0:43.90
100	Breast	Betty Christian	1992	1:39.18
200	Breast	Betty Christian	1992	3:36.00

Distance	Stroke	Men	Year	Time	Women	Year	Time
50	Fly	Birch Davidson	1989	0:31.95	Jeannette Eppley	1990	0:40.34
100	Fly	Andrew Holden	1990	1:18.88	Jeannette Eppley	1990	1:39.75
200	Fly	Anton Cerer	1987	2:58.78	Jeannette Eppley	1990	3:54.84
100	IM	Ray Taft	1989	1:13.66	Betty Christian	1993	1:33.02
200	IM	Birch Davidson	1989	2:47.68	Dorothy Donnelly	1992	3:31.04
400	IM	Birch Davidson	1989	6:14.18	Maxine Merlino	1982	7:36.45

Men / **Women**

75–79

Distance	Stroke	Men	Year	Time	Women	Year	Time
50	Free	Kelley Lemmon	1987	0:28.73	Lenore Wingard	1987	0:36.17
100	Free	Kelley Lemmon	1988	1:04.28	Lenore Wingard	1986	1:21.57
200	Free	Kelley Lemmon	1988	2:30.58	Lenore Wingard	1987	3:05.04
500	Free	Aldo DaRosa	1993	7:12.60	Louise Donovan	1993	8:53.70
1,000	Free	Aldo DaRosa	1993	14:37.47	Louise Donovan	1993	18:18.21
1,650	Free	Aldo DaRosa	1993	24:48.25	Jean Durston	1990	31:01.55
50	Back	Edward Shea	1991	0:37.10	Marie Wicklun	1989	0:46.51
100	Back	Al VandeWeghe	1992	1:21.83	Anne Walker	1992	1:42.30
200	Back	Edward Shea	1992	3:02.98	Marie Wicklun	1991	3:42.11
50	Breast	Paul Krup	1993	0:37.59	Gertrud Zint	1993	0:48.53
100	Breast	Aldo DaRosa	1993	1:25.80	Gertrud Zint	1993	1:53.48
200	Breast	Aldo DaRosa	1993	3:13.37	Gertrud Zint	1993	4:07.40
50	Fly	Kelley Lemmon	1987	0:35.44	Gertrud Zint	1993	0:47.97
100	Fly	Paul Krup	1993	1:27.99	Gertrud Zint	1993	2:00.42
200	Fly	Anton Cerer	1992	3:17.53	Maxine Merlino	1988	4:19.43
100	IM	Kelley Lemmon	1987	1:16.57	Gertrud Zint	1993	1:43.76
200	IM	Kelley Lemmon	1987	2:58.90	Maxine Merlino	1988	3:56.09
400	IM	Aldo DaRosa	1993	6:36.29	Maxine Merlino	1988	8:10.40

Men / **Women**

80–84

Distance	Stroke	Men	Year	Time	Women	Year	Time
50	Free	Kelley Lemmon	1992	0:32.10	Julia Dolce	1991	0:44.25

Time (Men)	Year	Name (Men)	Stroke	Distance	Name (Women)	Year	Time (Women)
1:17.82	1990	Gerson Sobel	Free	100	Julia Dolce	1990	1:39.96
2:49.94	1992	Kelley Lemmon	Free	200	Julia Dolce	1990	3:51.76
8:03.55	1985	Gus Langner	Free	500	Ruth Switzer	1988	10:45.81
16:54.23	1985	Gus Langner	Free	1,000	Marie Kelleher	1993	22:33.79
28:04.21	1985	Gus Langner	Free	1,650	Dorothy Hopkins	1990	38:35.07
0:41.09	1993	David Malbrough	Back	50	Aileen Soule	1989	0:52.35
1:33.96	1993	David Malbrough	Back	100	Aileen Soule	1989	1:56.19
3:34.08	1993	David Malbrough	Back	200	Aileen Soule	1991	4:16.57
0:41.39	1992	Kelley Lemmon	Breast	50	Helmi Meise	1993	0:59.02
1:32.72	1992	Kelley Lemmon	Breast	100	Helmi Meise	1993	2:17.42
4:03.66	1984	Al Kallunki	Breast	200	Elsa Mattila	1992	5:03.19
0:40.94	1990	Jesse Coon	Fly	50	Katherine Pelton	1986	1:06.25
1:50.88	1991	Jesse Coon	Fly	100	Katherine Pelton	1986	2:36.36
4:20.25	1990	Jesse Coon	Fly	200	Elsa Mattila	1991	5:33.46
1:40.18	1988	Jim Penfield	IM	100	Elsa Mattila	1990	2:14.16
3:48.22	1987	Herb Eisenschmidt	IM	200	Jewel Cooke	1989	4:51.27
8:27.54	1989	Herb Eisenschmidt	IM	400	Elsa Mattila	1990	9:53.28

Men

Women

85–89

Time (Men)	Year	Name (Men)	Stroke	Distance	Name (Women)	Year	Time (Women)
0:39.38	1993	F. K. Brasington	Free	50	Aileen Soule	1991	0:48.59
1:27.45	1990	Gus Langner	Free	100	Aileen Soule	1991	1:51.05
3:17.83	1990	Gus Langner	Free	200	Aileen Soule	1991	4:08.66
9:00.31	1990	Gus Langner	Free	500	Marian McKechnie	1990	14:15.17
18:18.29	1990	Gus Langner	Free	1,000	Marian McKechnie	1992	30:28.48
31:02.36	1990	Gus Langner	Free	1,650	Ella Peckham	1985	50:54.73
0:52.83	1990	Peter Jurczyk	Back	50	Aileen Soule	1991	0:49.59
1:54.21	1990	Peter Jurczyk	Back	100	Aileen Soule	1991	1:55.84
4:13.75	1993	Jim Penfield	Back	200	Aileen Soule	1991	4:09.33

Men			Event		Women		
Name	Year	Time	Dist.	Stroke	Name	Year	Time
Jim Penfield	1993	0:52.09	50	Breast	Marj Pollock	1992	1:17.90
Jim Penfield	1993	2:03.10	100	Breast	Katherine Pelton	1991	2:47.87
Al Kallunki	1990	4:34.29	200	Breast	Katherine Pelton	1991	6:12.44
Al Kallunki	1990	0:59.14	50	Fly	Ella Peckham	1985	1:16.00
Herb Eisenschmidt	1992	2:32.32	100	Fly	Ella Peckham	1984	3:01.71
			200	Fly	Katherine Pelton	1991	6:39.85
Al Kallunki	1990	2:00.04	100	IM	Ella Peckham	1984	2:41.31
Tom Curetont	1987	4:40.51	200	IM	Ella Peckham	1985	5:57.63
Herb Eisenschmidt	1992	9:47.85	400	IM	Martha Keller	1986	17:13.92

90–94

Men			Event		Women		
Name	Year	Time	Dist.	Stroke	Name	Year	Time
Joseph Reiners	1993	0:46.53	50	Free	Luella Tyra	1983	1:27.65
Paul Spangler	1989	2:24.60	100	Free	Anna Bauscher	1993	3:12.36
Paul Spangler	1990	5:22.61	200	Free	Anna Bauscher	1993	6:26.12
Paul Spangler	1989	13:13.36	500	Free	Anna Bauscher	1993	15:48.03
Paul Spangler	1989	28:04.65	1,000	Free	Anna Bauscher	1993	32:53.76
Paul Spangler	1989	51:31.39	1,650	Free			
Tom Lane	1989	1:15.02	50	Back	Anna Bauscher	1993	1:29.44
Tony Lopez	1992	3:17.90	100	Back	Pearl Miller	1988	3:32.00
Tony Lopez	1990	6:40.23	200	Back	Anna Bauscher	1993	6:29.37
Joseph Reiners	1993	1:10.74	50	Breast	Luella Tyra	1984	2:26.52
			100	Breast	Luella Tyra	1983	5:30.32
			200	Breast	Luella Tyra	1983	11:48.36
			50	Fly	Anna Bauscher	1993	4:13.58
			100	IM	Anna Bauscher	1993	5:22.45
			200	IM	Anna Bauscher	1993	10:43.74

AGE-GROUP SWIMMING AMERICAN RECORDS: SHORT COURSE (YARDS)

1994 U.S. SWIMMING NATIONAL AGE-GROUP RECORDS
Short Course—Yards

10 and Younger

	Girls		Dist.	Event		Boys	
1983	Grace Cornelius	25.47	50	Free	25.06	Ben Davidson	1991
1989	Lee Ann Gathings	56.11	100	Free	54.74	Chas Morton	1982
1989	Lee Ann Gathings	1:59.22	200	Free	2:00.70	Chas Morton	1982
1992	Beth Botsford	28.72	50	Back	29.06	Chas Morton	1982
1992	Beth Botsford	1:01.71	100	Back	1:02.21	Chas Morton	1982
1992	Jilen Siroky	32.66	50	Breast	32.31	Michael Milano	1989
1992	Jilen Siroky	1:11.63	100	Breast	1:11.11	Chas Morton	1982
1992	Katie Kochman	27.91	50	Fly	27.07	Chas Morton	1982
1984	Stephanie Rosenthal	1:02.54	100	Fly	59.97	Zachary Ferguson	1992
1984	Stephanie Rosenthal	1:03.23	100	IM	1:03.33	Chas Morton	1982
1984	Stephanie Rosenthal	2:17.53	200	IM	2:12.29	Chas Morton	1982

11–12

	Girls		Dist.	Event		Boys	
1983	Trina Radke	23.71	50	Free	22.69	Jay Martin	1987
1985	Grace Cornelius	23.71					
1985	Grace Cornelius	50.89	100	Free	49.46	Chas Morton	1984
1982	Michelle Richardson	1:50.40	200	Free	1:47.72	Jeff McPherson	1985
1977	Cynthia Woodhead	4:49.51	500	Free	4:47.96	Austin Lindsey	1986
1993	Beth Botsford	26.62	50	Back	25.32	David Chan	1992
1993	Lauren Stinnett	56.61	100	Back	54.79	David Chan	1992
1992	Suzy Nicoletti	30.61	50	Breast	28.37	Anthony Robinson	1992

11–12

Girls / Boys

Year	Girls	Time	Dist.	Stroke	Time	Boys	Year
1991	Erica Frykberg	1:05.23	100	Breast	1:02.21	Steve VonGluekiat	1989
1993	Michelle Griglione	26.01	50	Fly	24.50	Chas Morton	1984
1984	Grace Cornelius	26.01					
1993	Whitney Phelps	55.68	100	Fly	51.85	Chas Morton	1984
1989	Darby Chang	58.18	100	IM	55.93	David Chan	1992
1993	Emily Martin	2:06.10	200	IM	1:56.61	Chas Morton	1984

13–14

Girls / Boys

Year	Girls	Time	Dist.	Stroke	Time	Boys	Year
1982	Dara Torres	22.44	50	Free	20.82	Ugur Taner	1989
1987	Grace Cornelius	49.65	100	Free	45.75	Ugur Taner	1989
1978	Stephanie Elkins	1:45.91	200	Free	1:39.50	Ugur Taner	1989
1978	Cynthia Woodhead	4:39.94	500	Free	4:30.74	Paul Budd	1980
1984	Michele Richardson	9:33.39	1,000	Free	9:15.39	Paul Budd	1980
1981	Tiffany Cohen	15:54.86	1,650	Free	15:28.92	Paul Budd	1980
1986	Beth Barr	55.73	100	Back	52.05	Robert Brewer	1989
1986	Beth Barr	2:00.05	200	Back	1:52.63	Greg Burgess	1987
1991	Anita Nall	1:02.70	100	Breast	57.01	John Moffet	1979
1991	Anita Nall	2:12.54	200	Breast	2:03.89	John Moffet	1979
1987	Grace Cornelius	53.99	100	Fly	50.07	Chas Morton	1986
1979	Mary T. Meagher	1:56.58	200	Fly	1:51.77	Brian Alderman	1984
1978	Tracy Caulkins	2:00.27	200	IM	1:52.00	Ugur Taner	1989
1992	Allison Wagner	4:16.07	400	IM	3:57.30	Chas Morton	1986

15–16

Girls / Boys

Year	Girls	Time	Dist.	Stroke	Time	Boys	Year
1983	Dara Torres	22.60	50	Free	20.36	Byron Davis	1987
1979	Tracy Caulkins	49.03	100	Free	43.83	Joe Hudepohl	1990

15–16

Year	Girls	Time	Distance	Stroke	Boys	Year
1979	Cynthia Woodhead	1:44.10	200	Free	Eric Diehl	1990
1979	Tracy Caulkins	4:36.25	500	Free	Jeff Kostoff	1982
1990	Jane Skillman	9:30.35	1,000	Free	Jeff Kostoff	1982
1983	Tiffany Cohen	15:46.54	1,650	Free	Jeff Kostoff	1982
1991	Janie Wagstaff	54.37	100	Back	Derek Weatherford	1989
1990	Janie Wagstaff	1:56.14	200	Back	Derek Weatherford	1989
1989	Mary Ellen Blanchard	1:00.66	100	Breast	John Moffet	1981
1989	Mary Ellen Blanchard	2:09.06	200	Breast	John Moffet	1981
1981	Mary T. Meagher	53.00	100	Fly	Brad Bailey	1986
1981	Mary T. Meagher	1:52.99	200	Fly	Melvin Stewart	1985
1979	Tracy Caulkins	1:57.86	200	IM	Dave Wharton	1986
1979	Tracy Caulkins	4:08.09	400	IM	Dave Wharton	1986

17–18

Year	Girls	Time	Distance	Stroke	Boys	Year
1986	Jenna Johnson	22.46	50	Free	Tom Jager	1983
1991	Nicole Haislett	48.45	100	Free	Tom Jager	1983
1991	Nicole Haislett	1:45.05	200	Free	Troy Dalbey	1987
1990	Janet Evans	4:34.39	500	Free	Dan Jorgensen	1987
1989	Janet Evans	9:25.49	1,000	Free	Jeff Kostoff	1983
1990	Janet Evans	15:39.14	1,650	Free	Jeff Kostoff	1984
1992	Janie Wagstaff	53.68	100	Back	Brian Retterer	1991
1992	Janie Wagstaff	1:55.49	200	Back	Brad Bridgewater	1992
1981	Tracy Caulkins	1:01.13	100	Breast	Tyler Mayfield	1991
1980	Tracy Caulkins	2:11.46	200	Breast	Tyler Mayfield	1991
1982	Mary T. Meagher	53.22	100	Fly	Tom Jager	1983
1982	Mary T. Meagher	1:53.37	200	Fly	Melvin Stewart	1987

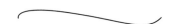

THE SWIMMER'S ADDRESS BOOK

For information about learning how to swim:

American National Red Cross
Seventeenth and D Streets, NW
Washington, DC 20006
Telephone: 202-737-8300

Y's of U.S.A.
101 North Wacker Drive
Chicago, IL 60606
Telephone: 312-977-0031

National Jewish Welfare Board
15 East Twenty-sixth Street
New York, NY 10010
Telephone: 212-532-4949

National Spa and Pool Institute
2111 Eisenhower Avenue
Alexandria, VA 22314
Telephone: 703-838-0083

For information about Masters swimming:

United States Masters Swimming, Inc. (USMS)
2 Peter Avenue
Rutland, MA 01543
Telephone: 508-886-6631
Fax: 508-886-6265

For information about age-group, open, and Olympic swimming:

United States Swimming, Inc. (USS)
One Olympic Plaza
Colorado Springs, CO 80909
Telephone: 719-578-4578
Fax: 719-578-4669

International Swimming Hall of Fame
One Hall of Fame Drive
Fort Lauderdale, FL 33316
Telephone: 305-462-6536

For information about teaching young children to swim:

National Swim School Association
1158 Thirty-fifth Avenue
St. Petersburg, FL 33704

For information about synchronized swimming:

United States Synchronized Swimming, Inc.
201 South Capitol Avenue, Suite 101
Indianapolis, IN 46225
Telephone: 317-237-5700
Fax: 317-237-5705

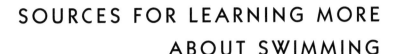

SOURCES FOR LEARNING MORE ABOUT SWIMMING

THIS APPENDIX PROVIDES annotated lists of magazines, books, and videos that are both helpful and inspirational.

SWIMMING MAGAZINES

SWIM Magazine, leading magazine for fitness and Masters swimmers. 6 issues/year. Newsstand: $2.95/issue. One-year subscription: $15.00. P.O. Box 91870, Pasadena, CA 91109-9769. Telephone: 800-538-9787 throughout North America except California (in California: 800-345-SWIM). Ask for Operator 4.

Swimming World, the "Bible" of competitive swimming, for competitive swimmers from age eight through college. 12 issues/year. Newsstand: $2.50/issue. One-year subscription: $19.00. P.O. Box 91870, Pasadena, CA 91109-9769. Telephone: 800-538-9787 throughout North America except California (in California: 800-345-SWIM). Ask for Operator 4.

Swimming Technique, for swim coaches, trainers, and exercise physiologists. 4 issues/year. Newsstand: $3.50/issue. One-year subscription: $13.00. P.O. Box 91870, Pasadena, CA 91109-9769. Telephone: 800-

538-9787 throughout North America except California (in California: 800-345-SWIM). Ask for Operator 4.

Splash! newsletter of United States Swimming (USS). For competitive age group through college swimmers. 6 issues/year. Free with membership in USS ($20.00/year). United States Swimming, 1750 East Boulder Street, Colorado Springs, CO 80909-5770. Telephone: (719) 578-4578.

SWIM Canada, for Canadian age-group through college competitive swimmers. 12 issues/year. One-year subscription: $30.00 Canadian. 402 King Street East, Toronto, Ontario M5A 1L3

BOOKS ABOUT SWIMMING AND HEALTH

The books described briefly in this section fall into seven categories:

- Places to swim
- Swimming and health
- Advanced swimming technique
- Inspirational
- Nutrition
- Aging and longevity
- Water Aerobics

Places to Swim

American Lap Swimmers Association, *ALSA Swimmers' Guide* (annual editions), 352 pages.

United States Masters Swimming, Inc., *Places to Swim* (revised annually) 42 pages.

Most swimmers have experienced the frustration of being away on business or vacation and not knowing where to go to get in our regular swim workouts. The American Lap Swimmers Association and United States Masters Swimming have stepped forward to solve that predicament.

Oriented primarily toward the lap swimmer, the *ALSA Swimmers' Guide* lists roughly 1,200 facilities—almost all over twenty yards long—in over 750 cities and towns in all fifty states plus the District of Columbia. These include municipal, YM/YWCA, YM/YWHA, college, school, club, and hotel pools.

Along with a listing you'll find the following valuable information about each pool: hours of availability, admission policies and fees, pool temperature, whether to bring your own lock and towel, even whether you can expect to have a lane to yourself or you'll have to share. The book also boasts some fifty-five maps and an index to find hotels with pools or discounted access to nearby pools.

Each edition of U.S. Masters Swimming's *Places to Swim* updates and expands its earlier versions. The most recent edition catalogs over 1,000 pools, many with coached Masters workouts, throughout the fifty states. It also features information about when workouts take place and when lap swim times are available, length of each pool, and whom to contact. (A valuable plus available from USMS free of charge, upon request, is a supplement listing places to swim in various foreign countries.)

The *Swimmers' Guide* is available for $14.95 plus $4.00 from the International Swimming Hall of Fame, Mail Order Company, One Hall of Fame Drive, Fort Lauderdale, FL 33316. Or call (800) 431-9111.

Places to Swim is available for $5.00 from the United States Masters Swimming National Office, 2 Peter Avenue, Rutland, MA 01543.

Swimming and Health

Alice Feinstein and the Editors of *Prevention* Magazine Health Books, *Training the Body to Cure Itself.* Emmaus, PA: Rodale Press, 1992, 516 pp.
A readable compendium of the benefits of exercise—including swimming—for making you more youthful looking, boosting your energy, enhancing your creative powers, warding off disease, and extending your life.

Nancy Hogshead and Gerald S. Couzens, *Asthma & Exercise.* New York: Henry Holt, 1990, 239 pp.
For generations, people with asthma have been encouraged to lead inactive lives. Today, thanks to new medical research and new medications, we know that if you have asthma, exercise—particularly swimming—can greatly enhance your physical and emotional well-being. Nancy Hogshead is an asthmatic who won four medals in swimming at the 1984 Olympic Games in Los Angeles. In this book she offers clear and detailed advice and instruction on how adults and children with asthma can participate safely in exercise and sports activities.

Judy Jetter and Nancy Kadlec, O.T.R., *The Arthritis Book of Water Exercise.* New York: Holt, Rinehart and Winston, 1985, 131 pp.
No exercise is more beneficial for treating arthritis and a host of physical ailments than swimming. If you have difficulty moving muscles because of pain, this book will help you out. Useful both for the chronic arthritis sufferer and for people who have undergone surgery, who have

had severe accidents, or who have impaired use of their limbs as a result of a stroke.

Jane Katz, Ed.D., *Swimming Through Your Pregnancy*. New York: Dolphin, Doubleday, 1983, 260 pp.

Swimming is the perfect exercise for pregnant women because of the buoyancy and protection the water provides both mother and fetus. In consultation with an obstetrician and childbirth instructor, Jane Katz, a top Masters swimmer, outlines a week-by-week, trimester-by-trimester program for keeping fit during pregnancy. The book is designed for women who have never swum before as well as experienced fitness swimmers.

Advanced Swimming Technique

Cecil M. Colwin, *Swimming into the Twenty-first Century*. Champaign, IL: Leisure Press, 1992, 255 pp.

Colwin, a world-renowned Canadian coach, has written a comprehensive volume, complete with user-friendly explanations of stroke mechanics and training, that focuses on swimming as an artistic expression.

David L. Costill et al., *Swimming* (an International Olympic Committee Medical Commission Publication). London: Blackwell Scientific Publications, 1992, 214 pp.

The first book in a projected series of handbooks of sports medicine and science, *Swimming* is written primarily for coaches, athletic trainers, family physicians, health-related professionals, and athletes. It covers biology, mechanics, and training.

Ernest W. Maglischo, *Swimming Even Faster*. Mountain View, CA: Mayfield Publishing, 1993, 755 pp.

This book, a successor to the author's earlier volume, *Swimming Faster,* is the most comprehensive text on the science of swimming. It emphasizes the biomechanics that are the foundation for efficient swimming and explains in detail the process of conditioning. It is highly technical, analytical, and dense, and of far more value to coaches and exercise physiologists than fitness or competitive swimmers.

Inspirational

John Jerome, *Staying with It: On Becoming an Athlete*. New York: Viking Penguin, 1984, 224 pp.

At the age of forty-seven, Jerome decided to become an athlete. He began training seriously for Masters swimming competition—swimming lap after lap, lifting weights, even attending adult swim camp (with hilarious results). In the process, he came to realize that swimming actually works in opposition to the aging process. He passed through the stages of pain and growth to a joyful mental and physical reawakening. *Staying with It* is the story of that passage—a fascinating, lyrical, funny, suspenseful, and personal exploration of the idea of athleticism and of its seeming obverse, the idea of aging.

Nutrition

Jacqueline R. Berning and Suzanne Nelson Steen, eds., *Sports Nutrition for the Nineties.* Gaithersburg, MD: Aspen Publishers, 1991, 302 pp.

Written for health professionals, this book is an up-to-date compendium of the latest information on sports nutrition.

Rachel F. Heller and Richard F. Heller, *The Carbohydrate Addict's Diet.* New York: Dutton, 1991, 283 pp.

Do you have a compelling hunger, craving, or desire for carbohydrate-rich foods; a recurring need to consume starches, snack foods, or sweets? If so, you are a carbohydrate addict, and you are not alone. Countless dieters have experienced the "yo-yo syndrome"—after weeks or months of dieting, they find themselves cheating, at first just a little, then more and more. The weight comes back, often containing more fat than before they began dieting. Doctors Rachel and Richard Heller of the Mt. Sinai School of Medicine in New York have discovered the cause of carbohydrate addiction and have developed a new diet, similar to the one in Appendix H, that helps carbohydrate addicts overcome their craving and control their eating and weight permanently.

Stanley Hershoff, Ph.D., *The Tufts University Guide to Total Nutrition.* New York: Harper & Row, 1990, 312 pp.

We live in a time of unprecedented health awareness. Current fascination with nutrition underscores this interest, yet most people do not have the knowledge to sort through conflicting food health claims and nutritional advice. *Total Nutrition* addresses virtually every nutrition issue and offers expert evaluation of current knowledge and research.

Aging and Longevity

Deepak Chopra, M.D., *Ageless Body, Timeless Mind: The Quantum Alternative to Growing Old.* New York: Harmony Books, 1993, 342 pp.

Contrary to our traditional notions of aging, Chopra argues, we can learn to direct the way our bodies metabolize time. In this book, the author combines mind-body medicine with current antiaging research to show why—and how—the effects of aging are largely preventable.

Kathy Keeton, *Longevity: The Science of Staying Young.* New York: Viking Penguin, 1992, 332 pp.

In this book, journalist Keeton takes you on a guided tour of the latest in antiaging science. At the same time she provides a long list of promising strategies—all emphasizing the importance of exercise—that may enable you to look, act, and feel younger than your years.

Linus Pauling, *How to Live Longer and Feel Better.* New York: W. H. Freeman, 1986, 322 pp.

Written by a two-time Nobel laureate, this book presents an easy-to-follow, inexpensive regimen for adding vigorous, healthy years to your life. Pauling, a nonagenarian, explains how vitamins work and how to make them work for you, and he emphasizes the importance of regular exercise in maintaining lifelong health.

Water Aerobics

Lynda Huey and Robert Forster, P.T., *The Complete Waterpower Workout Book.* New York: Random House, 1993, 373 pp.

Millions of people—from cardiac rehab patients to pregnant women to Olympic athletes—are discovering the benefits of working out in water. Written by one of the nation's leading water exercise trainers and a well-known sports physical therapist, this book covers waterpower workouts and water healing.

Swim Videos

After reading this book, the best way to learn to swim—or to swim better—is to get yourself down to your local pool, slip on your swimsuit, and start swimming. Under the watchful eye of a coach, or a knowledgeable swimming buddy, you can make progress quickly if you stick to it. But swim videos can help immensely: they can show you how the experts swim the four basic strokes; how a variety of drills will make you a smarter and more efficient swimmer; common mistakes to avoid; and so on.

Fortunately, there has been a profusion of excellent swim videos produced in recent years. Many of these videos claim to be useful for swimmers at all levels—from rank beginner to fitness and Masters swimmer and top-flight collegian. In fact, with a few exceptions, most videos assume that the viewer already knows the fundamentals of stroke mechanics in the four competitive strokes. And they assume that the viewer is basically familiar with training terms and procedures.

Most Masters swimmers and many fitness swimmers and triathletes *do* know these fundamentals, so the videos can be very useful indeed to them. The quality of the videos listed here is uniformly professional and, in most cases, state-of-the-art. However, they differ significantly in focus and intensity. Keep these differences in mind when choosing a video for yourself, or for a friend. Information on how to order the videos is at the end of this section.

The Fundamentals of Swimming (50 minutes, $32.00) is one of a small number of videos suitable for a novice. Produced by SwimAmerica, and developed by the American Swim Coaches Association, it is designed to help swimmers of all ages and various skill levels, from beginner to triathlete. The serious swimmer will find the other videos more useful. Hosted by "Madame Butterfly," Mary T. Meagher, it emphasizes health, safety, fun, and fitness. A ten-step progression helps you develop better fundamental swimming skills.

Olympic gold medalist Donna DeVarona guides you through an instructional swimming program in **Swimming for Fitness (53 minutes, $39.95)**. Suitable primarily for beginners, DeVarona's pointers will help increase your efficiency in the water.

The 1988 and 1992 U.S. Olympic swimming coaches, Richard Quick and Skip Kenney, have produced a gem with **Swim Smarter/Swim Faster II (50 minutes, $32.00)**. Underwater photography reveals the carefully orchestrated drills and stroke techniques needed to master the four strokes. Age-group as well as world-class swimmers are used to demonstrate these drills and techniques, while Quick and Kenney offer incisive, helpful, easily understood commentary.

Gettin' Better (50 minutes, $53.95) is what Olympic superstar John Naber hopes you'll be doing after viewing his video. Naber's offering is for the serious competitive swimmer who is interested in improving. But it is somewhat less intense than *Swim Smarter,* and it emphasizes more of a lifetime perspective than do most other videos: as long as you continue to learn and improve, Naber says, you are a winner. One unique aspect of this video is the use of simple but effective graphics to complement the stroke techniques demonstrated on tape. Naber's folksy analogies also assist the understanding of stroke mechanics.

Backstroke from the Bottom Up, Breaststroke from the Bottom Up, Butterfly from the Bottom Up, and **Freestyle from the Bottom Up (24 minutes, $42.00 each)** offer a unique perspective on all four strokes. Dave Bottom, former American record holder in the backstroke, takes the viewer from the basics of backstroke body position through the mental secrets of a champion. Susan Rapp, a 1984 and '88 Olympian, illustrates the fundamentals of the "wave-action" breaststroke, a technique she helped pioneer. Top freestylers and butterflyers demonstrate their techniques in the other two videos. Cinematographically, all four videos are exquisite.

There are four separate videos in **Don Gambril's Gold Medal Series (60 minutes, $48 each)**: **Freestyle**, **Breaststroke**, **Backstroke**, and **Butterfly**. Gambril, the 1984 U.S. Olympic coach, has America's '84 Olympic heroes demonstrate and comment on their techniques: Rowdy Gaines on freestyle, Steve Lundquist on breaststroke, Mary T. Meagher and Pablo Morales on butterfly, and Rick Carey on backstroke. The videos feature slow-motion analyses of stroke technique and provide tips on swim drills and dry land exercises. They also feature rare footage from the early days of swimming. Because the videos were made in 1985, they do not include information on the underwater backstroke popularized by Dave Berkoff in the 1988 Olympics, the new backstroke turn, or the wave-action breaststroke. Also available is **Swimming Techniques (60 minutes, $48.00)**, an authoritative view of swim techniques that uses computer graphics to illustrate its concepts.

Swimming Fastest II (100 minutes, $53) was produced by John Trembley, head coach at the University of Tennessee. Although Trembley states that the video is for swimmers at all levels, it really is for the sophisticated, accomplished athlete. Clear and concise, with a great deal of slow-motion and underwater footage, the video demonstrates drills to improve every aspect of each stroke plus starts and turns. This video is especially valuable for the Masters swimmer who does not have a regular coach.

These swim videos can be ordered by sending a check for the amount of the video (price includes postage and handling) to:

Swimming World
Mail Order Dept.
P.O. Box 45497
Los Angeles, CA 90045
Fax: (818) 304-7759

Basic Technique: From the Fast Lane; Basic Training: From the Fast Lane; and Advanced Technique: From the Fast Lane. Swim video series produced by LMH/Moffet Productions, $39.95 each; $99.95 for the series.

In *Basic Technique* (56 minutes), each of the four strokes is analyzed by the experts using the same easy-to-follow format: arm pull, kick, body position, and timing. The video offers outstanding slow motion cinematography and state-of-the-art underwater photography. In *Basic Training* (48 minutes), Moffet offers practical advice to help make your training both more interesting and more effective. It illustrates interval training and explains the use of various pool toys, including paddles, pull buoy, kick board, and Zoomers. Unlike most swim videos, *Basic Training* highlights the importance of cross training, emphasizing weight training in particular, as well as biking, running, surfing, and exercises to enhance flexibility. *Advanced Technique* (47 minutes) is really a continuation of the first tape. Here the emphasis is on perfecting your stroke. The video explains that working on stroke technique is an integral part of *every* practice session and demonstrates several stroke drills for each stroke. Finally, it illustrates how to execute efficient, powerful, streamlined turns and starts.

To order, call: 800-822-1105 (operator 52).

Water (57 minutes, $24.95), produced by Dr. Marty Hull, has as its subtitle "How to be safe in it, have fun in it, move powerfully in it, swim fast in it." Quite a claim, but Dr. Hull has the credentials to back up his expertise: he is the inventor of Zoomers swim fins, stroke consultant to the NCAA championship Stanford University men's and women's swim teams, and a national champion Masters swimmer in his own right. He is also a talented film producer. In the video, Hull puts together a sequence of ideas, techniques, and drills that will help you understand how to swim and move in the water more efficiently. The sequences progress from simple to complex, so swimmers of all ability levels can benefit.

To order, call 800-852-2909 or send a check to D'Zign, 1755 East Bayshore Road, Redwood City, CA 94063

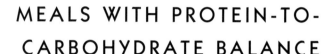

MEALS WITH PROTEIN-TO-CARBOHYDRATE BALANCE

CHAPTER 4 EXPLAINED the importance of maintaining a 4-to-3 ratio between carbohydrates and proteins. Here are some guidelines that will help you achieve this goal:

1. *Each meal* should contain the appropriate balance of protein and carbohydrate. Do not eat most of your daily carbohydrates at one meal and almost all your protein at another.
2. For most people, a reasonable meal contains about 30 grams of protein and 40 grams of carbohydrate, with 30 grams or less of fat. Even elite athletes should eat no more than 45 grams of protein and 60 grams of carbohydrate at each meal.
3. Try to make sure that most of the carbohydrates you eat come from those listed in the desirable carbohydrates table. *Desirable* here refers primarily to carbohydrates that are fiber-rich fruits and vegetables. These foods do not affect blood-sugar levels as quickly, or as much, as less desirable carbohydrates, which should be eaten in moderation.
4. Eat a meal or snack every four to six hours. Appropriate snacks include a cup of plain yogurt, or a half cup of cottage cheese with a piece of fruit.
5. Generally, do not eat more than 500 calories at a single meal. Excess calories are converted to fat.

Low-fat Protein Sources
(use as your foundation for each meal)

Item	Serving Size	Protein (grams)	Carbohydrate (grams)
Beef, lean	4 oz.	29	0
Chicken breast	4 oz.	32	0
Cod fish	4 oz.	20	0
Cottage cheese, 2%	1 cup	28	8
Egg white	1 each	3	0
Lamb, lean	4 oz.	28	0
Milk, low-fat	8 oz.	8	11
Shrimp	5 oz.	29	0
Tofu	8 oz.	17	5
Tuna (in water)	4 oz.	28	0
Turkey, white	4 oz.	33	0
Yogurt, plain	8 oz.	9	12

Desirable Carbohydrates
(use as your main source of carbohydrate)

Item	Serving Size	Carbohydrate (grams)
Apple	1 each	18
Asparagus, cooked	1 cup	8
Broccoli, cooked	1 cup	9
Cantaloupe	1/4 melon	11
Cauliflower, cooked	1 cup	6
Celery	1 stalk	1
Cucumber	1 each	3
Grapefruit	1/2 each	18
Grapes	1 cup	28
Green pepper	1 each	4
Kidney beans, cooked	1 cup	40
Lettuce, shredded	1 cup	1
Mushrooms	1 cup	6
Oatmeal (dry)	1 oz.	16
Onion	1 each	11
Orange	1 each	16
Peach	1 each	12
Pear	1 each	24
Peas, cooked	1 cup	25
Spinach, cooked	1 cup	7
String beans, cooked	1 cup	10
Tomato	1 each	6

Less Desirable Carbohydrates
(use in moderation)

Item	Serving Size	Carbohydrate (grams)
Bagel	1 each	30
Banana	1 each	27
Bread	1 slice	11
Bread crumbs	1 cup	65
Carrots, cooked	1 cup	16
Cereal, dry	1 oz.	25
Corn, cooked	1 cup	42
Granola	1 cup	49
Hamburger bun	1 each	26
Muffin	1 each	27
Pasta, cooked	1 cup	39
Pasta, dry	1 oz.	21
Popcorn, popped	1 cup	5
Potato, med., baked	1 each	51
Potato, mashed	1 cup	36
Potato, instant	1 cup	28
Raisins	1 cup	115
Rice, brown, cooked	1 cup	40
Rice, brown, dry	1 oz.	23
Rice cakes	1 each	8
Roll, hard	1 each	31
Roll, soft	1 each	20
Tortilla, corn	1 each	11
Tortilla, flour	1 each	24

INDEX

A

academic success, and swimming,
 203–4
adolescence
 obesity in, 201
 and swimming, 203–4
age-group swimming, 205–7
 described, 205–6
 origins of, 206–7
 records in, 342–44
aging process, xv, 78–83
 and body fat, 43
 and Masters swimming, 80–83,
  84, 207–14
 and sexuality, 176–77
Alexis, Kim, 15
Allen, Woody, 10
American College of Sports
 Medicine, 34

American Health magazine, 11, 41
American Heart Association
 (AHA), 22, 29, 30, 34, 36, 57
*American Journal of Clinical
 Nutrition,* 191
American Sociological
 Association, 39–40
American-style breaststroke,
 135–36
American Swim Coaches
 Association, 208
antioxidants, 57
apoplexy (stroke), 11, 21, 30, 60,
 69, 201
Armbruster, Dave, 157
arm pull
 backstroke, 95, 122–25, 282
 breaststroke, 96, 97, 135–36,
  141–45, 284–85

arm pull *(cont'd)*
  butterfly, 96, 159–61, 287
  drills, 279, 282, 284–85, 287
  freestyle (crawl), 95, 104–7,
    108, 112–14, 279
  and hand position, 99, 122,
    248, 249–50
  patterns of, 95–99
  workout, 234
arthritis, 201
Arthur, Ransom, 208
Association for Male Sexual
    Dysfunction, 184
atherosclerosis, 35, 37, 201
audio equipment, underwater, 297
Australian crawl, 102–3, *see also*
    freestyle (crawl)

B
babies, 201–2
back crawl, *see* backstroke
backstroke, 42, 80, 101, 116,
    119–33, 139
  arm pull, 95, 122–25, 282
  body position, 121–22
  body roll, 125–26, 283
  breathing, 127, 283
  distance per stroke, 228
  drills, 281–83
  flip turn, 127–31
  history of, 120–21
  kick, 126–27, 131
  putting it all together, 127, 128
  start, 131, 132
  thumb position, 250
  tips, 131–33
backstroke flags, 128–29
Bailey, Covert, 41, 42
Barrowman, Mike, 153
Bauer, Carl, 206–7, 208

Becker, Peter, 138
Benson, Herbert, 24
Bergen, Paul, 141
Berkoff, David, 120–21
Berkoff blastoff, 121, 131, 222
Bernardi, Oronzio de, 120
Berscheid, Ellen, 184
beta carotene, 57, 191–92
Bibbero, Marquis, 120
Biondi, Matt, 40, 103, 109, 112,
    228
Biosyn Technical Manual (Sears),
    49, 52
Bird, Larry, 16
blood pressure, *see* high blood
    pressure
body fat, 19, 42–52
  and aging process, 43
  and breast cancer, 190, 192–93
  and high blood pressure, 25
  loss of, with swimming, 31–32,
    34, 41, 43–45
  measuring, 45–52, 305–17
  of men, 42, 50–52, 310–17
  reducing, 42–52
  of women, 42, 46–49, 190,
    192–93, 201, 305–9
  see also obesity
body image, 184
body position
  backstroke, 121–22
  basic principles of, 94–95
  breaststroke, 139–41
  butterfly, 158–59
  freestyle (crawl), 104
body roll, 94
  backstroke, 125–26, 283
  drills, 279–80, 283
  freestyle (crawl), 107–9, 279–80
Bogues, Muggsy, 16
Bonning, Judy, 189

Bragg, Paul, 3, 4–5
breast cancer, 190–93
  and body fat, 190, 192–93
  and diet, 191–92
  and family history, 191
breaststroke, 80, 101, 116, 134–55
  arm pull, 96, 97, 135–36,
    141–45, 284–85
  body position, 139–41
  breathing, 139–41, 286
  broken, 230
  butterfly-breaststroke, 157,
    170–71
  butterfly versus, 158, 164
  distance per stroke, 228
  dolphin, 136, 140, 141, 155,
    222
  drills, 284–86
  history of, 135–36
  inverted, 120
  kick, 136, 145–47, 157, 225,
    285
  "natural," 136–39
  putting it all together, 147, 148
  start, 152
  tips, 152–53
  turn, 149–52
  wave-action, 136, 153–55, 222
  workout, 255–58
breathing
  backstroke, 127, 283
  breaststroke, 139–41, 286
  butterfly, 164–66, 286–87
  drills, 280, 281, 283, 286–87
  freestyle (crawl), 109–11, 280,
    281
Brecher, Edward M., 179, 180
broken swims, 230
Brown, Mardie, 10, 212
Brown, Nellie, 4, 5
Browning, Lisa, 176

butterfly, 80, 101, 116, 120, 134,
    135, 137, 156–71
  arm pull, 96, 159–61, 287
  body position, 158–59
  breaststroke versus, 158, 164
  breathing, 164–66, 286–87
  butterfly-breaststroke, 157,
    170–71
  distance per stroke, 228
  drills, 286–89
  history of, 157–58
  kick, 120, 156, 157, 158, 159,
    162–64, 288
  putting it all together, 166–68
  start, 168
  tips, 170
  turn, 168, 169
butterfly-breaststroke, 157, 170–71

C

calcium, 195
Callan, Murray, 202
cancer, 21, 43, 56, 60, 201
  breast, 190–93
  colon, 29, 201
  lung, 30
Cancer Research, 191
Can You Live to Be 100?
    (Woodruff), 76
carbohydrates, 53–55, 56–58, 191,
    356–59
Casey, Katherine, 195–97
Caulkins, Tracy, 140, 206, 208
Cavill, Charles, 103
Cavill, Syd, 103
Centers for Disease Control, 84,
    193
Cheever, John, 10
children
  lack of exercise, 200–201

children *(cont'd)*
    obesity of, 200–201
    sports injuries of, 204–5
    and swimming, 201–7
cholesterol, 25–29
    of children, 200
    defined, 26
    HDL (high-density lipoprotein),
        27–29, 69
    LDL (low-density lipoprotein),
        27–29
    readings, 26
    reducing total, 34, 35
circle swimming, 231–32
Circulation magazine, 34
clot busters, 35
coffee, 38
Collins, Judy, 3, 6–7, 40
colon cancer, 29, 201
Colwin, Cecil, 114, 162–63, 166
Connors, Jimmy, 80
Cook, James, 102
Couch, Don, 137, 138
Counsilman, James E. "Doc," 94,
        95, 99, 121, 125, 136, 145,
        224
Craven, Leslie, 188
crawl, *see* backstroke; freestyle
        (crawl)

D
David (statue), 40
Dean, Penny, 103
depression, 183–84, 185
descending rest interval, 227
descending set, 227
    negative splitting each repeat,
        227–28
DeVarona, Donna, 211
De Villers, Linda, 182, 184

diabetes, 43, 56, 60, 78
diastolic (resting) pressure, 23, 24
diet, 11, 53–58
    and atherosclerosis, 37
    and breast cancer, 191–92
    carbohydrates in, 53–55, 56–58,
        191, 356–59
    and cholesterol levels, 28–29
    and dietary endocrinology,
        53–58, 356–59
    and exercise, 33
    fat in, 25–29, 34, 35, 54, 55, 57,
        69, 191–92, 200
    and hormones, 53–58, 356–59
    ideal, 56–58
    protein in, 55–58, 191, 356–59
    salt in, 25, 38
    vitamins and minerals in, 57,
        191–92
dietary endocrinology, 53–58,
        356–59
distance per stroke (dps), 228–29
distance workouts, 269–73
diving
    drill set, 260, 261–62
    see also start
dolphin breaststroke, 136, 140,
        141, 155, 222
dolphin (fishtail) kick
    butterfly, 120, 156–59, 162–64
    with flip turn, 114
    reverse, 129, 222, 224
double-dolphin kick, 158
Douglas, Marjory Stoneham, 213
drag
    and arm pull, 97
    and body position, 94
    and swimsuit, 91, 224, 293
drag suits, 224, 293
drill set, 234
    arm pull, 279, 282, 284–85, 287

backstroke, 281–83
breaststroke, 284–86
butterfly, 286–89
catch-up freestyle, 270–72
diving, 260, 261–62
flip turn, 275, 277–78
freestyle (crawl), 270–72,
    279–81
push-off, 244, 245–46
stroke, 252–53, 256–58, 265–68
thumb, 248–50
Dunbar, Barbara, 215
Dybdahl, Thomas, 200

E

earplugs, 293–94
Ederle, Gertrude, 103
education
    academic success in, 203–4
    and life expectancy, 63, 66
Ekelund, Lars-Goran, 34
electrical impedance, 45
elementary backstroke, 101, 120
Elliot, Herb, 11
Elsenius, Mary Lou, 207
endocrinology, dietary, 53–58,
    356–59
endorphins, 32, 185
equipment, training, 90–92,
    217–25, 291–97
    earplugs, 293–94
    fins, 221–24, 294–95
    flume, 225
    goggles, 91–92, 93, 293–94
    hand paddles, 220–21, 294–95
    kick board, 92, 112, 162–63,
        218–19, 294–95
    nose clips, 92, 293–94
    pace clock, 217, 232
    parachutes, 224, 294–95

pull buoy, 92, 219–20, 294–95
    sources, 291–97
    swim caps, 92, 291, 293–94
    swimsuits, 90–91, 224, 292, 293
    webbed gloves, 225
    weights, 224
essential hypertension, 25
estrogen, 182, 186, 192, 193, 194
etiquette, swimming pool, 231–33
Evans, Janet, 103, 111, 112, 206,
    214
Evans, Linda, 185
exercise, lack of
    and body fat, 43
    in children, 200–201
    and heart disease, 29–30, 43

F

Fagan, Kimberly, 188–89
Farmer, George, 103
Farragher, Peter, 227
fat
    body, *see* body fat
    dietary, 54, 55, 57, 191–92, *see
        also* cholesterol
fiber
    and breast cancer, 192
    and cholesterol levels, 28–29
fins, 221–24, 294–95
    training, 223–24
fishtail (dolphin) kick, 114, 120,
    156–59, 162–64
fitness boom, 11–12
Fitness in America, 11
Fixx, Jim, 64
flags, backstroke, 128–29
Fletcher, Gerald F., 30
flip turn, 149
    backstroke, 127–31
    drill, 275, 277–78

flip turn *(cont'd)*
    freestroke (crawl), 114–16
    in practice session, 236
flumes, 225
flutter kick
    backstroke, 131
    four-beat, 103
    in freestyle (crawl), 103, 104,
        111–12, 224
    six-beat, 112, 118, 126, 127
    two-beat, 103, 112, 118
Foreman, George, 80
four-beat flutter kick, 103
Franklin, Benjamin, 135
Fraser, Dawn, 103
Freedman, Laurence S., 191
freestyle (crawl), 41, 80, 94, 99,
        101–18, 137, 165
    arm pull, 95, 104–7, 108,
        112–14, 279
    body position, 104
    body roll, 107–9, 279–80
    breathing, 109–11, 280, 281
    distance per stroke, 228–29
    drills, 279–81
    flip turn, 114–16
    history of, 102–3
    interval training, 226–28
    kick, 103, 104, 111–12, 224
    putting it all together, 112–14
    start, 116–18
    tips, 118
Frisch, Rose, 192, 193
frog (wedge) kick, 136, 145
front crawl, 101
FSH, 181

G
Gaines, Rowdy, 112–14
Geoghegan, Jack, 212

gloves, webbed, 225
glucagon, 55–58
glucagon-to-insulin ratio, 56–58
glycogen, 55
goggles, 91–92, 93, 293–94
Goldberg, Barry, 204–5
Goldstein, Esther, 194
grab start, 116, 117
Gregg, Steven, 41
Griffith, William, 184

H
Hale, Jack, 157
half fly, 168
hand paddles, 220–21, 294–95
hand position, 99
    backstroke, 122
    thumb drill, 248, 249–50
Harris, T. George, 11
Hayden, Jack, 197
HDL (high-density lipoprotein),
    27–29, 69
heart attacks, 21–22, 35, 64, 69,
    201
    death from, 34
    and high blood pressure, 24
    and smoking, 30
    swimming after, 37–38
heart disease, 11, 20–38, 43, 60
    death from, 21–22, 30, 34
    and diet, 56
    and dietary endocrinology, 53
    and exercise, lack of, 29–30, 43
    and high blood cholesterol,
        25–29
    and high blood pressure,
        23–25
    and modern life, 32–33
    and obesity, 31–32
    risk factors for, 22–23

and smoking, 30–31
and swimming, 33–38
heart rate, 35–37
Hebner, Harry, 120
Henricks, Jon, 230
heredity
    and breast cancer, 191
    and life expectancy, 60, 63, 66
Higdon, Hal, 41–42
high blood pressure, 23–25
    of children, 200
    controlling, 24–25, 34
    death from, 24
    measuring, 23–24
Hines, Emmett, 166, 168
Holmes, Larry, 80
Hong, Qian, 165
hormones
    and breast cancer, 192
    and dietary endocrinology,
        53–58, 356–59
    estrogen, 182, 186, 192, 193,
        194
    FSH, 181
    human growth (hGH), 78–79,
        183, 226
    insulin, 55, 56–58, 78, 192, 193
    and sexuality, 181–83, 185–86
    testosterone, 182, 186
Horner, Matina, 195
House, Carl, 16–17
Hull, Marty, 223
human growth hormone (hGH),
    78–79, 183, 226
Human Nutrition Research Center
    on Aging, 201
Hurt, Mary Beth, 9–10
Hussein, Saddam, 4
hydrostatic weighing, 45
hypertension, *see* high blood
    pressure

I
impotence, and obesity, 185–86
injuries, and children, 204–5
insulin, 55, 56–58, 78, 192, 193
interval training, 226–28
    holding repeats in, 226–27
    LOFO (last one, fast one),
        227–28

J
Jackson, Bo, 16
Japan
    blood cholesterol in, 26–27
    breast cancer in, 192
Jastremski, Chet, 136
John Paul II, Pope, 15
*Journal of the American Medical
    Association, The,* 195

K
Kahanamoku, Duke, 103
Kaplan, Helen Singer, 183
Karan, Donna, 15
Katz, Jane, 189
Kaufman, Beth, 207
Kern, Herb, 8–9
Kerrigan, Nancy, 16
ketosis, 57
kick
    backstroke, 126–27, 131
    breaststroke, 136, 145–47, 157,
        225, 285
    butterfly, 120, 156, 157, 158,
        159, 162–64, 288
    dolphin (fishtail), 114, 120,
        156–59, 162–64
    drills, 285, 288
    fins, 221–24, 294–95
    flutter, 103, 104, 111–12, 131

kick *(cont'd)*
    freestyle, 111–14
    sprints, 224
    workout, 234
kick boards, 92, 112, 162–63, 218–19, 294–95
King, Stephen, 15
Kinsey, Alfred, 177
Klein, Herbert, 157–58
Klyde, Barry J., 181, 185–86
Kraemer, William, 226
Kresch, Roberta, 7–8, 9

L

"lactic acid" workouts, 259–62
Lane, Tom, 214–15
lane designations, pool, 231
Langner, Gus, 212
Larson, James, 221
LDL (low-density lipoprotein), 27–29
life expectancy, 11, 57, 59–86
    and actuarial tables, 64, 304
    and aging process, 78–83
    and education and occupation, 63, 66
    and health, 63, 67
    and heredity, 60, 63, 66
    life-expectancy test, 62–67, 69, 70–77, 298–304
    and life-style, 60–61, 63, 66
    and smoking, 61, 62, 83–85
life-style
    and heart disease, 32–33
    and life expectancy, 60–61, 63, 66
Livingstone, Susan, 197–98
Louis Harris Polling Company, 11–12, 200
lung cancer, 30

M

Malone, Dan, 8
Manfredi, Thomas G., 37
Masters swimming, 207–14
    described, 209–10
    growth of, 209
    origins of, 208
    records in, 322–41
    research on, 80–83, 84
maximum heart rate (MHR), 36–37
meditation, 24–25, 37
Melpomene Institute, 189
men
    body fat of, 42, 50–52, 310–17
    swimming records of, 319–41
    swimsuits of, 90
menopause, 182, 191
    and osteoporosis, 194–95
Men's Health magazine, 41
minerals, 57
Moffit, Bill, 8
Moore, Jane A., 79
Morales, Pablo, 161, 165, 206
Mulliken, Bill, 225
Munzer, Martha, 213–14
Must, Aviva, 201
Myers, Henry, 157
Myers, Lynda, 60, 61–62, 65–67, 68, 85

N

Nagy, Jozsef, 136, 153
National Association for Sport and Physical Education, 200
National Cancer Institute, 191
National Institutes of Health, 26
National Swim School Association, 202
negative split, 227

Nelson, Richard C., 228–29
New England Journal of Medicine, The, 28, 34, 192–93, 194, 201
New Fit or Fat, The (Bailey), 41
Newton, Isaac, 94–95, 104
nose clips, 92, 293–94
nutrition bars, 297

O

obesity
    adolescent, 201
    and breast cancer, 192–93
    of children, 200–201
    defined, 26
    and heart disease, 31–32
    and impotence, 185–86
    of women, 192–93, 201
    see also body fat
O'Brien, Parry, 16
occupation, and life expectancy, 63, 66
Olanoff, Abe, 100, 212–13
open-water swimming, 267–68, 269–73
Ornish, Dean, 37
Orwoll, Eric S., 194
osteoporosis, 194–95
overarm stroke, 135

P

pace clock, 217, 232
paddles, hand, 220–21, 294–95
Paffenberger, Ralph S., 30
parachutes, 224, 294–95
Parish, Robert, 80
Perrier, 11–12, 84
Physician and Sportsmedicine, The (Larson), 221

plaque, 27
polio, 4, 5
Ponce de León, Juan, 59, 68, 85–86
pregnancy, 188–90
Prevention magazine, 200
Prince, Richard L., 194
Pritchard, Bob, 109
propulsive force, 99
prostaglandins, 192
protein, 55–58, 191, 356–59
pull, *see* arm pull
pull buoys, 92, 219–20, 294–95
Purdin, Bill, 43
push-off drill, 244, 245–46
pyramid interval set, 228

R

Rabelais, François, 135
Rademacher, Erich, 157
Redford, Robert, 185
Reid, Walt, 196
"relaxation response," 24–25
resistance, 18, 116–18, 224, 296
    and drag suits, 224, 293
rest, in training, 247–50
resting heart rate (RHR), 35–37
reverse dolphin kick, 129, 222, 224
Revolution from Within: A Book of Self-Esteem (Steinem), 195
Rhodes, Bonnie Glasgow, 188
Richard, Pat, 16
rolling, *see* body roll
Rothe, Desider, 189
Rouse, Jeff, 228
Rubinstein, Carin, 179
Rudman, Daniel, 78

running, 16–17, 18–19, 32, 41, 64, 95
Ryan, Nolan, 80

S

Salnikov, Vladimir, 103
salt, 25, 38
Saltza, Chris von, 207
Samuelson, Joan Benoit, 16
Sanders, Summer, 40, 62, 89, 165, 206
Sanguily, Manuel, 35, 208, 210–11
Sassoon, Vidal, 15
Schuler, Alexa, 203
Schwarzenegger, Arnold, 40
scissor kick, 103
Sears, Barry, 49, 52, 53, 54–55, 192
self-esteem, 184, 194–98
Sellers, Thomas, 193
Senie, Ruby, 193
senior swimmers, records of, 319–21
sexuality, 175–86
    and aging, 176–77
    and hormones, 181–83, 185–86
    sexual activity, 179–81
    sexual enjoyment, 181
    sexual interest, 178–79
    swimming and, 177–86
shaving down, 230–31
shooters, 224, 281
sidestroke, 101
Silvia, "Red," 158
six-beat flutter kick, 112, 118, 126, 127
skin caliper test, 45
smoking, 7, 9, 10, 11, 38
    death from, 83
    and heart disease, 30–31

and life expectancy, 61, 62, 83–85
Somax Posture and Sports, 109
Spannuth, John, 208
S-pattern arm pull, 104, 106, 112, 118, 122–25
Spector, Arnie, 20–21, 38
sphygmomanometer, 23
Spitz, Mark, 40, 89, 103, 165, 206
sprints, 235
    kicking, 224
    workout, 263–73
Stanford University, 53
start
    backstroke, 131, 132
    breaststroke, 152
    butterfly, 168
    freestyle (crawl), 116–18
starting block, 116, 131
Steenburgen, Mary, 40
Steinem, Gloria, 195
Stewart, Melvin, 165
Stocks, Mike, 138
Stones, Dwight, 7, 16
straight-arm pull, 97–98
streamlining, 94–95, 104
stress, 183–84, 185
    aerobic exercise and, 32–33
    reduction of, 24–25, 37
stretching, 234
stroke (apoplexy), 11, 21, 30, 60, 69, 201
Suzuki, Daichi, 121
SWIM Canada magazine, 290
swim caps, 92, 291, 293–94
Swim Chute, 224
SWIM Magazine, 276, 290
swimmer's body, 40
swimming
    basic principles of, 93–100

benefits of, xiv–xv, 6, 15–19,
33–34, 40–44, 67–68
equipment, *see* equipment,
training
popularity of, 12, 14–15
time spent, 34–35, 235
training, *see* training
workouts, *see* workouts
swimming pattern, 231–32
Swimming Technique, 279, 290
*Swimming Through Your
Pregnancy* (Katz), 189
Swimming World magazine,
203–4, 290
swimsuits, 90–91, 224, 292, 293
systolic (pumping) pressure, 23
Szabo, Jozsef, 153

T
Tamoxifen, 193
tapering, 229–31, 259
testosterone, 182, 186
tethered swimming, 225
Thompson, Jenny, 206
thumb drill, 248–50
timed swim, 235
tissue plasminogen activator
(TPA), 35
training
distance per stroke (dps),
228–29
equipment, *see* equipment,
training
goals in, 237
interval training, 226–28
planning for, 235–36
pool etiquette for, 231–33
rest in, 247–50
sample programs, 239–89
tapering in, 229–31

tips, 236
see also workouts
training range, 36–37
treadmills, 38
trudgeon, 103
Trust Your Heart (Collins), 6
Tsongas, Paul, 15
turn
backstroke, 127–31
breaststroke, 149–52
butterfly, 168, 169
flip, 114–16, 127–31, 149, 236,
275, 277–78
freestyle, 114–16
two-beat flutter kick, 103, 112,
118

U
U.S. Department of Health and
Human Services, 64
United States Swimming, Inc., 206
United States Swimming (USS)
program, 205–7
Updike, Wynne F., 200–201

V
Vassallo, Jesse, 120
videos, 93
vitamin A, 57, 191–92
vitamin C, 57, 191–92
vitamin E, 57, 191–92
Vlasov, Yuri, 16

W
Wainer, Howard, 41
Walford, Roy, 57, 60
Walster, Elaine, 184
Ward, Ann, 35

warm-down, 235
warm-up, 234
wave-action breaststroke, 136,
    153–55, 222
Webb, Matthew, 135
webbed gloves, 225
wedge (frog) kick, 136, 145
weight loss, 7, 9, 16, 40–52
   and diet, 53–58
   and high blood pressure, 25
   reducing body fat, 42–52
   and swimming, 31–32, 34, 41,
     43–45
   see also body fat
weights, 224
Weissmuller, Johnny, 103
whip kick, 136, 146–47
Whiteleather, Tom, 8–9
Wickham, Harry, 103
Wilkie, David, 140
Wilmore, Jack H., 45–46
Winwood, Steve, 107
women, 187–98
   body fat of, 42, 46–49, 190,
     192–93, 201, 305–9
   and cancer, 190–93
   and menopause, 182, 191,
     194–95
   and osteoporosis, 194–95
   overweight, 192–93, 201

   and pregnancy, 188–90
   and self-esteem, 184, 194–98
   and sexuality, 182, 186
   swimming records of, 319–41
   swimsuits of, 90–91
Woodruff, Diana S., 62–63, 69, 76
workouts, 239–89
   for beginners, 240–42
   breaststroke, 255–58
   distance, 269–73
   early season, 243–46
   joining, etiquette of, 232
   lactic acid, 259–62
   New Year's, 251–54
   off-season, 274–78
   planning, 235–36
   rest in, 247–50
   sprint, 263–73
   structure of, 233–35
   see also training

Y

Yorzyk, William, 158

Z

Zahn, Paula, 15
Zoomers, 223–24, 281
Zussman, Shirley, 184

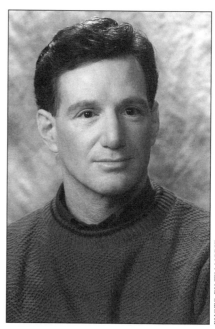

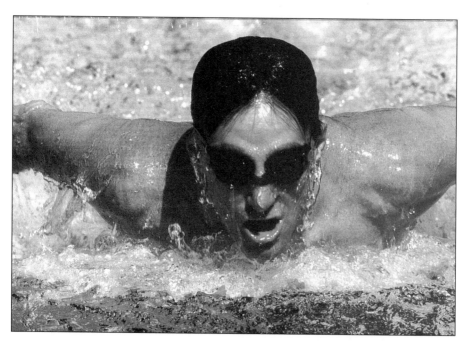

ABOUT THE AUTHOR

PHILLIP WHITTEN, author or coauthor of eighteen books and over one hundred major articles on a wide variety of topics, has lectured throughout the United States and several foreign countries on swimming and on fitness, health, and the aging process. He has published pioneering studies on exercise, aging, and sexuality, and on the effects of exercise in forestalling biological and psychological aging.

The editor-in-chief of *Swimming World* and *SWIM* magazines, Dr. Whitten is acknowledged as one of the world's leading authorities on swimming. He is also a top Masters swimmer, having set several national and world records.

An anthropologist and gerontologist, Whitten earned an interdisciplinary doctorate from Harvard University and has taught at Harvard University, Bentley College, and Endicott College.

ABOUT THE TYPE

This book was set in Garamond, a typeface designed
by the French printer Jean Jannon. It is styled after
Garamond's original models. The face is dignified, and
is light but without fragile lines. The italic is modeled
after a font of Granjon, which was probably cut in the
middle of the sixteenth century.